Cancer Research

IMPACT OF THE COOPERATIVE GROUPS

EDITED BY

BARTH HOOGSTRATEN, M.D.

American Cancer Society Professor of Clinical Oncology
Professor of Medicine, Department of Internal Medicine
University of Kansas Medical Center

ASSOCIATE EDITORS

PAUL P. CARBONE, M.D.
JOHN R. DURANT, M.D.
BERNARD FISHER, M.D.
G. DENMAN HAMMOND, M.D.
JAMES F. HOLLAND, M.D.
SIMON KRAMER, M.D.

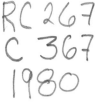

MASSON Publishing USA, Inc.
New York • Paris • Barcelona • Milan • Mexico City • Rio de Janeiro

Cherri Stadalman, Production Editor
Judy Daniels, Assistant
Eileen Wilson, Assistant

ISBN 0-89352-092-6

Library of Congress Catalog Card Number 80-82668

Printed in the United States of America

PREFACE

The Cooperative Group Program began in 1955 with the establishment of three groups; the Acute Leukemia Group A, which was to study childhood leukemia; the Acute Leukemia Group B which undertook the study of acute leukemia in adults; and the Eastern Solid Tumor Group. Together with two groups formed in 1956, the Southeastern Cancer Study Group and the Southwestern Cancer Study Group, these five groups have formed the backbone of the Cooperative Group Program during the past 25 years. Eventually a total of 36 groups were formed, but only 14 survived in 1977.

The Veterans Administration hospitals formed five groups in the 1950's and two, the VA Surgical Adjuvant and the VA Lung Cancer Groups are still active today. Of special interest is the very early formation of seven surgical adjuvant groups at a time when only very few drugs were available. Two of these groups are left, the National Surgical Adjuvant Breast Project and the VA Surgical Adjuvant Group.

During the first decade the Program consisted largely of chemotherapy in patients with advanced solid tumors and of the treatment of hematologic malignancies. A combination of radiotherapy and chemotherapy was inaugurated in Stage III Hodgkin's disease in 1966 and Wilms' tumor soon became a model for interdisciplinary collaboration. When the Program was transferred to the Division of Cancer Treatment, NCI, emphasis was placed on the incorporation of surgical oncology and pathology in the activity of most groups. The evolution of the Cooperative Groups from the chemotherapy for disseminated neoplasia, which was primarily of interest to hematologists and some progressive surgeons, to the multimodal treatment of cancer is now complete. The overall impact of the Program in terms of research, cancer care and education is documented in the various chapters of this book.

Probably no other program undertaken by the National Institutes of Health has been criticized and reviewed as much as the Cooperative Group Program. As early as 1959, when very few anticancer drugs were available, did Gellhorn question the usefulness of Cooperative Clinical Group studies.[1] He considered these embodied empiricism and repetition which neither optimally promoted the program of chemotherapy nor fully utilized the talent of involved participants. Gellhorn failed to recognize that the empiric approach would play a major role in the development of most therapeutic agents and that the involved participants were few indeed. A critical mass of clinical scientists needed to be developed. But the Gellhorn critique was deserved at least in part and led to significant changes.

Strong criticism of the Chemotherapy Program was also voiced in 1965 by the Wooldridge Committee.[2] The Committee concluded that the operations of the Cancer Chemotherapy National Service Center needed to be put on a sounder scientific footing and recommended a thorough review of the administration and management of collaborative programs. The NCI countered underserved criticism with the Richardson report[3] and answered the deserved portion of the critique with an acceleration of the execution of projected plans.

The Williamsburg Conference in 1968 and the Potomac Conference in 1975 both led to certain recommendations which were submitted to the National Cancer Advisory Board. However, both conferences testified to the viability of the Cooperative Group Program, and when in May, 1979, the Board of Scientific Counselors of the Division of Cancer Treatment met, the Groups had an opportunity for the first time to present their views and accomplishments.

The Cooperative Groups have endured despite all the criticism and reviews. One may ask why these many reviews and conferences took place. In part they result from intramural changes in the National Cancer Institute, in part they are motivated by monetary reasons: the basic science community is always vocal about the extent of basic research funding; the Organ-Site Programs are in competition with the Cooperative Group Program; the contract supported disease groups compete for funds and in part overlap with Group activities; and the Cancer Centers need to perform treatment research. However, the most important reason for the continuing scrutiny is the fact that the Cooperative Groups are so very much in the public eye. No aspect of cancer therapy has been left untouched by the Groups, nearly every medical school participates in the Program, the medical literature is replete with the results of its many studies. A program as visible as this is bound to be subjected to suggestions for improvements. And throughout these 25 years the Groups have been receptive to changes, have continued a healthy evolution and have been responsive to needs of the NCI, the medical schools and the cancer patient.

This book has been written to review the accomplishments of the Clinical Cooperative Groups during the past 25 years, to present a state of the art in the management of cancer in 1980 and to outline some of the problems facing the multidisciplinary approach to cancer treatment.

Barth Hoogstraten, M.D.

---

1. Gellhorn, A: Invited remarks on the current status of research in clinical cancer chemotherapy. Cancer Chemother Rep 5:1-12, 1959.

2. Biochemical science and its administration. A study of the National Institutes of Health. Report of Wooldridge Committee to the President. Washington, DC, US Government Print Office 1965.

3. Richardson Report. NIH, unpublished.

CONTRIBUTORS

Raymond Alexanian, M.D.
Department of Medicine
M.D. Anderson Hospital &
Tumor Institute
Houston, Texas

Laurence Baker, D.O.
Department of Oncology
Wayne State University
Medical Center
Detroit, Michigan

Charles M. Balch, M.D.
Department of Surgery
University of Alabama
Medical Center
Birmingham, Alabama

John M. Bennett, M.D.
Department of Medicine
Division of Oncology
University of Rochester
Cancer Center
Rochester, New York

Ernest C. Borden, M.D.
Division of Clinical Oncology
University of Wisconsin
Clinical Cancer Center
Madison, Wisconsin

James Butler, M.D.
Department of Pathology
M.D. Anderson Hospital &
Tumor Institute
Houston, Texas

William Caldwell, M.D.
Department of Radiation
  Therapy
University of Wisconsin
Radiotherapy Center
Madison, Wisconsin

Paul P. Carbone, M.D.
Department of Medicine
University of Wisconsin
Clinical Cancer Center
Madison, Wisconsin

Contributors

Chu H. Chang, M.D.
Department of Radiation
    Therapy
Columbia Presbyterian
Medical Center
New York, New York

Ronald L. Chard, M.D.
Department of Pediatric
    Oncology
Children's Orthopedic Hospital
    and Medical Center
Seattle, Washington

Harvey J. Cohen, M.D.
Department of Hematology/
    Oncology Division
Durham VA Hospital
Durham, North Carolina

Charles A. Coltman, Jr., M.D.
Division of Oncology
University of Texas Health
Science Center
San Antonio, Texas

John J. Costanzi, M.D.
Division of Hematology/
    Oncology
University of Texas
Medical Center
Galveston, Texas

James D. Cox, M.D.
Department of Radiation
    Therapy
Medical College of Wisconsin
Milwaukee, Wisconsin

Thomas J. Cunningham, M.D.
Division of Oncology
Department of Medicine
Albany Regional Cancer Center
Albany, New York

Giulio D'Angio, M.D.
Department of Radiation
    Therapy and Department
    of Pediatric Oncology
Children's Hospital of Philadelphia
Philadelphia, Pennsylvania

Hugh L. Davis, M.D.
Department of Medicine
University of Wisconsin
Clinical Cancer Center
Madison, Wisconsin

Lawrence W. Davis, M.D.
American College of Radiology
Philadelphia, Pennsylvania

Robert C. Donaldson, M.D.
Surgical Service
VA Medical Center
St. Louis, Missouri

John R. Durant, M.D.
Department of Medicine
Division of Hematology/
    Oncology
University of Alabama
School of Medicine
Birmingham, Alabama

Brian Durie, M.D.
Department of Internal
    Medicine
Section of Hematology/
    Oncology
University of Arizona
Health Sciences Center
Tucson, Arizona

Lawrence H. Einhorn, M.D.
Department of Medicine
Indiana University
School of Medicine
Indianapolis, Indiana

Contributors

Rose Ruth Ellison, M.D.
Department of Oncology
Columbia University
New York, New York

Audrey E. Evans, L.R.C.P., S.E.
Department of Pediatric
  Oncology
Children's Hospital of
  Philadelphia
Philadelphia, Pennsylvania

Bernard Fisher, M.D.
Department of Surgery
University of Pittsburgh
Pittsburgh, Pennsylvania

Edwin R. Fisher, M.D.
Department of Pathology
Shadyside Hospital
Pittsburgh, Pennsylvania

Emil J Freireich, M.D.
Department of Developmental
  Therapeutics
M.D. Anderson Hospital &
Tumor Institute
Houston, Texas

Richard A. Gams, M.D.
Division of Hematology/
  Oncology
University of Alabama
Medical Center
Birmingham, Alabama

Bernard Gardner, M.D.
Department of Surgery
Downstate Medical Center
Brooklyn, New York

Edmund Gehan, Ph.D.
Department of Biomathematics
University of Texas
M.D. Anderson Hospital &
Tumor Institute
Houston, Texas

Gerald S. Gilchrist, M.D.
Department of Pediatric
  Hematology/Oncology
Mayo Clinic
Rochester, Minnesota

John H. Glick, M.D.
Hematology/Oncology Section
Department of Medicine
University of Pennsylvania
  Hospital
Philadelphia, Pennsylvania

Oliver Glidewell
Department of Neoplastic
  Disease
Mt. Sinai School of Medicine
New York, New York

G. Denman Hammond, M.D.
Department of Pediatrics
University of Southern
  California
Los Angeles, California

Daniel M. Hays, M.D.
Department of Pediatric
  Surgery
Children's Hospital of
  Los Angeles
Los Angeles, California

George A. Higgins, Jr., M.D.
Department of Surgery
VA Hospital
Washington, D.C.

Contributors

Robert Hilgers, M.D.
GYN Oncology
University of New Mexico
Cancer Research &
Treatment Center
Albuquerque, New Mexico

James F. Holland, M.D.
Department of Neoplastic
  Disease
Mt. Sinai School of Medicine
New York, New York

Barth Hoogstraten, M.D.
Department of Medicine
Division of Clinical Oncology
University of Kansas
Medical Center
Kansas City, Kansas

John B. Horton, M.D.
Division of Oncology
Department of Medicine
Albany Medical College
Albany, New York

R.D.T. Jenkin, M.D.
Department of Radiation
  Therapy
Princess Margaret Hospital
Toronto, Ontario, Canada

Barbara Jones, M.D.
Department of Pediatrics
West Virginia School of
  Medicine
Morgantown, West Virginia

Simon Kramer, M.D.
Department of Radiation
  Therapy
Thomas Jefferson University
  Hospital
Philadelphia, Pennsylvania

Stephen A. Landaw, M.D., Ph.D.
Department of Medicine &
Department of Radiation
  Oncology
University of New York Upstate
Syracuse, New York

Sanford L. Leikin, M.D.
Department of Hematology/
  Oncology
Children's Hospital National
Medical Center
Washington, D.C.

Harvey J. Lerner, M.D.
Department of Surgery
Pennsylvania Hospital
Philadelphia, Pennsylvania

Brigid G. Leventhal, M.D.
Department of Pediatric
  Hematology/Oncology
Johns Hopkins Hospital
Children's Oncology Center
Baltimore, Maryland

George C. Lewis, Jr., M.D.
Department of Obstetrics &
  Gynecology
Jefferson Medical College
Philadelphia, Pennsylvania

Robert B. Livingston, M.D.
Department of Hematology/
  Oncology
Cleveland Clinic
Cleveland, Ohio

Albert F. LoBuglio, M.D.
Division of Hematology/
  Oncology
University of Michigan
Ann Arbor, Michigan

Contributors

Virgil Loeb, Jr., M.D.
Department of Medicine
Washington University
School of Medicine
St. Louis, Missouri

Robert McDivitt, M.D.
Department of Pathology
Jewish Hospital of St. Louis
St. Louis, Missouri

O. Ross McIntyre, M.D.
Department of Medicine
Hematology Section
Dartmouth-Hitchcock
Medical Center
Hanover, New Hampshire

Mary Matthews, M.D.
National Cancer Institute
VA Oncology Service
Washington, D.C.

Arnold Mittelman, M.D.
Department of Surgery
Roswell Park Memorial Institute
Buffalo, New York

Charles G. Moertel, M.D.
Department of Medicine
Graduate School
University of Minnesota
Rochester, Minnesota

Larry Nathanson, M.D.
Department of Hematology/
  Oncology
New England Medical Center
Boston, Massachusetts

Joseph Newall, M.D.
Department of Medicine
New York University
Medical Center
New York, New York

Mark E. Nesbit, M.D.
Department of Pediatrics
University of Minnesota
School of Medicine
Minneapolis, Minnesota

Carlos A. Perez, M.D.
Division of Radiation Oncology
Washington University
School of Medicine
St. Louis, Missouri

Ruheri Perez-Tamayo, M.D.
Department of Radiation
  Therapy
Loyola University
Medical Center
Maywood, Illinois

Theodore Phillips, M.D.
Department of Radiation
  Oncology
University of California
San Francisco, California

Cary A. Presant, M.D.
Department of Medical
  Oncology
City of Hope
National Medical Center
Duarte, California

George R. Prout, Jr., M.D.
Department of Surgery
Urological Service
Massachusetts General Hospital
Boston, Massachusetts

Lewis M. Schiffer, M.D.
Cell and Radiation Biology
  Laboratory
Allegheny General Hospital
Pittsburgh, Pennsylvania

Thomas W. Shields, M.D.
Department of Surgery
Northwestern University
Medical School
Chicago, Illinois

Robert E. Slayton, M.D., F.A.C.P.
Department of Medicine
Rush Medical College
Chicago, Illinois

James Snow, M.D.
Department of Otolaryngology
University of Pennsylvania
Medical Center
Philadelphia, Pennsylvania

Kenneth A. Starling, M.D.
Division of Pediatric Oncology
Texas Children's Hospital
Houston, Texas

Ronald Stephens, M.D.
Department of Medicine
Division of Clinical Oncology
University of Kansas
Medical Center
Kansas City, Kansas

Leo L. Stolbach, M.D.
Pondville Hospital
Walpole, Massachusetts

Wataru W. Sutow, M.D.
Department of Pediatrics
M.D. Anderson Hospital &
Tumor Institute
Houston, Texas

Douglass C. Tormey, M.D., Ph.D.
Department of Medicine
University of Wisconsin
Clinical Cancer Center
Madison, Wisconsin

Bill L. Tranum, M.D.
500 South University
Little Rock, Arkansas

Frederick A. Valeriote, Ph.D.
Department of Radiology
Division of Radiation Oncology
Washington University
School of Medicine
St. Louis, Missouri

Jan van Eys, M.D.
Department of Pediatrics
M.D. Anderson Hospital &
Tumor Institute
Houston, Texas

Ralph W. Vogler, M.D.
Department of Medicine
Emory University,
Atlanta, Georgia

V.K. Vaitkevicius, M.D.
Department of Oncology
Wayne State University
Detroit, Michigan

Peter H. Wiernik, M.D.
Clinical Oncology Branch
Baltimore Cancer Research
  Program
National Cancer Institute
Baltimore, Maryland

Julius Wolf, M.D.
Professional Services
VA Medical Center
Bronx, New York

Raymond Yesner, M.D.
Department of Pathology
VA Hospital
West Haven, Connecticut

Contributors

Marvin Zelen, Ph.D.
Department of Biostatistics &
  Epidemiology,
Sidney Farber Cancer Institute
Boston, Massachusetts

CONTENTS

Pediatric malignancies

Denman Hammond, Ronald L. Chard, Jr., Giulio J. D'Angio, Jan van Eys,
Gerald Gilchrist, Barbara Jones, Sanford Leikin, and Kenneth Starling

INTRODUCTION

The progress that has been made in the treatment and successful cure
of many cancers of infants and children over the past two decades is
one of the most gratifying accounts in the entire field of cancer
therapy. There is no better illustration of the advances that have been
made and the successes that have been realized than to recall that
twenty-five years ago when the pediatrician met to counsel the parents
of a child in whom the diagnosis of cancer was just established, one
attempted to give them an insight into the difficulties that lay ahead,
and explain the severe limitations in outcome that had to be faced.

Today, it is enormously more gratifying to be able to counsel such
parents, and to realize that the conversation is entirely different. In an
increasing proportion of instances, one can be sincerely optimistic
about the prognosis. It is now recognized that the survival rates for all
pediatric cancers have been significantly improved, and many cures
have been achieved.

The advances have not come from "breakthroughs". They are the
products of the carefully planned acquisition of data from clinical
research and the utilization of that data in successive generations of
clinical investigation to obtain additional answers to new questions
about improvements in therapy and the achievement of cure.

The state of the art of pediatric cancer therapy today is the result of the contributions of many such studies, many institutions and many investigators. Notable among these contributions have been those of Cooperative Groups of clinical cancer investigators. Many of the facts, and much of the knowledge and skill, upon which the current state of the art rests, could not have been accomplished in any other way nearly so effectively, or by this point in time.

One of the major achievements which has led to the successful treatment of the cancers of children is the fact that in major pediatric medical institutions throughout the nation there has been an almost total reorientation of the manner in which patients with cancer are managed. The cancers of children are now managed by teams of physicians, scientists, nurses and technologists who represent the scientific disciplines contributing to diagnosis, patient management and treatment, including all of the therapeutic and supportive care modalities that may be required for quality patient care.

It is remarkable that most of the nation's pediatric patients with cancer are no longer subjected to treatment by one specialist after another, but are managed by teams of specialists which include the variety of skills required for determining a complete diagnosis, and developing a treatment plan optimized for the patients. This is only one of the observations concerning the modern management of cancers of children that seems to serve well as a model for the management of many adult cancers.

Figure 1 shows the frequency of the major cancers among a population of over 10,000 infants and children with cancer. There are significant

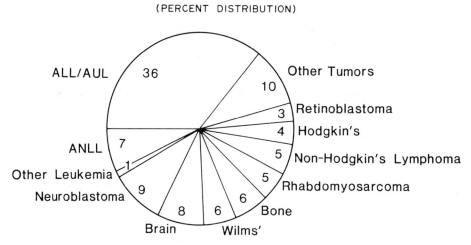

Fig. 1. Frequency of the major cancers among a population of 10,409 infants and children with cancer registered between 1974 to 1978

differences from the common cancers of adults.   The cancers of
children usually are not carcinomas, and do not usually involve epithelial tissues.   They are not usually superficial cancers, and most do
not permit early diagnosis.   The cancers of children are frequently
deep-seated, and are often diagnosed after spread beyond the local
area.   The most common cancers are the leukemias, followed by the
cancers of the central and sympathetic nervous systems.   The remainder are solid sarcomatous tumors of kidney, muscle and bone.

The variety of diagnostic and therapeutic disciplines represented among
the investigators of a typical children's Cooperative Group is shown in
Figure 2.   While cooperative management of cancer among specialists
in all relevant fields is a current goal in many of the nation's major
health care institutions, it has become an established fact in the
nation's major pediatric medical institutions caring for significant
numbers of patients with cancer.   This began prior to 1970, and in the
seventies there has been increasing participation in Cooperative Group
investigation, and in contributions to the science and governance of
Cooperative Groups, in the development of new study protocols, in the
conduct of clinical investigation and in the evaluation of clinical
research.   This is not simply an illustration of the organization of a
Cooperative Group.   This is indicative of the creation and development
of new multidisciplinary teams of physician-investigators at each
member institution.

The Cooperative Groups with a major commitment to childhood malignancies are the Childrens Cancer Study Group, the Southwest Oncology
Group and Cancer and Leukemia Group B.   The 58 member institutions

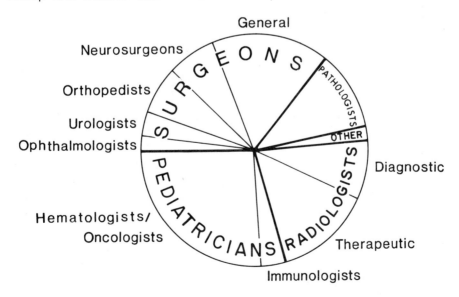

Fig. 2. Group membership by discipline

of these Groups are located in all of the large metropolitan areas of the country. The institutions involved are generally the major pediatric medical centers of our nation, including many departments of pediatrics of medical schools, major children's hospitals and many of the nation's large cancer centers.

In addition to the pediatric institutions participating in these three Cooperative Groups studying the cancers of children, there are more than 250 additional hospitals and institutions that are affiliated in some formal and effective manner with the member institutions, and which are substantially influenced in their management of pediatric cancer by their affiliation with the members of Cooperative Groups. The membership in Cooperative Groups, at least in pediatrics, involves generally very large institutions that have sizeable populations of children with cancer coming to them for management. It is in such institutions that one finds surgeons, radiation therapists, pathologists and others who deal exclusively with pediatric patients, and many of them exclusively with the cancers of pediatric patients. Moreover, since many of these are in major metropolitan areas, they see a broad cross section of pediatric cancer patients, who have not been pre-selected.

TREATMENT OF ACUTE LYMPHOCYTIC LEUKEMIA

It is instructive to review the important chronologic milestones in the successful treatment of acute lymphocytic leukemia (ALL).

It begins with the first demonstration that a chemotherapeutic agent could induce a remission, a disappearance of the clinical and laboratory manifestations of acute lymphocytic leukemia.[1] Successful induction therapy by a variety of single agents, and then by combinations of two or more agents quickly followed.[2-4] During that period it became more important to be able to identify subtypes of acute leukemia, some of which were clearly not responsive to some of the agents which were showing success in acute lymphocytic leukemia. The initial studies of leukemia by Cooperative Groups included all varieties of acute leukemia.

After the achievement of successful induction of remission in greater proportions, continuation of therapy to maintain the duration of remission became the central focus of therapeutic strategy.[5-7] Once induction of remission was successful, refinements in maintenance therapy, and in the dose and schedule of induction and maintenance therapy, became important strategies.

Another important milestone was the development of therapeutic strategies based upon the concept that if one made optimal use of the variety of chemotherapeutic agents known to be active, one might conceivably design chemotherapy for cure. This involved multiple drugs, and sequencing of the therapeutic regimens, to try to eliminate the minimal, residual population of leukemia cells that had thus far failed to be destroyed by the therapy. That concept had an enormous impact on improving induction and maintenance therapy, and in allowing cures to emerge.

Another important concept that has led to therapeutic innovation, and has contributed to the success of long-term survival and cure, is the recognition of the importance of the persistence of leukemia cells in certain sites of the body, which appear to be pharmacologic sanctuaries, such as the central nervous system[8] and testes[9]. These complications began to be recognized as major clinical problems only after there were a significant number of long-term survivors. First, therapy was designed to treat these complications, and subsequently the importance of prophylactically pretreating these areas was demonstrated.[10-12]

As soon as single agents capable of inducing complete remission were found, an occasional patient was encountered who achieved long-term survival in complete remission. These events were initially seen only occasionally, however, as induction and multiagent maintenance therapy became more successful, an increasing number of long-term survivors continued to be observed. It should not be forgotten that the many patients now known to be alive and well 10 to 20 years since their initial diagnosis received therapies which, by today's standards, were far less than optimal. It is not unreasonable to expect that among the much larger proportion of patients achieving three to five year continuous complete remissions are many more who may never relapse.

Throughout these years of significant advance, there were many improvements in supportive care. The provision of replacement therapy for bone marrow failure, more aggressive and more effective antibiotic therapy for infections, improved ability to recognize and deal with drug related toxicity and the recognition of the need for effective psychosocial support for patients, as well as for parents and siblings have been identified as essential factors in a complete program of supportive care.

During the period of development of reliable and successful therapies for acute lymphocytic leukemia, there also developed an environment which invited multidisciplinary teamwork in more accurate diagnosis and clinical staging, and in the definition of the important roles of participation, not only of pediatric hematologist/oncologists, but of radiation therapists and surgeons as well. The agents which had been so successful in the chemotherapy of leukemia were tried against a variety of the solid tumors of children.

It had long been recognized that certain clinical and laboratory features of acute lymphocytic leukemia were associated with poor response to therapy and poor outcome.[13,14] It came to be recognized that in order to appropriately analyze results of clinical investigations of ALL, some of the obvious factors which influenced prognosis had to be taken into account in order to appropriately assess the results of treatments under study. Such factors as the age of the child at the time of diagnosis, and the level of the initial white blood cell count enabled stratification into more homogeneous patient groups, so meaningful differences in thera- peutic regimens could be perceived. Subsequently, studies were de- signed which controlled these variables so other important factors which influenced outcome could be detected.

Finally, there have emerged many clinical and laboratory evaluations which have been applied to large populations of children with ALL. Some of these are strongly associated with good or poor outcome and, in addition, are of importance in identifying subgroups of patients which will one day be recognized as discrete diagnostic subgroups. It has become apparent that in order to compare one study with another, the specific composition of the patient populations must be known with respect to many important predictors of outcome. The leukemia

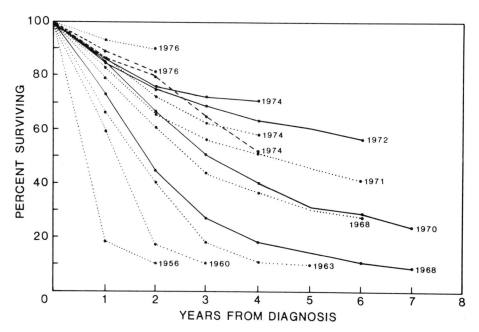

Fig. 3. Survival of children with ALL/AUL

studies of the future must be designed to control these clinical and biologic characteristics of patients so comparisons between regimens, as well as between studies can be done. This often requires more patients than any single institution has access to, in order to have sufficient numbers of appropriate analysis, once the population has been stratified into subgroups of appropriate homogeneity. Cooperative Groups were originally developed because of the efficiency and speed with which new therapies could be subjected to sophisticated clinical trials with appropriate controls. Cooperative Groups now have emerged as the only feasible mechanism by which certain clinical studies can be done.

There is progressive improvement in duration of survival of children with ALL (Figure 3). One can see the important progress in the survival duration of patients on studies from 1956 to 1976. Each Group has achieved major progress during this period of time. Beginning with a median survival of approximately six months in 1956, there was a series of studies begun in 1974 which gave a four-year survival between 50 percent and 70 percent. A study begun in 1972 has a six-year survival of approximately 60 percent. These are firm data, since there were 724 patients in the study. This population is large enough to be stratified into subgroups to permit definitive statistical analyses to determine the importance of clinical and biologic descriptors of acute lymphocytic leukemia, and their relative importance in predicting outcome.

What were the singular advances among the milestones which lead to this remarkable history of improvement in treatment outcome? Table 1 lists some of the initial Cooperative Group reports of the demonstration of antileukemic activity of single agents, the superior results using combinations of agents and the development of treatments which were increasingly effective in maintaining complete remission. The recognition and development of effective treatments for extramedullary involvement by leukemia, and the importance of treatment of such sites prior to evidence of their involvement by leukemia is shown in Table 2.

These tables are far from complete and only list some of the highlights. It is evident that the studies by Cooperative Clinical Investigation Groups have had a major and important role.

CLINICAL AND BIOLOGIC FACTORS THAT ARE ASSOCIATED WITH OUTCOME TO THERAPY

The recognition of a variety of clinical and biologic factors that have a high degree of association with therapeutic outcome has been made possible largely by the studies of acute lymphocytic leukemia by Cooperative Groups of clinical investigators.[13,14] Only by the careful

TABLE 1
Demonstration of Antileukemic Activity by Cooperative Groups

Single Agents

1962	Hydrocortisone vs. ACTH	Sutow
1962	Cyclophosphamide	Fernbach
1972	Adriamycin	Ragab
1973	L-ASP: Dose, Route, Schedule	Newton

Combinations

1958	6-MP + MTX ⟨Continuous / Intermittent	Frei
1961	MTX vs. 6-MP vs. MTX + 6-MP	Frei
1965	PRED + 6-MP	Frei
1965	PRED + VCR	Selawry
1966	PRED + 6-MP vs. PRED + MTX	Krivit
1972	DNM vs. DNM + PRED vs. DNM, PRED, VCR	Jones
1977	PRED, VCR, L-ASP	Ortega

Maintenance

1963	6-MP vs. Placebo	Freireich
1965	Methotrexate	Selawry
1968	PRED, VCR, MTX, 6-MP, CTX Cyclic vs. Sequential	Krivit
1969	6-MP + MTX vs. 6-MP (HN_2) + MTX (DACT)	Leikin
1969	VCR vs. ARA-C vs. VCR + ARA-C	Pierce
1970	MTX with VCR + PRED Reinforcement	Holland
1972	6-MP + MTX with VCR + PRED Reinforcement	Holland
1975	6-MP vs. 6-MP + PRED vs. 6-MP + PRED + VCR	Fernbach

TABLE 2
Treatment and Prophylaxis of Extramedullary Sites

Reported

1964	Clinical and Lab Manifestations, Response to IT MTX Therapy	Hyman
1965	6-MP + Oral MTX vs. 6-MP + IT MTX Prophylaxis	Frei
1971	IT MTX Maintenance Prophylaxis	Sullivan
1975	Controlled Trials of Prophylaxis: Craniospinal XRT + EFXRT vs. Craniospinal XRT vs. Cranial XRT + IT MTX vs. IT MTX	Hittle
1977	Prophylactic Testicular XRT	Nesbit
1979	1800 R vs. 2400 R Craniospinal Prophylaxis	Nesbit

analysis of large patient populations which have been stratified by one or multiple parameters has it been possible to examine more homogeneous subgroups of patients that are still sizable enough to permit valid statistical analysis. It has been determined that some of these prognostic predictors have such a strong association with outcome that they may select subpopulations of patients in which their influence on outcome is more powerful than the treatments under study. The next series of figures will illustrate many clinical and biologic observations which are associated with treatment outcome.

Figure 4 shows the duration of survival from diagnosis of 936 patients with acute lymphocytic leukemia, combined from a series of studies initiated between 1972 and 1975, all of which had essentially identical induction and maintenance therapy. The only variable used for stratifying this population into the four groups illustrated was the age at the time of diagnosis.

The 16 percent of patients over age 10 at diagnosis had the worst survival experience, and the 48 percent of patients between the ages of 3 and 7 years at diagnosis had the best. The five-year survival of patients over 10 years of age at diagnosis was approximately 50 percent, while the survival of the most favorable age group was approximately 70 percent. It is important to note that a median survival of five years for a large unselected population with acute lymphocytic leukemia would be considered, quite successful therapy, even in 1979.

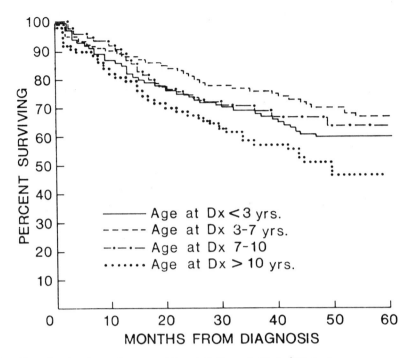

Fig. 4. Survival of patients with childhood ALL/AUL by age group

The survival of the same population of patients with ALL, but this time stratified according to the white blood cell count at the time of diagnosis is shown in Figure 5. It is apparent that the group with the least favorable outcome were those whose white count was greater than 100,000/mm^3. This group, which accounted for 11 percent of the total patient population, has only a 30 percent five-year survival. Fifty-three percent had a WBC less than 10,000, and an additional 15 percent had WBC between 10,000 and 20,000/mm^3. The five-year survival of these two groups was approximately 70 percent.

Clearly the level of the white blood cell count at the time of diagnosis of acute lymphocytic leukemia is an indicator of a fundamental biologic process, which has a powerful influence on the success and outcome of treatment. It is important to note that some of the other predictors of prognosis have a strong association with the white blood cell count, an association so strong in many cases that they do not make significant additional contribution to the prediction of outcome, once the white blood cell count has been considered.

These figures illustrate the ease with which clinical investigators can stratify an unselected population of children with ALL into more homogeneous populations with respect to anticipated outcome. This may often be advisable when devising clinical studies in order to permit

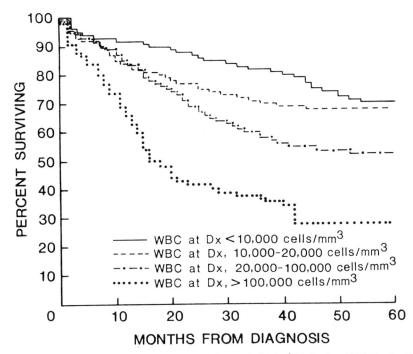

Fig. 5. Survival of patients with childhood ALL/AUL by WBC at diagnosis

the recognition and analysis of factors which are of additional significance, and which could not be perceived unless initial stratification according to important prognostic factors has been done. Stratification both by age and initial white blood cell count results in the creation of groups of patients, of which approximately 20 percent had very poor prognosis, based upon a high white blood cell count above 50,000/mm^3, approximately 25 percent had a very favorable prognosis having been selected with white blood cell count less than 10,000 and between 3 and 7 years of age. This group is likely to have a 5-year survival of at least 75 percent.

The influence of several factors on remission duration is shown in Table 3. Interestingly enough, patients with hemoglobin less than 7 grams percent at diagnosis have a more favorable outcome than those whose hemoglobin level is normal or increased. This unexpected observation has been confirmed in three successive studies, and is of considerable interest since the hemoglobin level is a variable which contributes to the prediction of outcome independently of the white cell count at diagnosis. Further analyses have shown a close association between normal to high hemoglobin levels with other features such as marked hepatosplenomegaly, marked lymphadenopathy and mediastinal mass in male patients over ten years of age. Currently it is hypothesized that

TABLE 3
Prognostic Factors Bone Marrow Remission Duration
Ranked by Multivariate Entry Criteria

PROGNISTIC FACTOR	CONTRIBUTION TO PREDICTION*
WBC	38.8%
Nodal Enlargement	19.0%
Age	17.7%
Hemoglobin	8.3%
Sex	7.0%
Platelets	5.2%
Splenomegaly	1.8%
Race	1.2%
Hepatomegaly	1.0%
Mediastinal Mass	0.01%

*Determined by the proportional increment in the log likelihood function compared to the amount of incremental change for all the variables included, using a stepwise entry procedure.

Several additional factors of importance were not studied in this particular patient population.

patients whose disease has a clinical presentation with major extra-medullary manifestations of involvement such as hepatosplenomegaly, lymphadenopathy, mediastinal mass, etc., may involve the marrow less by the time of diagnosis than those with a less lymphomatous presentation.

Patients with liver enlargement to the umbilicus or below have a much less favorable outcome. Similarly, patients with marked splenomegaly, palpable at or below the umbilicus, have a less favorable outcome. Patients with markedly enlarged, visible, lymph glands constitute 7 percent of the population, and had a much less favorable outcome. Seven percent of the patient population have a significant mediastinal mass, and their survival experience is less favorable.

It should be pointed out here that marked enlargement of liver, spleen, peripheral lymph nodes and mediastinal mass, are all closely associated with an elevated white blood cell count. If one selects a patient population on the basis of an elevated white blood cell count, one is simultaneously selecting most of the patients with marked hepato-splenomegaly, lymphadenopathy and mediastinal mass. In addition, patients with mediastinal mass tend not only to have high white blood cell count, but tend to be males over the age of ten. These variables appear to be of statistical significance when analyzed as if they were single variables. However, on multivariate statistical analysis, it becomes clear that the level of the white blood cell count is a stronger predictor of outcome, and that the closely associated factors do not make an additional significant contribution to prediction of outcome once the white blood cell count is taken into consideration.

Interestingly enough, the rapidity of the response to treatment as revealed by the percentage of lymphoblasts remaining in the marrow after the first two weeks of treatment is associated with the duration of the complete remission which is achieved. It seems to predict for events which occur years after the achievement of complete remission. Patients with a bone marrow rating of 3 at day 14 have a survival at 40 months of approximately 50 percent, compared to 68 percent of the study population with bone marrow cleared of blasts by day 14, 75 percent of which remained in continuous complete remission for 40 months. This observation is independent of the WBC at diagnosis, and is, therefore, a variable contributing additional information concerning prognosis, irrespective of the level of the initial white blood cell count. A statistical analysis of the significance of the difference between the three curves illustrated shows a p value equal to .001.

RELATIVE IMPORTANCE OF PREDICTORS OF OUTCOME

By multivariate statistical analysis, one can gain an insight into the relative contribution to the prediction of outcome of each of the factors that appear, when examined singly, to have a significant association with outcome. By this technique, it is possible to take into account the relative independence of each variable in predicting prognosis, as well as its association with one or more other variables, which appear to be importantly associated with outcome.

The rank order of prognostic factors as shown in Table 3 demonstrates that the WBC at diagnosis is the single most significant predictive factor in this analysis, when compared with all other factors. Marked enlargement of lymph nodes and age are other important contributors to prediction. The hemoglobin level, sex and platelet count are also of significant importance, while in this analysis splenomegaly, hepatomegaly and mediastinal mass are of no particular statistical value in predicting outcome once other factors have been taken into account.

The table does not include some of the prognostic variables that have been studied in other groups of patients, which are difficult to place within the rank order determined from studies of a different population. However, it would appear that blast cell morphology is a prognostic variable close to or equivalent to the white blood cell count in its contribution to prediction of outcome, that immunoglobulin status, the bone marrow rating after 14 days of therapy, and the presence or absence of CNS involvement at diagnosis, may be of roughly the same order of importance as the age in predicting outcome.

Some very important lessons have been learned from studies of clinical and biologic factors, which are associated with outcome. There can be no clearer demonstration that the population of children with the clinical diagnosis of acute lymphocytic leukemia is not homogenous. It is essential, therefore, to design studies employing reasonably homo-geneous groups of patients with respect to the factors strongly influ-encing outcome, in order to be able to detect significant differences among therapies being studied, and, also, it is essential when comparing one study to another to know the precise descriptors of the population involved, or which might have been excluded. The inescapable conclu-sion from these observations is that the populations available for study by single institutions are so small that the experimental design has severe limitations, since the population is not sufficiently large to permit the stratifications which are required for studying homogeneous populations.

The recognition of patient groups that have either favorable or unfavor-able prognosis invites speculation on the composition of patient groups that have the most favorable array of prognostic factors. Table 4 lists several factors that predict for most favorable prognosis. One might

TABLE 4
Best Prognosis - "Pure ALL"

1.	Initial WBC:	< 20,000
2.	AGE:	3 to 7 Years
3.	Cell Markers:	Non B, Non T
4.	Blast Morphology:	L1 or L1/L2
5.	IGG + IGA + IGM	Normal
6.	Extramedullary Involvement:	Minimal
7.	Response to Initial Therapy:	Rapid

euphemistically refer to this group as "pure" ALL. Such patients would have a low initial white blood cell count, an age between 3 and 7 years, cell surface markers that have neither T nor B lymphocyte character-istics, pure L_1 blast morphology, normal immunoglobulins, minimal extramedullary involvement, and a rapid response to initial chemo-therapy. It is tempting to speculate that if these were eligibility criteria for a homogeneous good risk population, the induction of remission would be close to 100 percent successful, the patients would enjoy continuous complete remission for 4 years of maintenance ther-apy, and after cessation of chemotherapy would have survival of 80 percent or better for six years, and eventually have a very high proportion of cures. This is certainly a reasonable expectation.

Conversely, Table 5 lists some of the factors predicting for poor prognosis and describes groups at high risk of induction failure, early relapse and death. It should be pointed out that this is not a homogeneous group, but simply a list of a variety of observations which occur among malignancies which manifest clinically as acute lympho-cytic leukemia. These include myeloid leukemia of M-1 blast cell morphology, which may be mistaken for ALL, L-2 or L-3 blast cell morphology, Philadelphia chromosome positive ALL, T-cell or B-cell ALL, patients with markedly reduced immunoglobulin levels, those with major extramedullary clinical presentation, those with other primarily lymphomatous presentations, congenital and infant ALL, and those that are either slow responders or nonresponders to induction chemotherapy.

TABLE 5
Some Factors Predicting Poor Prognosis

1. Myeloid Leukemia of M1 Blast Cell Morphology
2. Burkitt's Cell Leukemia
3. PH Chromosome Positive ALL
4. T-Cell ALL
5. Pure L2 Blast Cell Morphology
6. IGG, IGA, IGM Levels Below Normal
7. ALL With Major Extramedullary Presentations
8. ALL With Primary Lymphomatous Presentations
9. Congenital and Infant ALL
10. Slow Responders to Induction Chemotherapy
11. Nonresponders to Induction Chemotherapy

TABLE 6
Other Possible Descriptors of the Varieties of
Lymphoid Malignancies Manifesting Acute Leukemia

1. Antigen Markers

    a) Common ALL
    b) HTLA (T-Antigen)
    c) HBLA
    d) IA
    e) Anti-M

2. Pre-B Cell Studies

3. Terminal Transferase (TdT)

4. Complement and Fc Receptors, Mouse Rosettes

5. Acid Phosphatase, β Glucuronidase, Hexokinase,
    Hexosaminidase, Nonspecific Esterase

6. Glucocorticoid Receptors

There are a variety of other clinical and laboratory tests, either immunologic, biochemical, enzymatic or morphologic, which are under development and which are showing capability to define additional subsets of acute lymphocytic leukemia (Table 6). Certainly some of these, when applied to large populations of patients that have been concurrently characterized according to other known prognostic variables, will serve to provide greater biologic understanding of the variety of lymphoid malignancies that present clinically as what has been known to date as acute lymphocytic leukemia.

TREATMENT OF THE SOLID TUMORS OF CHILDREN

The improvements in survival and apparent cure rates of several of the common solid tumors of infants and children, which have been achieved during the past 25 years, have been no less spectacular than advances in the treatment of acute lymphocytic leukemia. Figure 6 is a chart which shows the dramatic improvements in the two-year survival percentage that has occurred between 1940 and 1977 for the common solid tumors of children. This time period covers the introduction and gradual widespread application of the principal therapeutic modalities.

In 1940, when surgery was the only available therapeutic modality, a time when the specialty of pediatric surgery had not yet emerged, the two-year survival rates for neuroblastoma, non-Hodgkin's lymphoma, brain tumors and Wilms' tumor were less than 10 percent. Several other

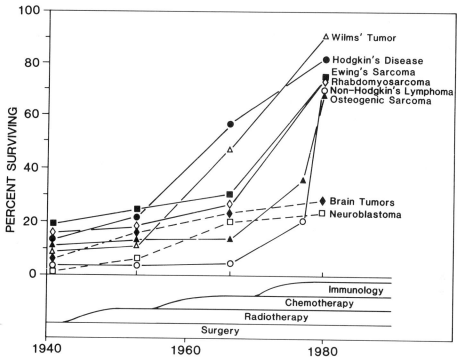

Fig. 6. Two-year survival of children with solid tumors

solid tumors of children, including osteogenic sarcoma, Hodgkin's disease, rhabdomyosarcoma and Ewing's sarcoma had two-year survival rates between 10 and 20 percent.

By 1950, orthovoltage radiation therapy for the treatment of solid tumors of children had been introduced, and was becoming more widely used, but in conservative doses. The two-year survival rates still ranged between 0 and 20 percent, and it was difficult to perceive that any significant change had occurred. By 1960, however, there had begun to be observed very significant improvements in the survival rates of Wilms' tumor and Hodgkin's disease in children. This was doubtless due to the more widespread use of radiation therapy as a principal modality of therapy, following attempts at surgical removal, and the beginnings of the use of megavoltage x-ray equipment to treat children. It would appear also that the survival rates for neuroblastoma and brain tumors had begun to improve.

By 1970, chemotherapy had been widely employed, using multiple agents with increasing frequency, in conjunction with radiation therapy and more careful surgery. Two-year survival rates for osteogenic sarcoma and non-Hodgkin's lymphoma were significantly improved, and by 1975, several of the major pediatric solid tumors, except for brain

tumors and neuroblastoma, had survival rates between 60 and 85
percent. By this time, immunotherapy had begun to be considered in
conjunction with other therapeutic modalities, however, its impact has
not been significant.

WILMS' TUMOR

Table 7 lists some of the important milestones in the successful
treatment of Wilms' tumor. It begins with the demonstration of the
effectiveness of dactinomycin by Farber in 1960, and follows the
introduction of additional chemotherapeutic agents,[15-17] the discovery
of characteristic histopathologic groups, and the evolution by pediatric
surgeons of new principles,[18] including the concept that total gross
resection to reduce the tumor burden is of considerable therapeutic
benefit, and permits more effective radiation therapy and chemotherapy in patients formerly considered to have tumors which were
surgically unresectable. In addition, surgical techniques for the management of bilateral Wilms' tumor were developed.[19]

Among the important lessons learned from extensive cooperative
studies of this tumor was the greater efficacy of multiple chemother-

TABLE 7
Milestones in Successful Treatment of Wilms' Tumor

Reported

1960	Dactinomycin Therapy	Farber
1963	Vincristine Therapy	Sutow
1968	Single Versus Multiple Courses of DACT	Wolff
1976	• DACT + VCR Superior to Single Agent	D'Angio
	• No XRT Needed in Group I < 2 Years of Age	
1978	Prognostic Importance of Histology	Beckwith
1978	• DACT + VCR + ADR Superior To 2 Drugs	D'Angio
	• Chemotherapy Duration: 6 Mos. = 15 Mos.	
1978	Definition of Surgical Principles	Leape

apeutic agents used concurrently, and the demonstration that patients less than two years of age, with tumor confined to the kidney, required no radiation therapy following surgical resection. Of considerable importance in the study of this tumor were the lessons that there were patients with favorable prognosis that could be treated adequately with less chemotherapy, less radiation therapy, and less extensive surgery.

It can be stated with conviction that the study of this tumor by the cooperative endeavors of Groups permitted investigators to conduct three successive multiregimen, multistage studies of this tumor, in a reasonably short span of years, which resulted in major advances in our understanding of the tumor and its successful management. This would not have been possible without the Cooperative Group mechanism. The two-year survival has improved from less than 10 percent to approximately 90 percent, and numerous patients, now considered cured, have survived for such lengths of time that there is concern about the late secondary effects of therapy that may appear in long-term survivors.

The thrust of the therapeutic strategy for this tumor now has become to ascertain how much less intensive radiation and chemotherapy such patients can be given,[20] particularly those within groups which can now be identified that have favorable prognosis, and which might lessen the undesirable late effects of successful treatment. This is a remarkable transformation of therapeutic concern from one of desperately attempting to find some way to have an impact on the relentless fatal course of this tumor to one of cautiously trying to reduce the intensity of therapy to achieve a better end result. Such a change would not conceivably have been possible had not multiinstitutional Cooperative Groups banded together. Clearly, such advances and such discoveries could not have been achieved by any single institution.

RHABDOMYOSARCOMA

It is surprising to note that the effectiveness of chemotherapy among patients with rhabdomyosarcoma was only first reported in 1965.[21] This resulted from a study employing three chemotherapeutic agents, each of which had shown some antitumor activity, in the hope that chemotherapy might contribute additional advantage to surgery in the control of this tumor.

Subsequently, additional agents were found to be effective, and it was recognized that the time was ripe for an intensified multimodality trial of therapy for this tumor. Representatives of the three Cooperative Groups treating significant numbers of children with cancer were convened on several occasions in order to explore concepts and areas of mutual interest in a study involving surgery, chemotherapy and radiation therapy. A new organization involving three different national, Cooperative Clinical Cancer Investigation Groups was nurtured into existence, which developed a multimodality therapeutic protocol with carefully specified guidelines for each.   The Intergroup Rhabdomyosarcoma Study constituted the first major national collaborative effort for the study of an uncommon, but important, tumor of children, which combined the resources of three existing Cooperative Groups.[22]

This organization has conducted three successive protocol studies of rhabdomyosarcoma, and has accumulated the largest body of clinical, pathologic and therapeutic information concerning this tumor that now exists.   This cooperative effort has resulted in a reclassification of histopathology, and the definition of new subgroups of prognostic importance, an accomplishment that would not have been possible were it not for a mechanism for central, independent review of specimens submitted from dozens of cooperating institutions.   Evaluation of reports of participating surgeons and descriptions of gross and microscopic pathology have led to entirely new concepts concerning the surgical management of this tumor, again a scientific advance that would have been impossible to accomplish at any single institution, simply because of restrictions on the patient material available for study.   This effort also resulted in the development of a new system for clinical staging of this tumor, its validation by the study, and adaptations of clinical management to the clinical staging of disease.

The Intergroup Rhabdomyosarcoma Study acquires an average of eleven patients per month, whereas even large institutions acquire only approximately seven patients per year. The cooperative study of large numbers of patients, made possible by the participation of many institutions, has led in a very short period of years to a new body of scientific information of considerable value.

It has been demonstrated that the survival of Group I patients is not improved by radiation therapy.   It has been demonstrated that it is possible to control gross residual tumor, which could not be surgically removed, by the combination of postoperative chemotherapy and radiation therapy.[23] It has been recognized that retroperitoneal nodes are frequently involved in genital, urinary and extremity rhabdomyosarcoma,[24] and this in turn has led to a revised surgical understanding and approach. Meningeal involvement by rhabdomyosarcoma has been discovered frequently in association with involvement of the nasopharynx, nasal sinuses and middle ear.[25] This in turn led to the use of craniospinal radiation therapy and intrathecal chemotherapy for patients with parameningeal involvement.

Two new histologic subtypes have been identified, including an alveolar cell type, which has a much less favorable prognosis. It has been documented that ultraradical, extirpative surgical procedures are rarely necessary in groups of patients that are likely to be responsive to chemotherapy and radiation therapy.

This new body of knowledge has led to successive improvements in chemotherapy, to significant changes in understanding of patho-physiology and patterns of metastasis, to changes in surgical manage-ment, to significant changes in radiation therapy management, and has highlighted the importance of accurate histopathologic diagnosis. These advances could not have been made without the availability of a large number of patients, and the pooling of talents, as well as patient resources, from a large number of cooperating institutions.

NEUROBLASTOMA

Since the 1960's there has been no change in the median survival of children with neuroblastoma[26] while the 5-year survival has increased only from about 5 to 20 percent (Fig. 7). A number of single agents and combinations have been shown to be effective in causing significant, and often complete regression, of detectable tumor; however, in this instance, we cannot be nearly so satisfied with the long-term results of treatment. Although this tumor appears to be highly responsive to a variety of chemotherapeutic agents, it is obvious that current therapies

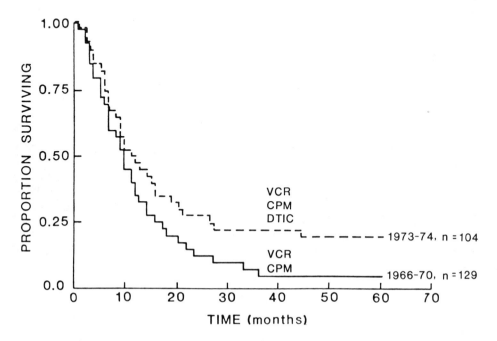

Fig. 7. Milestones in the successful treatment of Neuroblastoma

are not frequently successful in eliminating the tumor completely, since a large percentage of tumors recur, or metastasize, and the survival experience has not improved markedly.

There have, however, been several areas of important advance and new understanding. The histopathology of neuroblastoma has been well studied, utilizing the specimen resources of Cooperative Groups. A new clinical-pathologic staging system has been proposed, studied and validated.[27] The staging system has permitted the recognition that patients with Stage I neuroblastoma have a cure rate of 90 percent or more, and it has been demonstrated in this group that postoperative irradiation therapy is unnecessary, and, in addition, that this group does not benefit significantly from chemotherapy.

Multidisciplinary teamwork in studies of this tumor have led to the demonstration that some patients with surgically inoperable tumors can be made operable by the prior administration of courses of chemotherapy. Currently, a new therapeutic strategy, involving abdominal exploration of the site of the primary tumor, following courses of apparently successful chemotherapy, has been instituted. By this technique, it is becoming possible to identify patients whose tumor appears to have been eliminated by surgery and chemotherapy, as well as those for which additional surgery at the time of the postchemotherapy exploration may be of value.

Although one cannot be satisfied with the long-term results of treatment of neuroblastoma, it is of value to have documented the wisdom of eliminating traditional therapies, which have marked toxic effects, and which may cause late adverse effects on long-term survivors. This is true for not only neuroblastoma, but for rhabdomyosarcoma and Wilms' tumors also.

PHASE II STUDIES

The discovery of new chemotherapeutic agents during the past two decades has certainly been an area of major advance.[28] The Clinical Cooperative Groups studying the cancers of children have been responsible for the initial clinical trials, which demonstrated the activity of new chemotherapeutic agents against a variety of the cancers of infants and children. Many of the cancers of children occur in limited numbers compared to the principal cancers of adults. It appears that definitive Phase II studies of new anticancer agents can only by performed on significant numbers of patients with specific pediatric cancers by groups of institutions cooperating in such important clinical investigations.

1. Farber S, Diamond LK, Mercer RD, Sylvester RF, Wolff JA: Temporary remissions in acute leukemia in children produced by folic acid antagonist, 4-aminoptero VL-glutamic acid (aminop terin). N Engl J Med 238:787, 1948.

2. Heyn RM, Brubaker CA, Burchenal JH, Cramblett HG, Wolff JA: The comparison of 6-mercaptopurine with the combination of 6-mercaptopurine and azaserine in the treatment of acute leukemia in children; results of a cooperative study. Blood 15:350-359, 1960.

3. Frei E, Freireich EJ, Gehan E, Pinkel D, Holland JF, Selawry O, Haurani F, Spurr CL, Hayes DM, James GW, Rothberg H, Sodee DB, Rundles RW, Schroeder LR, Hoogstraten B, Wolman IJ, Traggis DG, Cooper T, Gendel BR, Ebaugh F, Taylor R: Studies of sequential and combination antimetabolite therapy in acute leukemia: 6-mercaptopurine and methotrexate. Blood 18:431-454, 1961.

4. Sullivan MP, Beatty EC Jr, Hyman CB, Murphy ML, Pierce MI, Severo NC: A comparison of the effectiveness of standard dose 6-mercaptopurine, combination 6-mercaptopurine and DON, and high loading 6-mercaptopurine therapies in treatment of acute leukemias of childhood: results of a cooperative study. Cancer Chemother Rep 18:83-95, 1962.

5. Freireich EJ, Gehan E, Frei E, Schroeder LR, Wolman IF, Anbari R, Burgert EO, Mills SD, Pinkel D, Selawry OS, Moon JH, Bendel BR, Spurr CL, Storrs R, Haurani F, Hoogstraten B, Lee S: The effect of 6-mercaptopurine on the duration of steroid induced remissions in acute leukemia: A model for evaluation of other potentially useful therapy. Blood 21:699-716, 1963.

6. Krivit W, Brubaker CA, Thatcher LG, Pierce M, Perrin E, Hartmann JR: Maintenance therapy in acute leukemia of childhood. Cancer 21:352-356, 1968.

7. Fernbach DJ, George SL, Sutow WW, Ragab AH, Lane DM, Haggard ME, Lonsdale D: Long-term results of reinforcement therapy in children with acute leukemia. Cancer 36:1552-1559, 1975.

8. Evans AE, Gilbert ES, Zandstra F: The increasing incidence of central nervous system leukemia in children. Cancer 26:404-409, 1970.

9. Land VJ, Askin FB, Ragab AH, Frankel L: Late occult leukemic infiltration of the testes. Blood (ASH) Supplement, 52:258, 1978.

10. Jones B, Holland JF, Glidewell O: Lower incidence of CNS leukemia using dexamethasone instead of prednisone for induction in acute lymphocytic leukemia. AACR 16:183, 1975.

11. Sullivan MP, Moon TE, Trueworthy T, Vietti T, Humphrey GB, Komp D: Combination intrathecal therapy for meningeal leukemia: two versus three drugs. Blood 50:471-479, 1977.

12. Nesbit M, Ortega J, Donaldson M, Hittle R, Hammond D, Weiner J: Prevention of testicular relapse by prophylactic radiation (XRT) in childhood acute lymphoblastic leukemia (ALL). ASCO 18:317, 1977.

13. Pierce M, Borges W, Heyn RM, Wolff JA, Gilbert E: Epidemiological factors and survival experience in 1770 children with acute leukemia. Cancer 23:1296-1304, 1969.

14. George SL, Fernbach DJ, Vietti TJ, Sullivan MP, Lane DM, Haggard ME, Berry DH, Lonsdale D, Komp D: Factors influencing survival in pediatric acute leukemia. The Southwest Oncology Group Experience, 1958-1970. Cancer 32:1542-1553, 1973.

15. Sutow WW, Thurman WG, Windmiller J: Vincristine (leurocristine) sulfate in the treatment of children with metastatic Wilms' tumor. Pediatrics 32:880-887, 1963.

16. Wolff JA, Krivit W, Newton WA Jr, D'Angio GJ: Single versus multiple dose dactinomycin therapy of Wilms' tumor. New Engl J Med 279:290-294, 1968.

17. D'Angio GJ, Evans AE, Breslow NE, Beckwith B, Bishop H, Feigl P, Goodwin W, Leape LL, Sinks LF, Sutow W, Tefft M, Wolff J: The treatment of Wilms' tumor: Results of the National Wilms' Tumor Study. Cancer 38:633-646, 1976.

18. Beckwith JB, Palmer NF: Histopathology and prognosis of Wilms' tumor: Results from the first National Wilms' Tumor Study. Cancer 41:1937-1948, 1978.

19. Leape LL, Breslow NE, Bishop HC: The surgical treatment of Wilms' tumor: Results of the National Wilms' Tumor Study. Ann Surg 187:351-356, 1978.

20. Tefft M, D'Angio GJ, Grant W: Postoperative radiation therapy for residual Wilms' tumor: Review of group III patients in the National Wilms' Tumor Study. Cancer 37:2768-2772, 1976.

21. Sitarz AL, Heyn R, Murphy M, Origenes M, Severo N: Triple drug therapy with actinomycin D (NSC-3053), chlorambucil (NSC-3088) and methotrexate (NSC-740) in metastatic solid tumors in children. Cancer Chemother Rep 45:45-51, 1965.

22. Maurer HM, Moon T, Donaldson M, Fernandez C, Gehan EA, Hammond D, Hays DM, Lawrence W, Newton W, Ragab A, Raney B, Soule EH, Sutow WW, Tefft M: The Intergroup Rhabdomyosarcoma Study - a preliminary report. Cancer 40:2015-2026, 1977.

23. Heyn R, Holland R, Joo P, Johnson D, Newton W, Tefft M, Breslow N, Hammond D: Treatment of rhabdomyosarcoma in children with surgery, radiotherapy and chemotherapy. Med and Pediatr Oncol 3:21-32, 1977.

24. Lawrence W Jr, Hays DM, Moon TE: Lymphatic metastasis with childhood rhabdomyosarcoma. Cancer 39:556-559, 1977.

25. Tefft M, Fernandez C, Donaldson M, Newton W, Moon TE: Incidence of meningeal involvement by rhabdomyosarcoma of the head and neck in children. Cancer 42:253-258, 1978.

26. Leikin SL, Evans AE, Heyn R, Newton W: The impact of chemotherapy on advanced neuroblastoma. Survival of patients diagnosed in 1956, 1962, and 1966-68 in Children's Cancer Study Group A. J Pediatr 84:131-134, 1974.

27. Evans AE, D'Angio GJ, Randolph J: A proposed staging for children with neuroblastoma. Children's CSGA: Cancer 27:374-378, 1971.

28. Ragab AH, Sutow WW, Komp DM, Starling KA, Lyon GM, George S: Adriamycin in the treatment of childhood solid tumors: A Southwest Oncology Group Study. Cancer 36:1561-1571, 1975.

2

Adult acute leukemia

Emil J Freireich, John M. Bennett, Ralph W. Vogler, and Peter H. Wiernik

INTRODUCTION

Acute leukemia has always been a major component of the Cooperative Group effort. The initial concept for the Cooperative Groups was to allow the accumulation of information on standardized treatment programs in a sufficiently large number of patients to permit precise estimates of effectiveness and to allow quantitative determination of differences between treatment programs. The major basis for the cooperative aspects of these studies was the attention to diseases which were relatively rare and therefore by pooling clinical experiences from a number of institutions, sufficient number of patients could be evaluated in a sufficiently short period of time. Acute leukemia was chosen as a prototype of cancer because the residual cancer problem revolves around the development of significant treatment for widely metastatic or systemic cancer. Since acute leukemia is a disease which is widespread at the outset, the localized forms of treatment play only a minor or an adjuvant role. Therefore, attention to systemic therapy was the essential component of the treatment of this disease from the time of diagnosis. A second important factor was the discovery that chemicals could induce substantial regression in these diseases and the early important drugs, the alkylating agents, the antimetabolites, the vinca alkaloids and the corticosteroids were all found to have anti-leukemic activity.

Two of the first Cooperative Groups were formed primarily to study acute leukemia. In the subsequent 20 years, acute leukemia continued to play a major leadership role in the Cooperative Group studies. It was in the acute leukemia groups that the development of objective, quantitative criteria for the evaluation of response were first introduced and widely agreed upon; [1] objective criteria for complete remission, partial remission, and less than partial degrees of improvement. The ready availability of objective quantitative data from blood and bone marrow led to the development of excellent data recording devices and of flow sheets which could be evaluated independently by the investigators. During the first ten years of the Cooperative Group Program, the important principles of combination chemotherapy with two drugs and subsequently with multiple drugs were developed; the importance of complete remission and its impact on prolongation of survival was appreciated; and the importance of therapy given to patients who were in complete remission was documented. Strategies of treatment during remission, such as rotational maintenance therapy, and intermittent reinduction, were developed. Studies relating to the role of meningeal leukemia as a sanctuary for residual leukemia and the first evidence of the curability of childhood acute leukemia were all developed by the Cooperative Groups.

By 1965 the progress in childhood leukemia, which is mainly in lymphoblastic leukemia, failed to be translated into the adult leukemias, which are predominantly a myeloblastic form of the disease. The frequency of complete remission was around 90 percent in childhood leukemia but still below 10 percent in the adult form of the disease. The discovery of the activity of cytosine arabinoside against adult acute leukemia and the documentation of the importance of schedule of administration on its effectiveness, began the era of rapid progress in the treatment of this disease. The subsequent discovery of the activity of anthracycline drugs and new combination regimens involving thiopurines, cytosine arabinoside, and anthracyclines were carefully worked out to the point where the frequency of complete remission is now in excess of 60 percent in many Cooperative Group studies.

For the majority of the time from 1958 to 1978 the major strategy in the management of acute leukemia has been directed toward increasing the frequency of complete remissions. The plan for accomplishing this goal has involved drug development, use of combination chemotherapy and improved supportive care. In each of these areas numerous spinoffs have contributed toward a better understanding of the biology of leukemia and normal marrow physiology.

The problem of increasing the frequency of complete remissions is beginning to be resolved. Consequently, the second major strategy, development of methods for indefinite prolongation of remission, is currently underway. The thrust is toward maintaining the first remission, since relapse bears a bad prognosis. The Cooperative Groups are well suited to execute this second strategy. They have the patient resources, clearly established criteria for diagnosis and assessment of treatment responses and superb statistical support.   This report concentrates on the studies conducted by the Groups.

Acute leukemia has also been important in the development of new principles for the chemotherapy control of systemic cancer.   Because the disease is relatively rare, progress in this area is a major justification for the continuation of Cooperative Group research as an important strategy for development of new methods for the control of systemic cancer.   Cooperative Group investigation of adult leukemia is an area where innovative treatment strategies are now under development in all the Cooperative Groups which have the potential for influencing research in the treatment of the more common forms of systemic cancer.   Important is the fact that the results of this research have directly benefited those patients who participated in it, reflected by the rapidly improving prognosis for this group of patients including the possibility that a small, but detectable fraction of patients are now being rendered disease-free or cured.   In addition, because of the rapidly progressive nature of the disease, the results of these cooperative investigations can be rapidly, quantitatively and objectively evaluated and information transmitted rapidly through the scientific meetings and abstracts to the academic community and subsequently to the community in general.   Thus, advances in treatment methods find rapid application throughout the country.

For the purposes of this review the acute leukemias are divided into 2 categories: 1) acute granulocytic leukemia (AGL) and 2) acute lymphoblastic leukemia (ALL).   Results will be restricted to adults.   Responses are considered as complete remissions (CR's), defined as 5 percent or less blast cells in the marrow, normal peripheral blood counts and absence of any detectable evidence of leukemia on physical examination (hepatomegaly, splenomegaly, adenopathy).

ACUTE GRANULOCYTIC LEUKEMIA

REMISSION INDUCTION

Single Agents

The agents available for clinical trials in the late 1950's consisted of corticosteroids, 6-mercaptopurine (6-MP) and the antifolate compounds, aminopterin, and methotrexate (MTX).   The use of these agents in acute granulocytic leukemia (AGL) yielded very poor results.   Remission induction rates were low and the median survival of all patients was a dismal 3 months.   The results of the first cooperative study appeared in

1958.[2]   It utilized 6-mercaptopurine (6-MP) and methotrexate (MTX) and was initially conducted in three institutions: National Cancer Institute, Roswell Park Memorial Institute and Children's Hospital of Buffalo. In a second study 6-MP and MTX were given in combination[3] and an 8 percent CR rate was found in 36 patients.

Several Group studies were conducted to evaluate the results of previous pilot studies arising from single institutions, many of which were Group members, and some significant misconceptions have been corrected by the Groups. For instance Huguley et al[4] reported a 40 percent CR rate with methotrexate given in 5-day courses. However, when the Group of which Huguley was a member used the same schedule only 3 percent complete remissions were seen.[5]

Changing the route of administration of 6-MP and of MTX from oral to intravenous led to no improvement. A randomized trial with two dose schedules each for the two drugs resulted in only 3 CR's in 67 patients treated with 6-MP and 2 CR's in 66 MTX treated patients,[6] hardly encouraging figures.   These and other experiences are summarized in Table 1.

TABLE 1
Composite Results of Single Agents in Acute
Granulocytic Leukemia

Drug	Number of Patients	Number of CR	Percent of CR
Corticosteroids	50	0	0
6-Mercaptopurine	142	9	6
Methotrexate	110	9	8
Cytosine Arabinoside	498	129	26
Daunorubicin	376	113	30

In 1964 Henderson and Burke introduced a new drug, cytosine arabino-side. Transient improvements were seen in a few leukemia patients. This drug proved to be more effective than its predecessors and extensive studies were conducted by the Groups to arrive at the best dose schedule (Table 2).

Thus these studies established the fact that cytosine arabinoside (CA) is an active agent. In trying to make use of what little is known of cell kinetics in acute leukemia one Group gave cytosar by continuous infusion 200 mg/M^2/day for 5 days and 35 percent of 26 patients achieved a CR.[8] Later this group even extended the infusions to 10 days. In order to confirm the greater efficacy of longer infusions patients were randomized between two schedules: 1,800 mg/M^2 for 48 hours or 1,000 mg/M^2 for 120 hours. The response rate was significantly better with the longer infusion[9] (Table 2).

TABLE 2
Cytosine Arabinoside in AGL

Dose & Schedule	Number Patients	Number CR	Percent CR	Reference
10 mg/M^2 x 12-24 hrs.	21	4	19	7
30 mg/M^2 x 12-24 hrs	77	12	16	
30 mg/M^2 x 1 hr	16	3	19	
30 mg/M^2 x 4 hr	26	3	12	
50 mg/M^2 x 1 hr	20	6	30	
100 mg/M^2 x 1 hr	20	5	25	
200 mg/M^2 per 24 hr day x 5	26	9	35	8
1,800 mg/M^2 x 48 hrs	53	12	23	9
1,000 mg/M^2 x 120 hrs	60	24	40	
100 mg/M^2 x 1 hr/day	49	7	14	10
200 mg/M^2 /day x 5	57	18	32	9

The second group of drugs developed in the 1960's and introduced into clinical trials were the anthracyclines. Daunorubicin given in doses up to 60 to 80 mg/M^2 daily for 3 to 7 days produced 20 remissions in 36 (56 percent) previously untreated adults with AGL. The European Organization of Research for the Treatment of Cancer (EORTC) treated 71 cases and obtained 25 percent complete remissions (Table 3). In promyelocytic leukemia Bernard et al[11] reported 43 percent complete remission in 40 adults treated with daunorubicin in doses of 60 mg/M^2 daily for 4 days. One Group studied varying schedules of daunorubicin and concluded that a daily schedule was more effective than semi-weekly or weekly, but was associated with severe toxicity. Clearly a dose of 60 mg/M^2 on 5 successive days was too toxic and a more cautious approach is preferable.

The related anthracycline, adriamycin, was studied in previously treated adult acute leukemia. Patients received a dose of 75 mg/M^2 every two to three weeks and 10 CR's in 55 patients (18 percent) were observed.[13] A third anthracycline, rubidazone, was introduced more recently. In early reports it appears to give a CR rate at least as good

TABLE 3
Two Anthracyclines in AGL

Daunorubicin	Number Patients	Number CR	Percent CR	Reference
60-80 mg/M² /d x 3-7	36	20	56	Boiron, et al
60-80 mg/M² /d x 3-7	71	18	25	EORTC
60 mg/M² /d x 3	20	3	15	12
60 mg/M² /d x 5	39	7	18	
60 mg/M² /d x 7	17	4	17	
60 mg/M² /d x 5	39	17	43	
60 mg/M² twice/weekly	45	8	17	
60 mg/M² /wk	47	8	17	
60 mg/M² /d x 4	40	17	43	11
Adriamycin				
75 mg/M² q 2-3 wks	55	10	18	13

as daunorubicin, but with less toxicity. In previously treated patients there were 13 of 67 (20 percent) complete remissions.[14]

Of the newer agents 5-azacytidine has been investigated by two Cooperative Groups. One reported 24 percent (11 of 45) CR's in refractory patients with AGL and the other observed similar results. However, responses are obtained at the expense of severe toxicity, particularly nausea and vomiting. When the agent is given by continuous infusion for 5 days it is better tolerated, but still very toxic.

Beta-deoxythioguanosine (β-TGdR) was given a Phase II trial in patients, most of whom were refractory to purine analogues.[16] One of 17 (6 percent) patients obtained a CR at a dose of 300 mg/M² daily x 5 and 6 of 49 (12 percent) obtained a CR at a dose of 400 mg/M² daily. These studies established the fact that β-TGdR had some, but limited activity as a single agent in treating AML.

The Groups have completed the Phase II evaluation of many other drugs (Table 4). Of these some have been forgotten, others had an incomplete evaluation, and a few are still being used in the management of leukemia, e.g. cyclophosphamide and vincristine. The Cooperative Groups obviously have played a major role in the evaluation of these and other components. In the current Drug Evaluation Program of the NCI the Groups continue to be important in the Phase II evaluation of new agents.

TABLE 4
Other Drugs Evaluated in AGL

Drug	Year	Drug	Year
6-Azauracil	1960	Dichloro-MTX	1965
BW 57-323	1960	Vincristine	1966
Cyclophosphamide	1960	BCNU	1968
Vinblastine	1961	L-asparaginase	1971
Methyl-GAG	1962	Emetine HCL	1971
Hydroxyurea	1963	Guanazole	1973
6-MP riboside	1964	Thioguanine	1978

Combination Chemotherapy

The previously mentioned combination of 6-MP and MTX was the first to be studied in acute leukemia.[3]   The results showed a greater efficacy of the two drugs when used in combination than when used sequentially. This very important finding formed the basis for future combination trials. The addition of prednisone (P), which as a single agent was inactive, to 6-MP did not lead to a higher response rate. VAMP, the 4-drug combination of vincristine (V), MTX, 6-MP and P, which was successful in children, was reshuffled and received the acronym POMP. It consists of the same 4 drugs but a somewhat different dose schedule was used. A complete remission rate of 27 percent has been reported.[17] This forms a distinct improvement over the earlier results, but the major push was not given until cytosine arabinoside arrived.

The efficacy of cytosine arabinoside as a single agent was such that many combinations with other agents at various dose schedules needed to be investigated. Reported here are only the Cooperative Group studies, without detracting from the importance of studies conducted in single institutions (Table 5). The improvement in CR rate is notable especially when the cytosine arabinoside infusions were extended to 5 and 10 days and when it was combined with oncovin and prednisone. The 50 percent CR mark was reached for the first time by the Groups in 1976.

When the anthracyclines were introduced the next important step forward could be made. Again several combinations had to be tried, dosages needed to be altered and drug interactions had to be evaluated. The Group experience is shown in Table 6.

TABLE 5
Combinations Including Cytosine Arabinoside and
Excluding Anthracyclines

Drugs CA +	Number Patients	Number CR	Percent CR	References
6-MP	56	15	27	10
Thioguanine (TG)	66	24	36	10
TG	162	71	44	18
TG q 12 h.	102	35	34	19
6-TG	69	16	23	20
6-TG q 12 h.	58	17	29	21
CCNU	60	18	30	20
CTX + MTX	55	18	33	21
OAP 5-day	73	31	43	22
OAP 10-day	158	81	51	23

TABLE 6
Combinations Including Cytosine Arabinoside
and Anthracyclines in AGL

Drugs and Days	Number Patients	Number CR	Percent CR	References
CA + D (5+2)	20	9	45	24
CA (int) + D (5+2)	38	14	37	25
CA (cont) + D (5+2)	41	17	41	
CA (int) + D (7+3)	83	43	52	
CA (cont) + D (7+3)	84	50	60	
CA + D (7+3)	52	31	60	26
CA + D + TG	154	77	50	18
CA + D + TG	104	40	38	19
CA + D + TG	122	58	48	26
CA + D + O + P	89	35	39	22
CIAL	337	194	58	27

The significant difference from Table 5 is the fact that now several studies led to a CR rate which exceeds the 50 percent mark. Thus after two decades of painstaking clinical research and after numerous disappointments we have finally arrived at a reproducible and acceptable response rate. One must remember that cytosine arabinoside was introduced in 1964, daunorubicin in 1968 and that the drug armamentarium is still very limited.

IMMUNOTHERAPY

Because of the successful use of BCG in prolonging remission duration in ALL reported by Mathe[28], various clinical trials have been underway. Powles[29] reported a statistically significant prolongation of survival in 25 AGL patients given BCG, allogeneic leukemic cells and chemotherapy during remission compared to 19 patients given only chemotherapy during remission. The prolongation of remission duration was of borderline significance. Subsequent analysis of the results after another 2.5 years of observation yielded similar findings. In addition, it was noted that the median duration of survival after relapse was significantly longer in the immunotherapy group.

One Cooperative Group conducted a study in which after six courses of consolidation 61 patients still in remission were randomized to receive twice weekly BCG (28 patients) administered by the TINE technique for 4 weeks followed by MTX, 30 mg/M^2 twice weekly until relapse, or MTX only (33 patients). Early studies reported a significant prolongation of remission duration from 9.7 to 20.4 weeks in the BCG group.[19] Subsequent followup of these patients revealed that the median survival was 93 weeks in the BCG group and 72 weeks in the MTX group, but that these were not statistically significant differences.[30] Subsequent remissions were longer in the BCG group.

Gutterman et al[31] studied 14 patients with AGL in complete remission following chemotherapy consisting of V, P + CA(OAP). Ten of the 20 patients received 3 intensive consolidation courses of OAP, the other 10 only one course. All patients then received BCG by scarification. They compared these patients with a historical group of 21 patients with AGL treated only with OAP prior to the onset of the study. The OAP group had a median remission duration of 60 weeks, the OAP + BCG group has not reached a median in this preliminary report.

One of the larger Cooperative Groups induced remissions with the 10-day OAP program, consolidated remissions with 3 courses of 5-day OAP and then randomized patients to receive either continued 5-day OAP courses or BCG + 5-day OAP.[32] The median duration of remission in

OAP (74 patients) was 75 weeks and on OAP+BCG (104 patients) 81 weeks (p = .87). The median duration of survival is also not different. Thus, this study refutes the uncontrolled results reported by Gutterman et al.

Another Group randomized patients between chemotherapy and chemo-therapy + Poly I:C during maintenance.[25]   Poly I:C had no effect. A randomized study conducted by this group using methanol-extraction residue of BCG(MER) showed no statistically significant differences in remission duration and survival with immunotherapy.[33]

Remission Maintenance and Survival

As already pointed out in the introduction, the median duration of remission is about one year and this requires maintenance therapy since the unmaintained remissions in AGL have a median duration of only 2 to 3 months.   Remissions induced with cytosine arabinoside (CA) and maintained with CA had a median duration of 58 weeks in one study. In another study the maintenance with COAP resulted in a median duration of 61 weeks. Patients induced with the 10-day OAP regimen and maintained with either 5-day OAP or 5-day OAP+BCG had an identical median duration of CR of 54 weeks.[23]

Until at least half of the patients achieve a CR little impact on the median survival time can be expected and it is too early for such observation.   However, just as the first survey of 5-year survival in children with acute leukemia served as an added stimulus to investi-gators, so will a survey of 5-year survival in adult AGL give new hope. A recent analysis in one Cooperative Group found 31 patients who had survived at least 5 years among 701 patients (4.4 percent).[34]   A substantially higher number of patients on more recent studies could potentially survive 5 years. There is a ripple in the surface.

ACUTE LYMPHOBLASTIC LEUKEMIA

Because of its relative infrequency there have been few therapeutic protocols for acute lymphoblastic leukemia (ALL) in adults.   The patients were usually included in studies designed for adult leukemia in general.   Results have been substantially less encouraging than in pediatric ALL.   Between 1965 and 1971 the CR rate in successive protocols was consistently 50 percent or less[35], but since that time there has been improvement as five Cooperative Group studies show (Table 7). POMP was not specifically designed for adult ALL, but it resulted in 63 percent complete remissions.   A treatment regimen similar to that used for childhood ALL gave 68 percent remissions[35] and

TABLE 7
Combination Chemotherapy in Adult ALL

Drugs	Number Patients	Number CR	Percent CR	References
POMP	32	20	63	17
PO + L-Asp. + CNS	50	34	68	35
PO + Adria	25	18	72	36
POM + CNS	85	69	81	37
COAP, OAP, DOAP	34	20	59	22

when adriamycin was added to prednisone and vincristine 72 percent CR's were obtained.[36]   The largest series with 85 patients have been treated with P+O+MTX.[37]   The CR rate is an encouraging 81 percent. The COAP, OAP, DOAP combinations resulted in 59 percent CR's.[22]

CNS prophylaxis appears necessary for prolongation of remission duration.   Without it the median duration was only ten months in one study.[36]   Using CNS prophylaxis a median duration of 18+ months is estimated with only six failures observed in 26 patients at risk.[35]   One study randomized patients between CNS prophylaxis or none.   The CNS relapse-free interval is significantly better for CNS prophylaxis. [37]

Adult ALL thus far appears to be a more heterogeneous group of diseases than its childhood counterpart.   Some cases may represent the leukemia phase of a lymphoma, others the blastic phase of chronic granulocytic leukemia.   Cell kinetics and metabolism of adult ALL may vary and drug resistance may occur more easily.   The heterogeneity could be important in the design of future protocols.

OTHER CONSIDERATIONS

The last decade of Cooperative Group research in adult acute leukemia has transformed the prognosis in this disease from a hopeless one with approximately 100 percent mortality in less than a year, to a circumstance where the palliative treatment is quite effective for the majority of patients and where a detectable fraction have prolonged disease-free periods, suggesting that a small fraction may actually enter the category of cured.

The process of remission induction in adult acute leukemia is still one fraught with a high degree of morbidity of the usual type, that is hemorrhage and infection. This high morbidity during a period of remission induction has drawn the Cooperative Groups' attention to new strategies of supportive therapy for the patients during the initial two to six week period of treatment, including leukocyte and platelet transfusion, treatment of disseminated intravascular coagulation, the use of prophylactic antibiotics and reverse isolation procedures and more recently a growing interest in the possibilities of allogeneic and autologous bone marrow transplantation.

With effective chemotherapy it is becoming evident that subgroups of the myeloblastic diseases require different strategies of treatment. Thus the elderly patients with the "oligoleukemic" blood picture are now being objectively and quantitatively identified and the current strategies of treatment are almost totally ineffective in this group of patients. In addition, in the patients who have chronic granulocytic leukemia and transform to an acute leukemic picture, a quarter to a third can be induced into complete remission, but these remissions tend to be extremely short in duration and poor in quality. Thus the chemotherapy which is highly effective in acute granulocytic leukemia is only marginally effective in the blast transformation of elderly patients with the oligoleukemic syndrome preceeding acute leukemia.

The Groups are now developing chemotherapy programs for other forms of adult acute leukemia which are less frequent, particularly those called acute lymphoblastic leukemia which make up between 15 to 20 percent of adult acute leukemia patients. These are a mixture of patients with disseminated B cell neoplasms which are identical to diffuse lymphomas, a small group of patients with T cell lymphomas, and a group of patients with highly undifferentiated acute leukemia. These subgroups of patients, like patients with the blast transformation of CML, tend to be susceptible to vincristine and prednisone remission induction therapy and tend to have a high proportion of complete remissions but have a comparably short remission duration when maintained on, for instance, arabinosyl cytosine in intermittent maintenance. Programs of cyclical or rotational maintenance analagous to programs developed in leukemias of childhood are beginning to show evidence of prolongation of survival.

1. Holland JF, Frei E, Burchenal JH: Criteria for evaluation of response to therapy of acute leukemia. VIth Int. Congr. Hemat., pp. 213-214, 1956.

2. Frei E, Holland JF, Schneiderman MA, Pinkel D, Selkirk G, Gold L, Regelson W, Freireich E, Silver R: A comparative study of two regimens of combination chemotherapy in acute leukemia. Blood 13:1126-1148, 1958.

3. Frei E, Freireich EJ, Gehan E, Pinkel D, Holland JF, Selawry O, Haurani F, Spurr CL, Hayes DM, James GW, Rothberg H, Sodee DB, Rundles RW, Schroeder LR, Hoogstraten B, Wolman IJ, Traggis DG, Cooper T, Gendel BR, Ebaugh F, Taylor R: Studies of sequential and combination antimetabolite therapy of acute leukemia: 6-mercaptopurine and methotrexate. Blood 18:431-454, 1961.

4. Huguley CM, Vogler WR, Lea JW, Corley CC, Lowrey ME: Acute leukemia treated with divided doses of methotrexate. Arch Intern Med 115:23-28, 1965.

5. Vogler WR, Huguley CM, Rundles RW: Comparison of methotrexate with 6-mercaptopurine-prednisone in the treatment of acute leukemia in adults. Cancer 20:1221-1226, 1967.

6. Ellison RR, Hoogstraten B, Holland JF, Levy RN, Lee SL, Silver RT, Leone LA, Cooper T, Oberfield RA, ten Pas A, Blom J, Jacquillat C, Haurani F: Intermittent therapy with 6-mercaptopurine and methotrexate given intravenously to adults with acute leukemia. Cancer Chemother Rep 56:535-542, 1972.

7. Ellison RR, Holland JR, Weil M, Jacquillat C, Boiron M, Bernard J, Sawitsky A, Rosner F, Gussoff B, Silver RT, Karanas F, Cuttner J, Spurr CL, Hayes DM, Blom J, Leone LA, Laurani F, Kyle R, Hutchison JL, Forcier RJ, Moon JH: Arabinosyl cytosine: A useful agent in the treatment of acute leukemia in adults. Blood 32:507-523, 1968.

8. Bodey GP, Freireich EJ, Monto RW, Hewlett JS: Cytosine arabinoside therapy for acute leukemia in adults. Cancer Chemother Rep 53:59-66, 1969.

9. Southwest Oncology Group: Cytarabine for acute leukemia in adults. Effect of schedule on therapeutic response. Arch Intern Med 133:251-259, 1974.

10. Carey RW, Ribas-Mundo M, Ellison RR, Glidewell O, Lee ST, Cuttner J; et al: Comparative study of cytosine arabinoside therapy alone and combined with thioguanine, mercaptopurine, or daunorubicin in acute myelocytic leukemia. Cancer 36:1560-1566, 1975.

11. Bernard J, Weil M, Boiron M, Jacquillat CL, Flandrin G, Gemon MF: Acute promyelocytic leukemia: Results of treatment by daunorubicin. Blood 41:489-496, 1973.

12. Weil M, Glidewell OJ, Jacquillat C, Levy R, Serpick AA, Wiernik PH, Cuttner J, Hoogstraten B, Wasserman L, Ellison RR, et al: Daunorubicin in the therapy of acute granulocytic leukemia. Cancer Res 33:921-928, 1973.

13. Wilson HE, Bodey GP, Moon TE, Amare M, Bottomley R, Haut A, Hewlett JS, Morrison F, Saiki JH: Adriamycin therapy in previously treated adult acute leukemia. Cancer Treat Rep 61:905-907, 1977.

14. Bickers J, Benjamin R, Wilson H, Eyre H, Hewlett J, McCredie K: Rubidazone in adults with previously treated acute leukemia and blast phase of chronic myelocytic leukemia. A Southwest Oncology Group study. Cancer Treat Rep, In press.

15. Vogler WR, Miller DS, Keller JW: 5-azacytidine: A new drug for treatment of myeloblastic leukemia. Blood 48:331-337, 1976.

16. Omura GA, Vogler WR, Smalley RV, Maldonado N, Broun GO, Knospe WH, Ahn YS, Faguet GB: Phase II study of β-2'-deoxythioguanisone in adult acute leukemia. Cancer Treat Rep 61:1379-1381, 1977.

17. Rodriguez V, Hart JS, Freireich EJ, Bodey G, McCredie KB, Whitecar JP, Coltman CA: POMP combination chemotherapy of adult acute leukemia. Cancer 32:69-75, 1973.

18. Wiernik PH, Glidewell O, Holland JF: Comparison of daunorubicin with cytosine arabinoside and thioguanine, and with a combination of all 3 drugs for induction therapy of previously untreated AML. AACR 16:82, 1975.

19. Vogler WR, Chan YK: Prolonging remission in myeloblastic leukemia by Tice strain Baccilus-Calmette-Guerin (BCG). Lancet 2:128, 1974.

20. Wallace HJ, Hoagland HC, Ellison RR, Glidewell O, Holland JF: CCNU plus cytosine arabinoside treatment of acute myelocytic leukemia compared with thioguanine plus ara-C. AACR 14:100, 1973.

21. Skeel RT, Costello W, Bertino JR, Bennett JM: Cyclophosphamide, cytosine arabinoside and methotrexate versus cytosine arabinoside and thioguanine for acute nonlymphocytic leukemia in adults. ASCO 17:301, 1976.

22. Coltman CA, Bodey GP, Hewlett JS, Haut AB, Bickers JN, Balcerzak SP, Costanzi JJ, Freireich EJ, McCredie KB, Groppe C, Smith TL, Gehan EA: Chemotherapy of acute leukemia: Comparison of vincristine, cytarabine, and prednisone (OAP) alone and in combination with cyclophosphamide (COAP) or daunorubicin (DOAP). Arch Intern Med 138:1342-1348, 1978.

23. Hewlett J, et al: In Immunotherapy of Cancer: Present Status of Trials in Man, Raven Press, pp. 383, 1978.

24. Holland JF, Glidewell O, Ellison RR, Carey RW, Schwartz J, Wallace HJ, Hoagland HC, Wiernik P, Rai K, Bekesi G, Cuttner J: Acute myelocytic leukemia. Arch Intern Med 136:1377-1381, 1976.

25. McIntyre OR, Rai K, Glidewell O, Holland JF: Polyribocytidylic acid as an adjunct to remission maintenance therapy in acute myelogenous leukemia. In Immunotherapy of Cancer: Present Status of Trials in Man, WD Terry, D Winthorst, eds, New York: Raven Press, pp. 423-440, 1978.

26. Omura GA, Vogler WR, Lynn MJ: A controlled clinical trial of chemotherapy versus BCG immunotherapy versus no further therapy in remission maintenance of acute myelogenous leukemia (AML). ASCO 18:272, 1977.

REFERENCES

27.   McCredie KB, Hewlett JS, Gehan EA, Freireich EJ: Chemoimmunotherapy of acute leukemia (CIAL). AACR 18:127, 1977.

28.   Mathé G: Approaches to the immunological treatment of cancer in man. Br Med J, 4:7, 1969.

29.   Powles R, Growther D, Bateman CJT, Beard MEJ, McElwain TJ, Russell J, Lister TA, Whitehouse JMA, Wrigley PFM, Pike M, Alexander P, Hamilton-Fairey G: Immunotherapy for acute myelogenous leukemia. Br J Cancer 28:365-376, 1973.

30.   Vogler WR, Bartolucci AA, Omura GA, Miller DS, Smalley RV, Knospe WH, Goldsmith AS, Chan YK, Murphy S: A randomized clinical trial of remission induction, consolidation and chemoimmunotherapy maintenance in adult acute myeloblastic leukemia. Cancer Immunol 3:163, 1978.

31.   Gutterman JU, et al: Chemoimmunotherapy of adult acute leukemia: Prolongation of remission in myeloblastic leukemia with BCG. Lancet 2:1405-1409, 1974.

32.   Southwest Oncology Group. Progress Report, 1977-1979.

33.   Cancer and Leukemia Group B. Minutes, June, 1978.

34.   Southwest Oncology Group. Minutes, November, 1978.

35.   Henderson ES, Glidewell O: Combination therapy of adult patients with acute lymphoblastic leukemia. AACR 15:102, 1974.

36.   Shaw MT, Raab SO: Adriamycin in combination chemotherapy of adult acute lymphoblastic leukemia: A Southwest Oncology Group Study. Med Pediatr Oncol 3:261-266, 1977.

37.   Omura GA, Moffitt S: The value of central nervous system prophylaxis in management of adult acute lymphoblastic leukemia: A randomized trial. ASCO 19:313, 1978.

3

Lymphoma

Charles A. Coltman, Jr., Richard A. Gams, John H. Glick,
and R. Derek Jenkin

INTRODUCTION

The Cooperative Group Program has had a definite and important impact on the care of patients with lymphoma in this country and others throughout the world. To date 15,024 lymphoma patients (6,312 Hodgkin's disease and 8,712 non-Hodgkin's lymphoma) have been entered into cooperative group clinical trials. These studies have helped to bring quality patient care to patients in small towns as well as large university medical centers. Through these clinical trials, the cooperative groups, using relatively unselected populations of patients, have simulated what goes on in the community practice of oncology.

The Cooperative Group program has made major contributions to our understanding of Hodgkin's disease and non-Hodgkin's lymphoma:

1. The groups established the activity of virtually all single agents in advanced Hodgkin's disease.
2. The groups confirmed the value of MOPP in advanced Hodgkin's disease with equivalent survival curves.
3. The groups have systematically explored drugs added to MOPP in an attempt to improve on the standard MOPP regimen (Bleomycin, Adriamycin).
4. The groups were the first to explore alternative regimens, with less toxicity, in direct comparison with MOPP (BCVPP).
5. The groups have systematically explored the role of maintenance therapy in advanced Hodgkin's disease, confirming the studies which have failed to show it to be of value.

6.   The groups have established the cost of remission in Hodgkin's disease in terms of complication. Both benign and malignant complications have been documented.

7.   The groups were the first to compare COP with single agents in advanced non-Hodgkin's lymphoma.

8.   The groups extensively explored the use of nitrosoureas in advanced non-Hodgkin's lymphoma.

9.   The groups explored the use of less intensive treatment in nodular non-Hodgkin's lymphoma.

10. The groups first documented the value of adriamycin alone and in combination in the management of non-Hodgkin's lymphoma.

11. The groups have, by their example, altered the standard care in the community.

This document is prepared as a detailed, but not exhaustive review of the group activities over the years in clinical trials involving Hodgkin's disease and non-Hodgkin's lymphoma.

HODGKIN'S DISEASE

HISTOPATHOLOGICAL REVIEW

Since the introduction of the Lukes and Butler classification of Hodgkin's disease and its modification at the Rye Conference in 1966, the prognostic importance of histological classification has been recognized. The development of the Pathology Panel and Repository Center for Lymphoma Clinical Studies (LPPR) in 1967 has gone a long way toward improving the precision and accuracy of histopathological classification in cooperative group clinical trials. Jones and associates showed that when LPPR reviewed diagnoses were compared to the contributing pathologist's diagnosis, Hodgkin's disease was confirmed in 94 percent of cases. In a comparison of 175 patients there was an overall 66 percent concordance for subtype classification (36 percent for lymphocyte depletion; 50 percent for lymphocyte predominance; 67 percent for mixed cellularity and 68 percent for nodular sclerosis). This panel has had an important impact on the quality control of Cooperative Group studies and such review is now mandatory for Hodgkin's disease studies in all groups.

A case in point is presented by Ward et al in which six patients (five diagnosed as HD and one NHL) were discovered to have immunoblastic lymphadenopathy. Their survival was uniformly poor and thus if they had not been properly identified they would have adversely influenced the survival ratio of patients in the studies to which they were assigned.

It is interesting, however, that with the introduction of extensive staging, high-dose intermittent combination chemotherapy and extensive high-dose radiotherapy, the prognostic significance of pathological classification has become less significant. In four cooperative group studies, one in localized Hodgkin's disease (Stage I and II)[3,4], one in intermediate stage (Stage III)[5,6], and two in advanced disease (Stage III B and IV)[7,8] there is no significant difference in survival between nodular sclerosis and mixed cellular Hodgkin's disease with followup to six, seven, and six years respectively. As a matter of fact, in the localized Hodgkin's study, there have been eight deaths among patients with nodular sclerosis while no patients with mixed cellular disease have died. This interesting inversion of prognostic impact dictates a reevaluation of the histopathological classification, with particular interest in the possibility of subclassifying nodular sclerosis Hodgkin's disease.

STAGING

The Cooperative Groups have been meticulous in demanding complete staging of patients with Hodgkin's disease prior to entry on study. This has permitted stratification of patients prior to therapy with regard to this important pretreatment variable. Information concerning methodology of staging as well as the prognostic implication of various stages of disease has resulted from consistent application of a standard method of evaluation to the large number of patients entered on cooperative group trials. Because of their access to large numbers of patients, the groups have been able to design broad Phase III studies for patients with specific stages of the disorder.

All of the cooperative groups currently use the staging schema defined by the Ann Arbor symposium adopted in 1971. Additional staging techniques have been explored in cooperative group settings. B-mode ultrasound[9] and computed tomography[10] have proven to be extremely valuable noninvasive techniques for the detection of abdominal disease. Of 35 patients shown to have abdominal involvement at laparotomy, B-mode ultrasound was correct in identifying 32 (91 percent correct). In the case of computerized tomography, 34 (85 percent) of 40 CT scans correctly reflected the presence or absence of lymphoma. Both techniques showed excellent correlation with lymphography without the attendant hazards and discomforts of this latter technique.

The routine use of staging laparotomies has resulted in a large cadre of patients who have had a diagnostic splenectomy. Although the initial data in these patients[11] suggested than an enhanced response rate might be expected in the splenectomized group because the asplenic patients tolerated delivery of greater amounts of drug in shorter periods of time, subsequent analysis[12] failed to show any difference in duration of remission or survival between the patients who had or had not undergone splenectomy. Thus, early splenectomy is felt to be important in the assessment of splenic disease but should not be considered a therapeutic measure. Long-term followup of 20 patients following staging splenectomy[12] failed to show more than a slight suggestion that there may have been impaired resistance to subsequent infections.

The importance of systematic restaging to assess the completeness of remission after therapy for advanced Hodgkin's disease has recently been investigated.[13] Restaging consisted of the meticulous repetition of all studies that had been abnormal prior to therapy, including peripheral lymph node biopsies, bone marrow biopsies, lymphangiograms, liver biopsies and in rare instances laparotomy. In 82 patients, thought to have achieved remission after systemic chemotherapy, occult disease was found in 10 (12 percent) predominantly in nodal sites (91 percent). In every instance these nodal sites had been involved prior to therapy. The most useful techniques were repeat chest radiography, 67-Gallium tumor scanning, and lymphography. These data emphasize the importance of careful evaluation of extent of disease during all phases of therapy to insure both the correctness of remission rates and the completeness of therapy, particularly in a disorder which is potentially curable.

Careful staging including the above mentioned techniques remains necessary in the clinical research setting of Cooperative Group trials. This will ensure continued uniformity of patient populations and accurate determination of response rates. Nevertheless, a review of this extensive experience with staging techniques has permitted suggestions concerning a practical approach to the question of staging laparotomies in the routine management of these patients. Jain suggests that laparotomy be performed only when the treatment regimen is stage-dependent and only if nonsurgical staging procedures have reliably failed to rule out disseminated disease.[14] He further suggests that staging laparotomy should not be done when the treatment plan is not altered by staging data, when there is a medical contraindication, or when evidence of disseminated disease has been reliably obtained by nonsurgical methods such as needle biopsy of liver or bone marrow, lymphography, scintigraphic studies and laparoscopy.

CHEMOTHERAPY OF ADVANCED HODGKIN'S DISEASE

Since the reports in 1969 and 1970 by DeVita and the National Cancer Institute that a combination of nitrogen mustard, vincristine, procarbazine and prednisone (MOPP) results in an 80 percent complete remission rate in Hodgkin's disease with sustained unmaintained remissions, therapy of the advanced stages of this disorder (IIIB and IV) has consisted of intensive combination chemotherapy. Further refinement of this therapeutic modality has subsequently taken place largely in the cooperative group setting. This section will explore the progressive refinement of MOPP chemotherapy on the one hand and the development of alternative regimens, particularly those including nitrosoureas, on the other.

Development of MOPP Regimens

Modern combination chemotherapy for advanced Hodgkin's disease is solidly based on the early exploratory studies by Cooperative Groups identifying active agents in this disorder. In 1962 Gold[15] reported on the response in Hodgkin's disease to alkylating agents administered as single drugs. Objective responses were found in 17 out of 26 patients treated with nitrogen mustard (66 percent response rate), 10 of 19 patients treated with cytoxan (53 percent response rate), but only 6 of 20 patients treated with uracil mustard (30 percent response rate). The duration of the responses was brief (30-95 days).

Further studies with alkylating agents were reported in 1964 by Brindley.[16] Nitrogen mustard given at two dosage schedules was compared with thiotepa also given at two dosage levels. High-dose nitrogen mustard (.1 mg/kg daily x 4 followed by weekly maintenance at the same dosage level) provided objective response rates in 5 of 10 patients (50 percent with a median duration of response at 44 days). The same drug given at half that dosage level provided objective responses in 4 of 7 patients (57 percent with a median duration of 33.5 days). Consequently, with nitrogen mustard there was little relation to dosage level, and duration of response remained brief. In the case of thiotepa, the high-dosage level (0.4 mg/kg) given on the same schedule resulted in similar response rates in 13 of 22 patients (59 percent) with similar median duration of remission (36 days). Half the dose of thiotepa, however, resulted in an objective response in only 1 of 9 patients (11 percent) with a shorter duration of remission (22 days).

Jacobs[17] compared a nitrogen mustard/chlorambucil regimen with cyclophosphamide. Response rates and duration of response rates were similar for the two agents and consistent with previous studies. Eleven of 19 patients (58 percent) treated with the nitrogen mustard/ chlorambucil regimen had objective responses with the median duration of response at 10 months. In those patients treated with cyclophosphamide 11 of 18 (61 percent) responded with a median duration response of 8 months.

Carbone[18] compared the alkylating agent cyclophosphamide with the vinca alkaloid vinblastine. For those patients who had no prior therapy, 10 of 54 treated with cyclophosphamide achieved complete remission, 19 of 54 a partial response, for an overall response rate of 54 percent. In the same group of patients treated with vinblastine, 15 of 56 achieved complete remission, 27 of 56 partial remission, for an overall response rate of 75 percent. For those patients who had received prior therapy only two of 32 treated with cytoxan achieved complete remission and three of 32 treated with velban achieved complete remission. This study documents the poor prognostic implications for patients who have had prior therapy and established vinca alkaloids as active agents in this disorder.

Solomon[19] compared nitrogen mustard with velban and introduced a crossover to determine whether the agents were cross resistant. Thirty of 44 patients (68 percent) treated with mustard and 15 of 26 (58 percent) treated with vinblastine achieved an objective response. When nonresponders were crossed over to the alternate regimen eight of 17 (47 percent) responded to nitrogen mustard while 11 of 21 (53 percent) responded to velban. These results continue to demonstrate the efficacy of both alkylating agents and vinca alkaloids in achieving responses in advanced Hodgkin's disease and further demonstrate a lack of cross resistance between these two classes of compounds. As in all previous studies with single agents, durations of response were brief and all patients who responded had relapsed by 36 months.

In 1970 Stilinsky[20] explored the efficacy of a new agent, procarbazine, in advanced Hodgkin's disease. When used as a single agent, procarbazine produced objective responses in 22 of 33 patients (67 percent) with a median duration of response of 98 days.

Preliminary combination studies were also investigated in the Cooperative Group setting. The combination of nitrogen mustard and velban[21] was found to produce an 85 percent response rate in 28 patients. Luce[22] explored the response of Hodgkin's disease to a three-drug regimen, cytoxan, vincristine and prednisone (COP). Thirty-six percent of patients with Hodgkin's disease achieved complete remission with remissions lasting 42 weeks if the patients received maintenance therapy or 19 weeks if no maintenance therapy was given.   Lenhard[23] explored the combination of cyclophosphamide, vinblastine, and prednisone and compared it to vinblastine alone. While the total response rates were similar in the vinblastine and combination arms, the combination of cytoxan, velban and prednisone achieved a higher complete remission rate (38 percent).   Again, the median time for disease-free remissions was brief (6.2 months for the combination, 4.2 months for vinblastine alone).

These studies from the Cooperative Groups during the decade prior to 1970 clearly established all the elements necessary for the development of the MOPP program.   Mustard-type alkylating agents, vinca alkaloids, procarbazine and prednisone were shown to be effective noncross resistant agents in the management of advanced Hodgkin's disease.   The major drawback for these agents used alone or in combination with one, two or three agents appeared to be a low complete remission rate and a brief duration of response.   The combination of all of these elements into the MOPP program, announced in preliminary form in 1969 and more detail in 1970, represented the culmination of these efforts and introduced for the first time the concept of possible cure, by chemotherapy, of advanced Hodgkin's disease.

The Cooperative Groups promptly incorporated MOPP into clinical trials to confirm its efficacy and explore its implications further.   In 1973 Luce[24] and later Frei[25] utilized a MOPP regimen consisting of mechlorethamine hydrochloride 6 mg/M^2 IV on days one and eight, vincristine sulphate 1.4 mg/M^2 IV on days one and eight, procarbazine hydrochloride 50 mg orally on day one, 100 mg orally on day two, and then 100 mg/M^2 orally each day for a total of 10 days; prednisone at a dosage of 40 mg/M^2 orally was given daily for 10 days on the first and fourth courses of therapy.   These doses are typical of MOPP regimens in other studies reported.   In this study the complete remission rate for all patients was 65 percent.   This complete remission rate has changed very little with increasing experience with the MOPP regimen.   While various factors such as age and stage appear to relate to the overall remission rate, the most important prognostic factor was whether or not the patient had had major prior chemotherapy or major prior chemotherapy and radiotherapy.   Responders were randomly allocated to alternate month chemotherapy for an additional 18 months or were followed in unmaintained remission after achieving complete remission.   The study concluded that duration of remission was approximately doubled in those patients who received continued maintenance therapy although the survival was not different.   In this study the dramatic difference in survival between those patients who achieved complete response and those who achieved less than complete response signaled the importance of achieving complete remission, an observation that has been obtained repeatedly in subsequent studies (Fig.1).

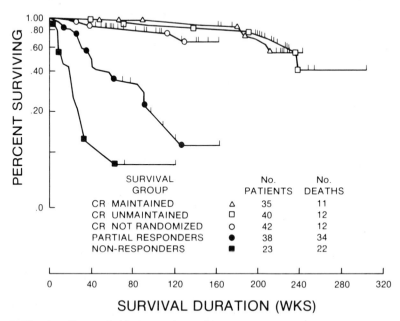

Fig. 1. Effect of remission and maintenance treatment on survival. CR = complete remission; marks on lines indicate date of follow-up examination

Huguley and associates[26] randomly allocated patients to induction with the MOPP regimen or with intensive nitrogen mustard alone. The complete remission rate of 47.5 percent with MOPP was significantly better than the 12.8 percent complete remission rate obtained with nitrogen mustard alone. In addition, the survival of all patients initially treated with MOPP was significantly better than that of those treated with nitrogen mustard alone, although the survival of complete responders to either was not different.

Stutzman[27] also compared MOPP with two other chemotherapeutic combinations: ALB consisting of vincristine and procarbazine alternating with chlorambucil, vinblastine and prednisone and a sequential (SEQ) schedule consisting of the same agents given individually in sequence. Complete response rates approaching 60 percent were found for both the MOPP and ALB regimens. The sequential regimen resulted in a response rate of only 50 percent. Although the MOPP regimen had the greatest toxicity, it also yielded the longest duration of response. Little difference in survival rates among patients on the three routines was found.

As experience with the MOPP regimen increased the next important question to be addressed was the optimal duration of induction therapy. Although earlier data[25] suggested superiority in the duration of remission for those patients who were continued on maintenance therapy after the completion of the induction regimen, subsequent followup failed to confirm this observation. Thus, after a followup period of over seven years, Coltman[7] demonstrated that differences in duration of remission had disappeared and that there was no difference in survival between the maintained and unmaintained patients. In a subsequent study[28] maintenance therapy with actinomycin D, methotrexate or vinblastine for 18 months following remission induced by MOPP failed to show any advantage over unmaintained remissions.

A series of experiments were then performed in which bleomycin was added to the MOPP induction regimen.[29] Bleomycin was given at two dosage schedules, the low dose being 2 IU/M^2 on days one and eight and the high dose being 10 IU/M^2 on days one and eight in each of the induction cycles. Patients with a compromise in pulmonary function were treated with MOPP alone. The death of three patients with irreversible myelosuppression on the high-dose bleomycin arm resulted in closure of that limb. The difference between the MOPP plus low-dose bleomycin and MOPP alone arms was almost but not quite statistically significantly different. In addition, MOPP plus bleomycin appeared to improve survival (Fig. 2); in this latter regimen, at seven years more than 50 percent of such patients are still alive.

It is of interest that in this latter study a consolidation arm of radiation therapy to areas of pretreatment bulk disease was compared with maintenance therapy. No difference in survival was found among these consolidation regimens. The latest analysis of the MOPP plus low-dose bleomycin therapy[30] continues to show suggestive evidence that bleomycin when added to MOPP in low dose enhances the CR rate ($P = 0.076$) and survival ($P = 0.06$) when compared to MOPP alone.

In a preliminary report in 1978[31] Jones reports a study comparing MOPP plus low-dose bleomycin, and two regimens in which adriamycin is given on day eight only or on days one and eight. The early results suggest that both adriamycin containing regimens have complete remission rates (76 percent and 77 percent) that are superior to the MOPP/low-dose bleomycin arm (54 percent). Nevertheless, a prognostic factor analysis suggests that more patients with unfavorable prognostic factors (cardiac disease and prior chemotherapy) were allocated to the MOPP/low-dose bleomycin arm. Continued analysis

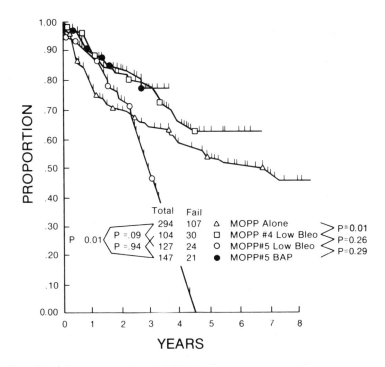

Fig. 2. Survival by regimen: MOPP alone versus MOPP low-bleomycin versus MOP-BAP

of this study will be necessary to determine whether or not the use of adriamycin in combination with a modified MOPP regimen will prove superior to the MOPP plus bleomycin regimen.

Development of Nitrosourea Containing Regimens

Soon after the introduction of a new class of chemotherapeutic agents - the nitrosoureas - the activity of these compounds was demonstrated for advanced Hodgkin's disease. In 1968 Lessner[32] found responses in 17 of 31 patients with advanced Hodgkin's disease (55 percent response rate) when treated with BCNU as a single agent. In 1973 Hoogstraten[33] found 6 of 19 responses (32 percent) in a group of lymphoma patients in a broad Phase II study of CCNU. Only some of these lymphoma patients had Hodgkin's disease. Tranum[34] subsequently found 9 of 16 patients with Hodgkin's disease to respond to Methyl CCNU (56 percent response rate), and Rege[35] again documented the responsiveness of advanced Hodgkin's disease to BCNU when 16 of 33 patients (48 percent) had a favorable result from treatment with this agent.

In 1975 Cooper[36] reported a study in which CCNU was substituted for nitrogen mustard in four-drug combinations. The programs evaluated included MOPP; CCNU, vincristine, procarbazine and prednisone; and CCNU, velban, procarbazine and prednisone. Complete remission rates ranged from 59 to 66 percent.

The duration of remission, however, was greater with either CCNU containing arm. In the CCNU, velban, procarbazine and prednisone arm there were 68 percent fewer relapses in three years than in those patients treated with MOPP. Durant[37] reported on the development of a number of four-drug combinations for advanced Hodgkin's disease, all of which included BCNU. These regimens included BCNU, cyclophosphamide, vincristine, vinblastine and procarbazine in various combinations. (The dosages and response rates are shown in Table 1.)

TABLE 1
Nitrosoureas in Hodgkin's Disease: 4-drug BCNU and Cyclophosphamide Combinations in Stages III and IV Refractory Hodgkin's Disease (1969-1971)

Drugs (route)	Dose (mg/m²) and schedule	No. of evaluable patients	Complete†	Partial	None	%	Hemo-globin	Granulo-cytes	Platelets	Gastro-Intes-tinal	Central nervous system
BCNU (iv) Cyclophosphamide (iv) Vincristine (iv) Procarbazine (oral)	100, q28d 600, q28d 1, q14d 100, × 10 days	31	9	14	8	74 (28/31)	2	16	9	12	13
BCNU (iv) Vincristine (iv) Vinblastine (iv) Procarbazine (oral)	100, q28d 1, q14d 5, q28d 100, × 10 days	8	3	2	3	62 (5/8)	1	2	3	5	1
BCNU (iv) Cyclophosphamide (iv) Vinblastine (iv) Procarbazine (oral)	100, q28d 600, q28d 5, q28d 100, × 10 days	22	9	8	5	77 (17/22)	4	8	1	10	2

Response (No. of evaluable patients, Complete, Partial, None, %); No. of patients with toxicity (Hemoglobin, Granulocytes, Platelets, Gastro-Intestinal, Central nervous system)

†Five patients continue in their original CR 5 years from start of study.

While the complete remission rates in none of these regimens were superior to MOPP, these regimens demonstrated the feasibility of combining BCNU with cyclophosphamide, a vinca alkaloid, and procarbazine.

Durant has recently reported the final analysis of a broad Phase III study employing a five-drug treatment regimen including BCNU, velban, cyclophosphamide, procarbazine and prednisone (BVCPP) in advanced Hodgkin's disease. The study was based on the earlier observations that nitrosoureas are active in advanced Hodgkin's disease and that the combination of BCNU and cytoxan is synergistic in a number of animal tumor systems. Drug dosages which are typical for nitrosoureas are shown in Table 2.

TABLE 2
Five-drug Regimen for Advanced Hodgkin's Disease (BCUPP)

		Day 1 Day 2 . . . . Day 10	Day 29
BCNU	100 mg/M² iv	X	X
Cytoxan	600 mg/M² iv	X	X
Velban	5 mg/M² iv	X	X
Procarbazine	100 mg/M² po	X ⟶ X	X ⟶
Prednisone	100 mg/M² po	X ⟶ X	X ⟶

Complete response rates were 68 to 73 percent for those patients who had not received prior chemotherapy and 28 percent for those who had. Thus, complete response rates for this alternative regimen are similar to those obtained with MOPP. Initial analysis of the study[3 9] suggested that 12 monthly cycles of BVCPP significantly prolonged complete remission in previously untreated patients. Multivariate analysis, however, did not demonstrate such therapy to be a significant prognostic factor. Subsequent analysis[4 0] showed that the maintenance and nonmaintenance groups of previously untreated patients were not strictly comparable and that the maintained group had more patients with favorable histologies who were less than 40 years of age. Thus, it

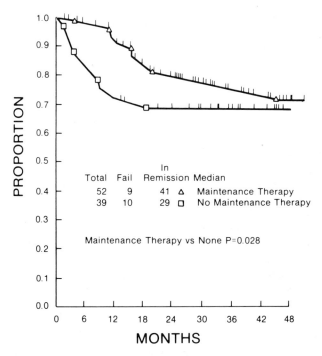

Fig. 3. Remission duration from end of induction for patients with no or minimal prior therapy who went on to maintenance and were evaluable. Maintenance therapy versus no maintenance

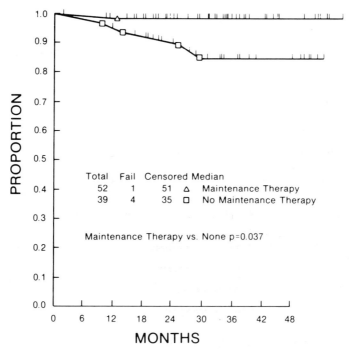

Fig. 4. Survival of complete responders from date on study for patients with no or minimal prior therapy who went on to maintenance and were evaluable. Maintenance therapy versus no maintenance

was concluded that maintenance therapy with BVCPP or MOPP did not significantly improve duration of complete remission or survival, a result similar to that described under the experience with MOPP induction chemotherapy. Duration of remission and survival after therapy with BVCPP are shown in Fig. 3 and 4. These figures demonstrate duration of remission and survival comparable to those found after MOPP chemotherapy.

Bakemeier[41] has reported a direct comparison between patients treated with BVCPP and MOPP chemotherapy. Complete remissions occurred in 73 of 106 (69 percent) treated with MOPP and 80 of 114 (70 percent) treated with BVCPP. It was felt that the gastrointestinal and neurologic toxicity were less with the BVCPP regimen. There was no significant difference in the duration of remission or survival among those patients who achieved complete remission maintained with six additional cycles of BVCPP after induction, with BCG immunotherapy after CR, or with no additional treatment.

In another study utilizing immunotherapy, Vinciguerra[42] found that the addition of MER (Methanol extraction residue of BCG) conferred no advantage on patients treated either with CVPP (CCNU, vinblastine, procarbazine and prednisone) or BAVS (bleomycin, adriamycin, vincristine and streptozotocin). All patients had received prior therapy with approximately 60 percent having received prior chemotherapy. Complete responses of 40 to 53 percent were found. This is a preliminary report that studies additional alternative regimens containing nitrosoureas.

Additional Studies in Advanced Hodgkin's Disease

The Cooperative Groups have demonstrated activity for a number of other single agents in advanced Hodgkin's disease. These include methyglyoxal-bis-guanylhydrazone[43], imidazole carboxamide[44], piperazinedione[45], hexamethylmelamine[46], dichloromethotrexate[47], VP-16[48] and VM-26[49]. These data have provided the basis for new regimens in the management of advanced Hodgkin's disease initially as salvage therapies for patients failing on the primary treatment with the possibility that some of these agents might be used in the initial management of patients with advanced disease.

O'Connell[50] reported a pilot study in which two adriamycin-based regimens were administered to patients with advanced disease. The first consisted of BCNU, adriamycin and prednisone (BAP) and the second VP-16 combined with adriamycin and prednisone (VAP). All patients treated had widespread disease and were refractory to other agents. Nine of 27 patients treated with BAP and 5 of 15 patients treated with VAP experienced objective tumor regressions, a 33 percent response rate in each case. It must be noted that not all of these patients had advanced Hodgkin's disease; some of them had other forms of malignant lymphoma.

Rossof[51] reported the use of the combination of bleomycin, vincristine, adriamycin and prednisone (BOAP) in patients with refractory lymphoma. Three of 3 patients with advanced refractory Hodgkin's disease achieved complete response.

The Cooperative Groups have been instrumental in developing intensive multiple agent chemotherapy for advanced Hodgkin's disease to the point that cures are expected in a majority of patients. There has been an orderly progression from the establishment of effectiveness of single agents to the use of combinations based on single agent data. It is clear that as long as complete response rates and disease-free survival are less than 100 percent, continued experimentation is necessary. Current Cooperative Group studies, including adriamycin as a first-line drug as well as the use of sequential alternating combinations of noncross resistant agents, remain too early to analyze but show promise of still further improvement in the therapy of advanced Hodgkin's disease.

QUALITY OF PATIENT CARE

Attempts are currently being made to improve the quality of patient care as well as to insure the quality of research results in the cooperative group setting. These efforts have potential application to the community and may represent a major methodology for the transfer of technology to the community setting. Wirtschafter[52] has recently reported the preliminary results of such an effort. A protocol for advanced Hodgkin's disease was rewritten as a clinical algorithm. This generated treatment advice rules and represented a computer simulation of how an investigator would follow the protocol for an individual patient specific visit considering his blood counts and prior response to therapy. Forms generated by the algorithms for each visit permitted investigators to evaluate how closely the protocol was followed at each individual treatment visit. Eight randomly selected medical centers in the cooperative group utilized the clinical algorithm method. The nine other members served as the control group. Those using the clinical algorithm method were found to follow the protocols 94 percent of the time as opposed to the control group which followed them 67 percent of the time (p < .001). Severe hematologic toxicity occurred significantly less frequently in those using the algorithm method (3% vs. 12% p <.005), suggesting the importance of careful protocol compliance. Such a clinical algorithm method has also been used in an adjuvant breast cancer trial among community physicians. The results again indicate that this methodology is capable of achieving higher protocol compliance and improved patient safety. This is as germane to community practice as it is to clinical research.[53]

RADIOTHERAPY ALONE

In an initial cooperative randomized trial, 22 centers combined to examine the radiation treatment of Stages I and II Hodgkin's disease. Four hundred sixty-seven eligible patients entered this trial during 1967-1973. Involved field radiotherapy (IFRT) was compared with extended field radiotherapy (EFRT).[54] At four years the survival rates of patients treated by these two methods were the same: IFRT - 82 percent and EFRT - 83 percent, but there was a significant difference in disease-free survival: IFRT - 47 percent and EFRT - 61 percent.

This important study pioneered the methodology to be used in collaborative trials of the radiation treatment of Hodgkin's disease, but in retrospect there were two principal design difficulties; the practice of staging laparotomy with splenectomy was introduced during the course of this trial and the treatment of first relapse was not precisely defined. Adequate time has still not elapsed for the hazard of relapse to be determined in this study, so that most investigators treat pathologic stage (PS) IIA disease with EFRT alone, despite the lesser morbidity and equal prospect for survival during the first four to five years provided by IFRT.

This study formed the basis for the subsequent comparison in PS I and II of IFRT plus MOPP and ERFT in SWOG-781.

COMBINED RADIOTHERAPY AND CHEMOTHERAPY

The earliest study of combined radiotherapy and chemotherapy of Hodgkin's disease was begun in 1965 by a cooperative group.[55] One hundred four clinical Stage III (lymphogram required) were randomly assigned to chemotherapy followed by involved field radiotherapy, chemotherapy alone, total nodal radiotherapy followed by chemotherapy, chemotherapy followed by total nodal radiotherapy and total nodal radiotherapy alone. The chemotherapy was nitrogen mustard and vinblastine. The seventy-two percent overall complete response (CR) rate was adversely influenced by a 45 percent CR rate with chemotherapy alone.

This study was innovative research conducted by a cooperative group but its ultimate value is limited by the small number of patients (11-24) randomized to each limb of the study as well as relatively ineffective chemotherapy. It must be recalled, however, that this study was initiated a year prior to the introduction of MOPP combination chemotherapy. The study did show a survival advantage (Fig. 5) for the chemotherapy-total nodal sequence (median 66 months) over radiotherapy-chemotherapy sequence (median 24 months) in IIIB disease.[56]

The second cooperative group combined-modality study in Hodgkin's disease involved the use of MOPP in 144 pathological Stage III A and B patients (74 patients received 3 cycles; while 70 patients received more than 3 cycles followed by total nodal radiotherapy). The relapse-free survival is 60 percent and overall survival is 70 percent at seven years.[5] There was no significant difference in toxicity, relapse-free and overall survival between the 74 patients who received only three

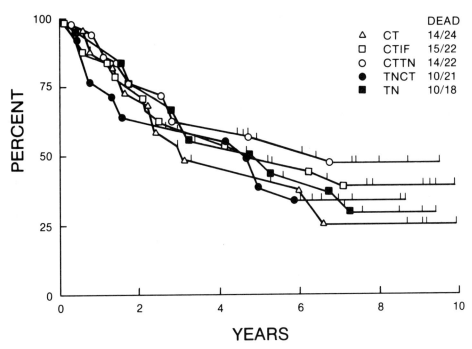

Fig. 5. Long-term followup of combination chemotherapy-radiotherapy of Stage III Hodgkin's disease

cycles of MOPP and the 70 patients who received more than three cycles of MOPP. This study showed that three cycles of MOPP could be administered safely prior to total nodal radiotherapy. This led to a followup study in pathological Stage III A and B patients randomized to ten cycles of MOPP plus bleomycin alone or followed by total nodal radiotherapy.[57] With 101 patients entered, the estimated two-year relapse-free survivals are 90 and 73 percent and overall survival 90 and 96 percent respectively. This study will ultimately answer an important question in the management of intermediate stage Hodgkin's disease.

Six years ago a cooperative group study was begun which compared extended field radiotherapy with involved field radiotherapy plus six cycles of MOPP in 206 previously untreated pathologically Stage I and II A and B Hodgkin's disease.[4] With followup to six years, a larger proportion of patients relapsed after extended field therapy alone than after involved field plus MOPP (p=0.01). A significantly larger proportion of patients who were Stage II (p=0.01) with mediastinal involvement (p=0.04), and who were symptomatic (p=0.002) relapsed on extended field than on involved field plus MOPP. In addition, a larger proportion of patients on extended field therapy alone have had extranodal relapse (p=0.004). In spite of this, no survival advantage has yet appeared (89 percent overall survival at six years). These data show that radiotherapy alone may not adequately control bulky mediastinal disease and that adjuvant MOPP is able to control inapparent or even microscopic extranodal disease. That there is yet no survival advantage for the combined modality treatment is a testimony to the success of salvage therapy in the extended field group, this despite a preponderance of extranodal relapses.

The report of Frei et al[25], in which patients with advanced Hodgkin's disease were treated with MOPP, demonstrated that there was a definite pattern of relapse. Eighty-five percent of relapses were in areas of prior bulky disease. Based on these data, a study was designed in which patients with advanced disease who achieved complete response were randomly assigned to treatment with chemotherapy (MOPP q 2 mo x 9) or to radiotherapy to bulk area of disease. With followup out to six years, there is no survival advantage for adjuvant radiotherapy. However, the study was flawed in that the radiotherapy was followed by additional chemotherapy, thus obscuring the radiotherapy effect.

COMPLICATIONS - MALIGNANT

Second malignancy complicating the therapy of Hodgkin's disease has become an important problem in combined modality management. Toland and associates[58] have performed an important confirmatory study regarding this problem. They reviewed some 643 patients treated on three concurrently run studies of Hodgkin's disease, including patients with all stages of disease and single (chemotherapy or radiotherapy) as well as combined modality therapy. These included all the eligible patients with Hodgkin's disease treated by one cooperative group, between 1971 and 1976. These data confirm the increased incidence of second malignancy in Hodgkin's disease, emphasize that the risk is primarily in the development of acute myelogenous leukemia, and confirm the correlation of that risk with intensity of treatment. The overall incidence density ratio is 10.33 while the incidence density ratio for acute leukemia in patients receiving intensive radiotherapy plus intensive combination chemotherapy is 1048.7. This observation of necessity puts the wholesale use of combined modality treatment for patients with all stages of Hodgkin's disease in a different perspective. Combined modality treatment, from the outset, must be limited to those subsets of patients in which a single modality followed by salvage therapy results in a survival disadvantage over combined modality treatment. Such limited combined modality (3 cycles MOPP + involved field XRT) versus single modality (chemotherapy alone) studies in Stage IIB patients with bulky mediastinal disease are now underway in the Cooperative Group setting.

COMPLICATIONS - NONMALIGNANT

All the therapeutic modalities involved in the treatment of Hodgkin's disease are associated with acute transient side effects. The occurrence of myelosuppression, nausea and vomiting, alopecia, peripheral neuropathy, oral mucositis, etc., have been well documented and the incidence of such toxic reactions can be found in any of the reports of the broad Phase II studies. This section will summarize, however, two reports which address themselves specifically to the complications of radiation therapy and one particular untoward effect of nitrosourea chemotherapy.

The complications of involved field or extended field radiation therapy have been described in a cooperative group trial involving 541 patients of whom 74 were excluded for varying degrees of ineligibility.[54] Out of the entire group a total of 35 patients treated with involved field radiotherapy and 64 patients treated with extended field radiotherapy were felt to have complications ranging in severity from mild and transient to severe and life-threatening. Patients with complications had an unfavorable survival experience, with death occurring in 11 of the 35 involved field patients and 16 of the 64 extended field patients. In 14 of these (five involved field and nine extended field) the treatment complication was considered to have contributed to death. Seven deaths (two IF and five EF), were attributed solely to the complications of radiotherapy.

The nature of the complications that occurred are shown in Table 3. Pulmonary and neurologic problems together constituted approxi-

TABLE 3
Complications by System

| | Numbers of Complications | | | | | | | | | | | | | |
| | Skin | | Lung | | Neur. | | CT* | | GI* | | Hemat. | | Other* | |
	IF	EF	IF	EF	IF	EF	IF	EF	IF	EF	IF	EF	IF	EF
Nondisabling	6	11	12	14	5	9	4	6	4	3	3	3	3	1
Minor, transient	1		1	1		1	2	1					1	
Minor, persistent		1		10	1	6	1			2	1	1	1	3
Major	1	1	3	5	1	1	2	3		3			2	2
Questionable				1										
TOTAL	8	13	16	31	7	17	9	10	4	8	4	4	7	6

*CT: connective tissue. GI: gastrointestinal. Other: genitourinary, thyroid, pericardium.

mately half of all untoward reactions. Most commonly the pulmonary lesions consisted of pulmonary fibrosis, often with pleural effusion. In approximately half the cases this radiographic finding progressed to severe disability and six of the seven deaths in which a complication of therapy was considered to be the cause of death were from pulmonary toxicity. The majority of neurologic disorders were mild consisting primarily of the presence of Lhermitte's sign; nine cases had persisting mild disability, and two had major disability with one of these patients dying with transverse myelitis, and paraplegia 44 months after completion of therapy.

Skin and connective tissue complications were the next most frequent adverse reactions and in five patients these were associated with major disability.

A variety of other systems were involved as seen from Table 3. The most severe other complication was a case of esophageal stenosis requiring bypass surgery with death occurring as a complication of surgery and residual or recurrent Hodgkin's disease.

The major finding of this study was the observation that there were an excess of complications of greater severity in the extended field series in most organ systems.

In a study currently in press[59], the incidence of a specific complication of nitrosourea chemotherapy was determined primarily because of the large number of cases seen in a cooperative group setting. This report describes the development of pulmonary fibrosis in ten patients following BCNU therapy for malignancy. The development was lethal in seven patients, four of whom had no evidence of tumor at autopsy. Onset of symptoms was usually insidious with the early development of cough and dyspnea. In some instances sudden respiratory failure occurred. Chest x-rays generally showed diffuse interstitial fibrosis. Both diffusion and restrictive defects were found on pulmonary function. No particular relationship was found between dose of drug received and the development of pulmonary toxicity, nor did there seem to be any relationship to prior radiation therapy. In one instance pulmonary symptoms occurred after the first treatment.

The Cooperative Group setting represents an ideal situation for the early recognition and characterization of untoward reactions to therapy, as well as the determination of their precise incidence.

In another study of this type, Chilcote et al[60] did a retrospective evaluation of septicemia and meningitis in 200 children who underwent laparotomy and splenectomy. They described 20 episodes in 18 children with primary gram positive, penicillin sensitive organisms with a high mortality. They suggested this might be attenuated by penicillin prophylaxis and/or bacteria vaccines.

PEDIATRIC HODGKIN'S DISEASE

Only about 15 percent of patients with Hodgkin's disease present in the pediatric age range. Fortunately there is no qualitative difference in the response to treatment for this disease in the child as opposed to the adult. Thus it has been possible to apply to children the treatment methods found to be successful in young adults, but with the proviso that treatment related morbidity is greater in the child so that more weight has been given to conservative treatment methods.

Because of the small number of cases no single cooperative group has undertaken a major treatment study in pediatric Hodgkin's disease, but an intergroup study (SWOG, CCSG, CALGB) opened for patient entry in December of 1976 and accessed 109 patients in PS I and II in the first 18 months (Fig. 6).

This study has two principal aims: 1) To assess the relative response to IFRT, IFRT plus MOPP, and EFRT with defined treatment for first relapse, and 2) to assess the relative morbidities of these treatments with regard to: growth defects; hypothyroidism; sterility; incidence of second tumor; the complications of laparotomy with splenectomy, and the effect of penicillin prophylaxis following splenectomy. While no results are available from this study, important questions are posed which the study has the power to answer.

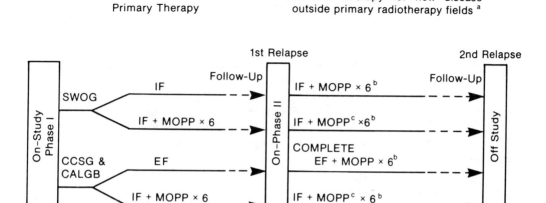

Fig. 6. CCG-541 Schema Hodgkin's disease Stages I & II

While these studies have provided valuable data they all have major limitations. The total numbers are small, about ten patients a year at each institution, and as a consequence anomalous results are evident, particularly with regard to the effect of standard dose EFRT in PS IIA. All studies have indicated a marked improvement in five-year survival rates to about 90 percent, so that comparisons of effectiveness and complications require at least ten years of followup.

NON-HODGKIN'S LYMPHOMA

PATHOLOGY REVIEW

Until recently, the management of non-Hodgkin's lymphoma (NHL) has been based on imprecise histopathologic criteria. Although Rappaport first formulated a working classification of NHL in 1956, only recently has it replaced the inadequate terminology of lymphosarcoma, reticulum cell sarcoma, and giant follicular lymphoma. This classification was first validated by a detailed retrospective review of 405 cases at Stanford. In 1967, the Lymphoma Pathology Review Panel was established under the direction of Dr. Henry Rappaport to aid the cooperative groups by providing more uniform and consistent interpretation of pathologic material from patients entered in various group studies.

The importance of this review has been documented by Jones, et al[1] who reported that 96 percent (162/168) of the patients studied could be confirmed to have NHL on review. However, complete agreement (type and subtype) between institutional pathologists and the Lymphoma Pathology Panel review diagnosis was found in only 58 percent of the confirmed cases of NHL. In 26 (16 percent) of 160 cases of non-Hodgkin's lymphoma, the initial interpretation of pattern (nodular vs. diffuse) differed: 20 (25 percent) of 81 nodular lymphomas had been thought to be diffuse and six (8 percent) of 79 diffuse lymphomas had been diagnosed as nodular. The diagnosis of a nodular lymphoma was more likely to be substantiated on review than the diagnosis of a diffuse lymphoma (P = 0.01). Furthermore, two distinct subtypes of NHL were most often correctly diagnosed at the institutional level: 86 percent of the cases of diffuse histiocytic lymphoma and 78 percent of the cases of nodular lymphocytic poorly differentiated lymphoma were confirmed on review. Significantly less agreement was noted for all other subtypes of NHL.

Ezdinli et al[61] found similar results. The diagnosis of non-Hodgkin's lymphoma was confirmed in 514/535 cases reviewed, giving an agreement rate of 96 percent between institutional pathologists and the Lymphoma Pathology Panel. However, the agreement rates as to cell type and pattern were much lower. Only 281/334 patients (81 percent) entered on a study for lymphocytic lymphoma were found on pathology review to have the eligible cell types. The corresponding rate on another study (histiocytic and mixed cell types) was somewhat lower (79 percent). When both studies are combined, it becomes evident that NHL randomization based on histiologic classification as to cell type by diverse institutional pathologists resulted in a 20 percent ineligibility rate. In more recent protocols, institutional pathologists were requested to determine primarily the pattern rather than the cell type. In this study concordance improved so that 88 percent entered appropriately into the favorable (NLPD, NM, NH, or DLWD) subgroups. The agreement rate with institutional pathologists as to both cell type and pattern was most acceptable for NLPD (82 percent).

Importance of histologic review has also been confirmed by Durant et al. In 205/406 cases (48 percent) the referee disagreed with the local pathologists concerning the specific Rappaport classification. However, if only changes from the broad categories of good risk (essen tially favorable histologies of the nodular subtypes) and poor risk (unfavorable histologies of the diffuse subtype) were considered, there was disagreement in only 56/406 cases (14 percent).

These results further support the need to have pathologic review of all cases in the major lymphoma studies so that comparability can be assured and the results placed in proper perspective. At the present time, mandatory submission of lymphoma pathology material is required by all the cooperative groups. In addition to the anticipated improved reliability of lymphoma diagnoses, the cooperative groups can expect improved communication between institutional and referral pathologists. We hope this will lead to improved rates of agreement between institutional and Lymphoma Pathology Panel diagnoses. It does appear that prospective stratification or separation of patients into prognostically favorable (nodular) or unfavorable (diffuse) histopathologic groups is feasible. However, the newer proposed histopathologic classifications of NHL may introduce a significantly higher rate of disagreement than that which has been noted with the Rappaport classification.

STAGING IN NON-HODGKIN'S LYMPHOMA

The frequency with which disseminated disease is present in non-Hodgkin's lymphoma suggests that there may be limited usefulness to the application of the Ann Arbor system of staging to this group of disorders. A major argument for careful staging has been the identification of true Stage I disease which has been said to be potentially curable by radiation therapy.

Even this concept has been called into question by a recent study utilizing chemotherapy alone in the management of localized histiocytic lymphoma.[63] In this study 18 patients with histiocytic lymphoma with Stages IA, I$_E$A, IIA and II$_E$A were treated with a combination of cyclophosphamide, adriamycin, vincristine and prednisone (CHOP), with or without involved field irradiation. All of the patients treated with chemotherapy alone (9 patients) achieved complete remission. Only a single patient relapsed in a site of previous involvement and was subsequently rendered disease free with involved field irradiation.

Nevertheless, staging in these disorders has provided useful information. In a group of over 300 patients with non-Hodgkin's lymphoma, Bartolucci, et al[64] found that lack of extranodal involvement proved to be an important prognostic factor. Herman et al[65] found that 90 percent of patients who developed central nervous system involvement with non-Hodgkin's lymphoma presented with Stage IV disease. The most common extranodal sites included bone marrow, gastrointestinal tract, skin, and lung.

Herman and Jones[66] investigated the question of systematic restaging in the management of non-Hodgkin's lymphomas. Eighteen of 100 patients with advanced non-Hodgkin's lymphoma, thought to have achieved a complete response, were found to have residual disease predominantly in lymph nodes and bone marrow. The importance of extranodal disease prior to the onset of therapy was again found since patients with persistent lymphoma at systematic restaging more often had Stage IV disease. In the majority of instances persistent disease was found in the sites of original involvement. Although it seems reasonable that therapy should continue in patients with persistent lymphoma, it may also be necessary in those who are in complete remission, since 20 of the 82 patients without demonstrable residual disease at restaging subsequently relapsed. In any event, the finding of a high percentage of clinically inapparent residual disease makes systematic restaging imperative for the accurate determination of response rates.

CHEMOTHERAPY

Chemotherapy of the non-Hodgkin's lymphomas has evolved over the past decade from the demonstration that single alkylating agents are active in the treatment of these diseases to the use of high-dose intermittent combination chemotherapy with curative potential.[63,67,68,69,70] Between 1966 and 1976, the Cooperative Groups completed 16 major Phase III studies involving more than 4,000 patients with Stage III and IV disease. Although these studies employed new and inventive therapeutic approaches, any analysis that attempts to compare one therapeutic program with another faces certain basic difficulties. These include differences in histopathologic interpretation and other prognostic factors including prior chemotherapy, as well as definition of complete response. Nonetheless, this analysis will demonstrate that there has been an overall improvement in response rate and survival from the initial studies with single agent chemotherapy to the current potential curability of diffuse histiocytic lymphomas.

Gold[67] first demonstrated in 1963 that single alkylating agents were active in the treatment of lymphosarcoma. Early comparative studies of the remission-inducing effect of single agent cyclophosphamide as compared to the vinca alkaloids in what was then called lymphosarcoma and reticulum cell sarcoma demonstrated that the cyclophosphamide-treated groups had a consistently higher remission induction rate when compared to vinca-treated patients.[18] The initial report by Hoogstraten[71] in 1969 was the first trial comparing single agent cyclophosphamide with both a high and low-dose combination of cyclophosphamide, vincristine, and prednisone. The low-dose combination was given at two-thirds of the high-dose program (Table 4).

TABLE 4
Remission Induction Therapy* for NHL

Drug (route)	Single agent (mg/kg/wk)	Combination treatment (mg/kg)	
		High CVP	Low CVP
Cyclophosphamide (iv)	15	15/wk	10/wk
Vincristine (iv)	——	0.025/wk	0.017/wk
Prednisone (oral)	——	1.0/day	0.67/day

*Treatment course = 6 weeks; maintenance = methotrexate or no treatment.

The response rates are indicated in Table 5. In lymphosarcoma, both combinations increased the percentage of remissions significantly when compared to cyclophosphamide alone (p < .01), but in reticulum cell sarcoma only the high-dose combination increased the response rate (p < .05). Significantly more complete remissions (CR) were

TABLE 5
Response by Disease and Therapy for NHL

	CR + PR (%)	
Treatment	Lymphosarcoma	Reticulum cell sarcoma
Cyclophosphamide	43	45
High-dose CVP	100 $P < 0.01$	85 $P < 0.05$
Low-dose CVP	90	54

achieved with the three-drug combinations (33 percent) than with the single agent (16 percent). The total percentage of complete and partial remissions obtained with the high-dose CVP combination was better than any previously reported in the literature.[7 1]

Subsequent generations of cooperative group studies were designed to confirm the effectiveness of intermittent combination chemotherapy utilizing cyclophosphamide-vincristine-prednisone (COP or CVP) in different dosages and schedules. Luce[22] reported an overall complete response rate of 35 percent and a partial response rate of 36 percent in 149 fully and partially evaluable patients with lymphosarcoma and reticulum cell sarcoma utilizing the COP 1 regimen (Tables 6 and 7).

The median duration of maintained response on monthly COP was longer than that of unmaintained response. All parameters of response, that is, complete remission rate, duration of remission, and survival were adversely affected by major prior treatment with radiotherapy and chemotherapy. Response to treatment correlated positively with survival. Although the complete response rate was clearly better than that described with use of most single agents at the time of initiation of this study, the median duration of complete response was still not significantly improved. A more protracted treatment program utilizing the same drugs in a four-week cycle (COP 2-Tables 3 and 4) was instituted in 1968 and achieved a complete response rate of 49 percent and a partial response rate of 35 percent in 154 patients. The overall duration of complete response was 109 weeks with those on maintenance therapy having a more prolonged response. The overall survival, 150.6 weeks, was significantly better than that achieved by the same cooperative group utilizing the same three drugs on a two-week schedule (p=0.003).[68]

The role of prednisone in the COP combination was examined by Lenhard et al[72] (Table 8). A complete response rate of 43 percent was demonstrated in patients treated with the three-drug COP program versus a 17 percent CR rate with cyclophosphamide-vincristine (CO) alone. COP was also associated with longer remission duration and improved survival. Survival was significantly higher for all patients who achieved a CR than for those who achieved a partial response. Cyclic maintenance therapy with CO extended the duration of remissions by approximately eight months regardless of the induction program.

The next generation of cooperative group studies investigated the addition of other active single agents to the COP regime. In SWOG-765 (COP 3 - Table 6), cytosine arabinoside (ARA-C) was added to the

TABLE 6
SWOG Dosage Schedules in NHL Studies

Regimen	Drug	Dose and Schedule	Interval (wks)
COP 1 (SWOG-753)	Cyclophosphamide	800 mg/m² iv Day 1	2
	Vincristine	2 mg/m² iv Day 1	2
	Prednisone	60 mg/m²/day po x 8 days	2
COP 2 (SWOG-760)	Cyclophosphamide	100 mg/m² day po x 14 days	4
	Vincristine	1.4 mg/m² iv Days 1 and 8	4
	Prednisone	60 mg/m² day po x 8 days	4
COP 3 (SWOG-765)			
Treatment 1	See COP 1		
Treatment 2	Cyclophosphamide	400 mg/m² iv Day 1	2
	Vincristine	1.4 mg/m² iv Day 1	2
	Prednisone	100 mg/day po x 5 days	2
	ARA-C	50 mg/m² iv Days 2-5	2
Treatment 3	Mechlorethamine	6 mg/m² iv Days 1 and 8	4
	Vincristine	1.4 mg/m² iv Days 1 and 8	4
	Prednisone	40 mg/m²/day po x 10 days	4
	Procarbazine	100 mg/m²/day po x 10 days	4
COP 4 (SWOG-780)	Cyclophosphamide	125 mg/m²/day po x 14 days	4
	Vincristine	1.4 mg/m² iv Days 1 and 8	4
	Prednisone	60 mg/m²/day po x 5 days	4
	Bleomycin	10 units/m²/day iv Days 2-5	4
CHOP/HOP (SWOG-7204)			
Treatment 1	Cyclophosphamide	750 mg/m² iv Day 1	2-3
	Adriamycin	50 mg/m² iv Day 1	2-3
	Vincristine	1.4 mg/m² iv Day 1	2-3
	Prednisone	100 mg/day po x 5 days	2-3
Treatment 2	Adriamycin	80 mg/m² iv Day 1	2-3
	Vincristine	1.4 mg/m²/day iv Day 1	2-3
	Prednisone	100 mg/m²/day po x 5 days	2-3

COP regimen and compared to COP alone and to standard MOPP chemotherapy as utilized in the treatment of Hodgkin's disease.[6][8] The overall complete response rate was 46 percent and the partial response rate was 27 percent (Table 7). No differences were noted in the complete response rates between the three regimens. The median duration of complete response was 220.5 weeks with an overall survival of 117.6 weeks. Thus, there were no advantages in the addition of ARA-C or the use of the more aggressive MOPP regimen.

A variety of investigators examined the role of the nitrosourea, BCNU, in non-Hodgkin's lymphomas. Ezdinli et al[7][3] (ECOG 1472 - Table 8) compared cyclophosphamide-prednisone (CP) induction chemotherapy to BCNU-prednisone (BP) induction chemotherapy in patients with both nodular and diffuse lymphocytic lymphoma.

TABLE 7
SWOG Studies in NHL

Study	Patients	Complete response (%)	Median duration of complete response* (wks)	Median survival duration* (wks)
Overall results				
COP 1	149	52(35)	——	80.9
COP 2	154	76(49)	109.3	150.6
COP 3	301	137(46)	220.5	117.6
COP 4	74	51(69)	109.7	176.2
CHOP/HOP	465	268(58)	123.3	NR
Stanford	255	——	——	165.0
Results in DHL				
COP 1	53	12(23)	——	29.7
COP 2	49	24(49)	60.7	71.1
COP 3 = ARA-C	65	22(34)	197.4	66.7
COP 3 - MOPP	36	34(29)	114.3	39.7
COP 4	16	10(63)	107.0	44.7
CHOP	68	32(47)	101.1	47.9
HOP	69	38(55)	95.5	87.5
Stanford	65	——	——	47.3
Results in NLPD				
COP 1	3	0	——	——
COP 2	17	9(53)	NR	154.4
COP 3 = ARA-C	20	14(70)	NR	198.7
COP 3 - MOPP	14	6(43)	NR	132.2
COP 4	15	10(67)	152.0	184.3
CHOP	62	48(77)	NR	NR
HOP	54	32(59)	NR	NR
Stanford	52	——	——	388.1

*NR = not reached.

TABLE 8
ECOG Studies in NHL

Regimen	Drug	Dose and Schedule		Interval (wks)	No. of Patients	Complete Response
EST 0168 Induction						
CO	Cyclophosphamide	10 mg/kg	iv Day 1	1	59	10 (17)
	Vincristine	0.017 mg/kg	iv Day 1	1		
COP	Cyclophosphamide	10 mg/kg	iv Day 1	1	54	23 (43)
	Vincristine	0.017 mg/kg	iv Day 1	1		
	Prednisone	1 mg/kg/day	oral daily	daily		
EST 1472 Phase One						
CP	Cyclophosphamide	1000 mg/m^2	iv Day 1	4	135	31 (23)
	Prednisone	100 mg/m^2/day po x 5 days		4		
BP	BCNU	120 mg/m^2	iv Day 1	4	138	26 (19)
	Prednisone	100 mg/m^2/day po x 5 days		4		
Phase Two	PR or CR at end of Phase One Re-Randomized for Phase Two;					
BCOP	BCNU	60mg/m^2	iv Day 1	4	38	(39)
	Cyclophosphamide	600mg/m^2	iv Day 1	4		
	Vincristine	1.4 mg/m^2	iv Day 1	4		
	Prednisone	100 mg/m^2/day po × 5 days		4		
CLB	Chlorambucil	18 mg/m^2	po	2	39	8(21)
EST 3472						
CP	See CP Above			3	66	14(21)
COP	Cyclophosphamide	1000 mg/m^2	iv Day 1	3	59	20(34)
	Vincristine	1 mg/m^2	iv Day 1	3		
	Prednisone	100 mg/m^2	po × 5 days	3		
BCOP	BCNU	60 mg/m^2	iv Day 1	3	62	21(34)
	Cyclophosphamide	1000 mg/m^2	iv Day 1	3		
	Vincristine	1.2 mg/m^2	iv Day 1	3		
	Prednisone	100 mg/m^2	po × 5 days	3		
EST 2474						
CP	Cyclophosphamide	600 mg/m^2	iv Days 1 and 8	4	45	23(52)
	Prednisone	100 mg/m^2	po × 5 days	4		
COPP	Cyclophosphamide	600 mg/m^2	iv Days 1 and 8	4	40	21(53)
	Vincristine	1.4 mg/m^2	iv Days 1 and 8	4		
	Procarbazine	100 mg/m^2/day po x 14 days		4		
	Prednisone	100 mg/m^2/day po x 5 days		4		
BCOP	See BCOP as in 3472			3	44	22(50)
EST 3474						
COPA	Cyclophosphamide	600 mg/m^2	iv Day 1	3	57	27(47)
	Vincristine	1.2 mg/m^2	iv Day 1	3		
	Prednisone	100 mg/m^2/day po x 5 days		3		
	Adriamycin	50 mg/m^2	iv Day 1	3		
CPOB	Cyclophosphamide	1000 mg/m^2	iv Day 1	3	47	20 (43)
	Prednisone	100 mg/m^2/day po ×5 days		3		
	Vincristine	1.2 mg/m^2	iv Day 15	3		
	Bleomycin	10 mg/m^2	iv Day 15	3		
COPB	Same as CPOB except Vincristine and Bleomycin Given on Day 1			3	48	17 (35)
BCOP	See BCOP as in 3472			3	38	12 (32)

Patients were treated with three cycles of chemotherapy and then crossed over to BCOP (BCNU, cytoxan, vincristine, prednisone) or chlorambucil. Complete responses with the combination of BP were 19 percent versus 23 percent with the CP treatment. These CR rates were inferior to that achieved by the same group with the COP program (43 percent) in a previous study. This trial also achieved a 37 percent partial remission rate with the BP program versus 44 percent with CP. Approximately half of the patients who failed to achieve at least a PR obtained a response with the crossover program, demonstrating a lack of cross resistance between BCNU and cyclophosphamide. The complete and overall response rate in NLPD of 47 percent and 81 percent was significantly superior to 25 percent and 59 percent obtained in DLPD.[74] The estimated two-year survival of 83 percent in NLPD was also significantly superior to the 47 percent two-year survival in DLPD (p < .001). A response to chemotherapy had a significantly favorable effect on DLPD patients with two-year survivals of 84 percent for complete responders, 58 percent for partial responders and 17 percent for those with progressive disease. In NLPD the effect of successful chemotherapy responsiveness on survival was less striking (91 percent of CRs, 85 percent of PRs and 72 percent of those with progressive disease surviving two years). These data confirmed the rationale for the use of more aggressive multiple agent chemotherapy regimens including adriamycin and bleomycin in DLPD, where achievement of complete response is the single most important factor in improving survivorship. Ezdinli[74] contrasted this to the histologic subgroup of NLPD where excellent survival rates, only partially dependent on chemotherapeutic responsiveness, were obtained. They recommended that this subgroup might serve as an ideal model for moderate (i.e., cyclophosphamide plus prednisone alone) or single agent chemotherapy.

Lenhard[75] compared CP, COP, and BCNU plus COP (BCOP) in histiocytic and mixed cell lymphomas, both nodular and diffuse (ECOG 3472 - Table 8). The observed complete remission rates were CP (21 percent), COP (34 percent), and BCOP (34 percent). Both COP and BCOP had significantly more complete remissions than CP, but survival following COP (118 weeks) was significantly longer than that following either BCOP (76 weeks) or CP (74 weeks). This study also confirmed that vincristine makes a significant contribution to the treatment of histiocytic and mixed lymphomas when added to a combination of cyclophosphamide and prednisone.

Prospective trials from all the cooperative groups have confirmed the better responsiveness and superior survival of the lymphomas with a nodular pattern (good risk or favorable histologies) versus those of the diffuse type (poor risk or unfavorable).[62,68,69,70] The distinction by histologic classification into good- and poor-risk categories appears to be not only important but also practical in terms of accurate histo-

TABLE 9
Response Rates of Non-Hodgkin's Lymphoma According to Histology
When Treated With COP or BCOP

Histology	No. of CRs/ No. treated	No. of CRs + good PRs/No. treated
Good risk	39/115 (34%)	94/115 (81%)
		P = < 0.005
Poor risk	59/185 (32%)	118/185 (64%)

pathologic review. Durant et al[62] demonstrated in a SECSG trial
(Table 9) that the response rate for good histologies is significantly
greater than for poor histologies at three months when patients were
treated with COP or BCNU plus COP (BCOP).

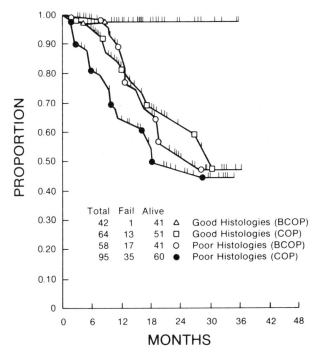

Significant Differences
BCOP Good Histologies versus BCOP Poor Histologies (p = 0.004)
COP Good Histologies versus COP Poor Histologies (P = 0.006)
BCOP Good Histologies versus COP Good Histologies (p = 0.046)

Fig. 7. Non-Hodgkin's lymphoma: Survival among responders (3
months induction). CR and good PR according to histologic treatment

This is due to a better partial response rate in the good-risk histologies because the CR rate in both groups was the same. Good-risk patients originally treated with either COP or BCOP survive longer than the similar poor-risk patients (Fig. 7), but the duration of these remissions (Fig. 8) was not different whether all remissions or only CRs were considered. Thus, it appears that histologic classification has an important effect on response rates and survival without influencing duration of response, suggesting again that the biology of the disease must be considered when assessing the value of any treatment. Furthermore, although the response and duration of remission of good-risk histologies to COP and BCOP were the same, subsequent survival was very different, regardless of the maintenance therapy, suggesting a value for BCNU in this group of patients reported by Durant.[62]

The above results were not confirmed by Ezdinli et al[76] who reported on 129 patients with favorable (good risk) histologies of non-Hodgkin's lymphomas randomized on ECOG 2474 to receive either cyclophosphamide plus prednisone (CP), COP plus procarbazine (COPP), or COP + BCNU (BCOP) (Table 8). Each of the above regimens gave a complete response rate of approximately 52 percent, with no significant differences noted in either the CR or overall response between regimens. Severe or life-threatening toxicity was significantly less on

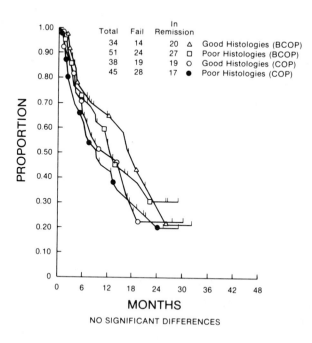

Fig. 8. Non-Hodgkin's lymphoma: duration of remission after COP and BCOP therapy by histology (3 months induction)

the least intensive chemotherapy program (CP). One-year survival was superior for the CP regimen (95 percent alive at one year) when compared to COPP (86 percent) or BCOP (77 percent). The authors concluded from their preliminary analysis that in favorable non-Hodgkin's lymphomas, moderate treatment with cyclophosphamide plus prednisone is the least toxic and is as effective as the more intensive COPP and BCOP regimens.

Nissen et al[70] have reviewed the extensive CALGB experience with streptonigrin in NHL (see Figure 9 and Tables 10 and 11). Their first study (6703) with this agent demonstrated a higher frequency of CRs obtained by day 42 when either streptonigrin or cyclophosphamide was added to vincristine and prednisone. Remission duration was significantly lower if patients were given maintenance therapy with daily oral cyclophosphamide rather than semiweekly methotrexate.

Their next study (6810) again clearly demonstrated the longer remission durations with daily oral cyclophosphamide maintenance.

Protocol 7051 demonstrated that the duration of remission and survival achieved with vincristine-prednisone induction followed by cyclophosphamide maintenance is prolonged if periodic "reinduction pulses" of vincristine and prednisone were given during maintenance therapy.

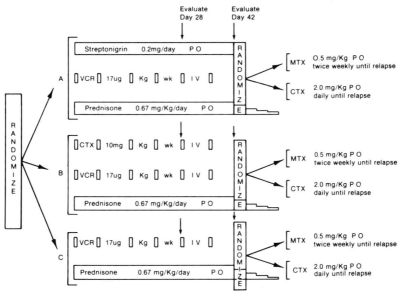

If progressive disease at day 28 or no response or progressive disease at day 42, patient goes off study

Fig. 9. Study design of CALGB-6703

The most recently completed study (7253) examined the remission induction potential of vincristine and prednisone alone or with the addition of streptonigrin and/or bleomycin. Maintenance treatment with daily oral cyclophosphamide plus monthly reinforcements of VP were given to all patients. Preliminary analysis suggests a higher frequency of complete remission in those patients with unfavorable histologies who received streptonigrin.

When the above trials are reviewed in perspective, it becomes apparent that the combination of cyclophosphamide-vincristine-prednisone (COP) represented an important contribution of the cooperative groups to the management of NHL in terms of improving overall complete response rates and survival. However, recent investigations

TABLE 10

Frequency of Best Response Throughout Study in 4 CALGB Protocols in Patients not Previously Treated with Chemotherapy

Study	Drugs*	Lymphocytic lymphoma			Reticulum cell sarcoma			Favorable			Unfavorable		
		No†	%CR	%PR	No†	%CR	%PR	No†	%CR	%PR	No†	%CR	%PR
6703‡	VPS	16	44	56	17	24	29	4	25	75	5	0	60
	VPC	24	8	63	16	31	31	5	20	80	8	13	63
	VP	24	17	67	12	8	67	9	22	78	8	13	75
6810	Combination VCR+ SN +CYT + PRED	49	41	29	38	45	21	18	56	22	27	52	19
	Sequential VCR + SN + CYT + PRED	46	46	35	35	45	17	20	50	35	22	55	23
	VP → CYT	53	47	36	38	47	32	16	50	31	23	43	35
7051	Low VCR	78	63	28	75	31	35	29	59	31	63	48	33
	High VCR	81	49	35	81	47	30	33	58	30	64	50	31
7253	VP	56	46	43	60	33	38	15	40	47	83	40	39
	VPB	48	54	33	50	34	36	13	38	46	71	48	31
	VPS	48	31	54	45	49	38	9	22	67	71	42	39
	VPBS	50	56	32	57	53	33	11	64	36	79	52	33

*See Text for explanation of drugs and combination.
†Total No. of patients.
‡6703 results are analyzed after 6 weeks of induction therapy; for the other 3 studies late CR's are included.

TABLE 11
Duration of CR in 3 CALGB Studies According to Study Regimens and Histology*

Study	Drugs†	Lymphocytic lymphoma		Reticulum cell sarcoma		Rappaport favorable		Rappaport unfavorable	
		No. of patients	Median duration of CR (mos)	No. of patients	Median duration of CR (mos)	No. of patients	Median duration of CR (mos)	No. of patients	Median duration of CR (mos)
6810	Combination VCR + SN + CYT + PRED	20	12.0	17	6.3	10	8.0	14	6.3
	Sequential VCR + SN + CY + PRED	21	8.0	16	8.0	10	13.0	12	5.0
	VP →CYT	25	25.0	18	14.0	8	7.5	10	12.0
7051	Low VCR	49	21.1	23	22.6	17	15.5	30	21.9
	High VCR	40	50.1	37	19.3	19	>24	31	40.5
	No reinforcement	34	17.4	21	10.1	13	>24	25	10.0
	Reinforcement	48	32.0	31	38.9	20	16.2	30	>36
7253	VP	25	> 22.0	19	19.4	—	—	31	25.3
	VPB	26	21.7	15	35.1	—		32	22.4
	VPS	14	> 17.0	20	11.4	—	—	29	16.8
	VPBS	27	> 24.0	27	12.5	—	—	37	>17.0

*6703 not included in this analysis due to small sample sizes.
†See Text for explanation of drugs and combinations.

suggest that less intensive chemotherapy regimens appear to achieve equivalent survival in the nodular lymphomas, while more aggressive combinations than COP will be required to improve CR rates and survival in the diffuse lymphomas.

The new anthracycline antibiotic, adriamycin, had been used both alone and in combination in patients with lymphoma of various types.[77] McKelvey first reported in 1973 the results of the CHOP versus HOP (Table 6) study in which adriamycin-containing combinations were systematically investigated.[78] Patients were randomly assigned to receive either one of these adriamycin-containing combinations. After achieving a complete response, the patients received three additional consolidation treatments at the same dosage. Those who remained in complete response were randomly assigned to maintenance therapy with COP or OAP (ARA-C substituted for cyclophosphamide). These data have been updated and an overall response rate of 58 percent and a partial response rate of 21 percent have been reported.[79] There were more complete responses with CHOP than HOP but the difference was not statistically significant.   The median duration of maintained remission was 114.0 weeks with CHOP, slightly superior to HOP (p=0.17).   The median survival has yet to be reached. Of 115 patients maintained on COP, 75 percent remained in complete response after one year. For the 108 patients maintained on OAP, 60 percent remained in complete response at one year.   The highest number of relapses have occurred in patients who never received cyclophosphamide. Figure 10 shows the overall survival curves of all patients with NHL who were treated on the SWOG regimens, COP, or CHOP/HOP, and also shows the Stanford survival experience (1960-71). There are no significant differences between these curves.

The overall complete response of 58 percent for all histologies on the CHOP/HOP study with a median duration of complete response of 123 weeks prompted Jones et al[80] to compare CHOP plus bleomycin versus CHOP plus BCG by scarification to COP plus bleomycin.   The background for this protocol was the SWOG single arm pilot study[68] conducted between November, 1971 and April, 1972 which observed a promising 69 percent rate of complete remission in 74 percent patients

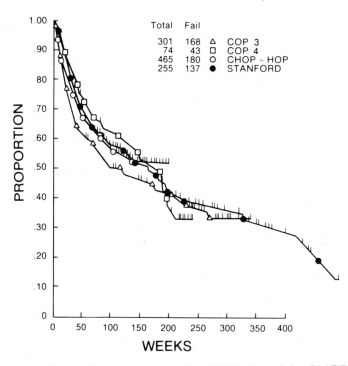

Fig. 10. Survival of all patients in the COP 3 and 4, CHOP/HOP, and Stanford studies

(all histologies) by adding bleomycin to a 14-day COP schedule (designated as COP 4 in Table 6). The study design of this most recent protocol emphasized mandatory histopathology review by the Lymphoma Panel and systematic restaging to define complete remission after eight courses of induction chemotherapy. There were no significant differences in response rates, remission duration or survival between treatment with CHOP-bleo and CHOP-BCG (eg, CR rates of 56 percent and 63 percent, respectively). Accordingly, the results of these two programs for remission induction were combined and compared to the results achieved with COP-bleo. Confirmed rates of CR for 433 evaluable patients were 59 percent for 286 patients receiving the CHOP regimens and 59 percent for the 157 patients receiving COP-bleo. Rates of CR were higher for patients with nodular lymphoma (69 percent) compared to those with diffuse lymphoma (54 percent) (p=0.005). For patients with nodular lymphoma there was no difference in CR rates according to treatment (68 percent with CHOP regimens and 70 percent with COP-bleo). For patients with diffuse lymphomas the CR rate was higher with the CHOP programs (68 percent) than with COP-bleo (44 percent) (p=0.10). Remission duration for patients with nodular lymphoma was similar regardless of whether the patient received the CHOP regimens or COP-bleo. However, remission duration for patients with diffuse lymphoma was significantly shorter if remission was induced with COP-bleo rather than the CHOP regimens (p< 0.01). Overall survival of patients on this study was significantly better if the patients had nodular lymphoma rather than diffuse lymphoma. Although there was no difference in survival for patients with nodular lymphoma according to the initial induction treatment, survival of patients with diffuse lymphoma was significantly worse (p=0.02) if the initial treatment was COP-bleo rather than the CHOP regimens. The study by Jones[80] established the value of an adriamycin-containing combination (CHOP) for the initial management of patients with Stages III and IV diffuse lymphoma. Not only was the time to complete remission considerably shorter, but the rates of complete remission favored the use of the adriamycin-containing combination, and the duration of remission induced with the CHOP program was distinctly longer than that produced by the COP-bleo regimen. Finally and most importantly, overall survival was significantly longer for patients treated with the CHOP regimens rather than COP-bleo as initial induction therapy.

Additional evidence to support the use of adriamycin-containing combinations in the diffuse lymphomas has been demonstrated in the recently completed study by Johnson et al.[81] One hundred ninety previously untreated patients with Stages III or IV unfavorable diffuse NHL have been evaluated on ECOG 3474 which randomized to COPA (similar to the CHOP regimen except the dose of cytoxan is 600 mg/M^2, BCOP, or one of two schedules of COP plus bleomycin (Table

8). This protocol investigated the schedule dependency of vincristine and bleomycin which were both given either on day 1 in the COPB regimen or on day 15 in the CPOB schedule. Complete remission rates were highest for the adriamycin-containing COPA regimen (47 percent) and for the day 15 vincristine and bleomycin regimen of CPOB (43 percent). Complete remission rates for the day one vincristine and bleomycin CPOB regimen of 35 percent and for the BCOP (32 percent) were similar to those that had been observed by Durant[62] with BCOP alone. Median response duration is longer, and median survival of patients treated with COPA (115 weeks) is significantly longer than for those treated with COPB or BCOP, but not for the day 15 vincristine and bleo CPOB schedule. This study demonstrated that the addition of adriamycin to COP is more effective than the addition of BCNU or bleomycin on day one, and that the schedule dependency of bleomycin and vincristine on day 15 should be explored in future NHL treatment programs containing adriamycin in diffuse lymphomas. The effect of prognostic variables on objective response rate was investigated and revealed significantly higher CR rates for patients with IIIA disease, good performance status, and no liver or marrow involvement.

The potential curability for poor-risk patients, particularly of those with diffuse histiocytic lymphoma has been demonstrated by the cooperative groups. In each SWOG study there is definite evidence of a plateau in the survival curve beyond two years.[82] Of the 356 DHL patients entered in the first five SWOG studies, 197 have died within the first two years, but only 21 patients (10 percent of the deaths) have died after two years. Forty-nine percent of the living patients (67 of 138 patients) remain alive from 2+ to 7+ years (Fig. 11).[68]

Indeed, the potential curability of DHL is not only demonstrated for adriamycin containing combinations but also for those patients who obtain a complete remission with BCNU plus COP. Durant reported in a pilot trial[83] that in previously untreated diffuse histiocytic lymphoma this combination produced a 50 percent CR rate (14 CRs among 28 patients) with approximately 32 percent of the CRs expected to persist for greater than two years. The recently completed SECSG study[62] making a direct comparison of COP with BCOP in diffuse histiocytic lymphoma did not produce as high a response rate (41 percent) but did produce 34 percent CRs. These remissions are durable with a 62 percent probability of remaining in CR 32 months. However, the recent results with adriamycin-containing combinations and their ability to produce complete response rates in excess of 50 percent indicate a limited role for the BCOP regimen in diffuse NHL lymphomas. These studies indicate that there is a population of DHL patients who have been cured by chemotherapy, and that adriamycin is a part of the most successful regimen.

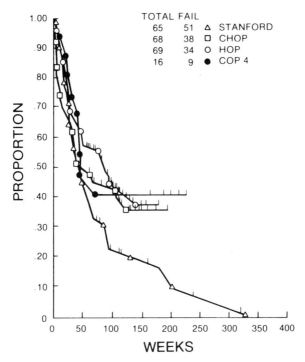

Fig. 11. Survival of DHL patients in the COP, 4 CHOP, HOP, and Stanford studies

In contrast to the documented value of aggressive combination chemotherapy in unfavorable histologies of NHL, the groups have demonstrated that more intense chemotherapy regimens for the nodular lymphomas do not seem to improve survival. Although complete response rates vary from 20 percent with cyclophosphamide alone to 77 percent with CHOP, survival of the NLPD group is not improved in comparison with the retrospective Stanford data (Fig. 12).[68]

The Cooperative Group studies in NHL have methodically attempted to define response rate, response duration and survival in a heterogeneous population of lymphoma patients with a general trend towards improvement in the past ten years. The absence of a uniform hematopathologic classification and the lack of centralized hematopathologic review have compromised the definitive review of these data. The failure to establish rigid criteria for the definition of completeness of response has been an additional problem which has been compounded by the many maintenance programs. These problems have been remedied in all the current cooperative group studies in which mandatory hematopathologic review is required for patient eligiblity,

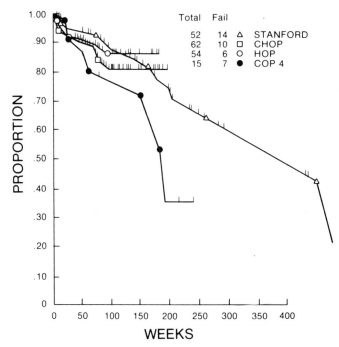

Fig. 12. Survival of NLPD patients in the COP 4, CHOP, HOP, and Stanford studies

and clear definitions of the determination of completeness of response have been established.

Current investigations in Cooperative Group protocols include the further investigation of immunotherapy and of low-dose radiotherapy to all sites of pretreatment involvement once a complete remission has been obtained with combination chemotherapy. Protocols to evaluate newer Phase II agents once a patient becomes refractory to potentially curative chemotherapy are currently in progress. Recently completed Phase II trials have identified hexamethylmelamine,[46] VM-26,[3] and piperazinedione [45]as drugs deserving further investigation.

PEDIATRIC NON-HODGKIN'S LYMPHOMA

Prior to 1970, data from single institutions was in agreement that approximately 10 to 20 percent of all children with non-Hodgkin's lymphoma could be cured. It was clear that only in the localized or regional forms of this disease was there some prospect for cure and this was obtained with various combinations of resection and irradiation. More recently, single institutions piloted the use of intensive systemic treatment in all patients with non-Hodgkin's lymphoma and were able to show marked improvement in survival rates. Of major importance was Wollner's demonstration at Memorial Hospital that the ten-drug LSA_2-L_2 regimen increased the overall two-year survival rate to 81 percent.

In American Burkitt's lymphoma Ziegler at the NCI demonstrated the value of short term intensive combination chemotherapy.

Against this background of improved results, the relative importance of histology, anatomical site and extent, age, meningeal or bone marrow involvement is uncertain. Because of the rarity of this disease and its remarkable variation in clinical spectrum the Cooperative Group mechanism has been ideal to mount a comprehensive study of the disease and its biology in children.

The Childrens Cancer Study Group opened a randomized study (CCG-554) (Fig. 13) in April of 1977 that has accessed 150 children in 18 months. It is a simple two-arm study in which the LSA_2-L_2 ten-drug regimen is compared to a four-drug treatment program (cyclophosphamide, methotrexate, vincristine, prednisone).[84] Radiation for bulk disease and CNS prophylaxis with intrathecal methotrexate are standardized. In more favorable anatomical locations, radical irradiation is delivered to all known disease. In this study there is appropriate stratification for histologic type, extent of disease, site, age, CNS disease and bone marrow involvement at diagnosis.

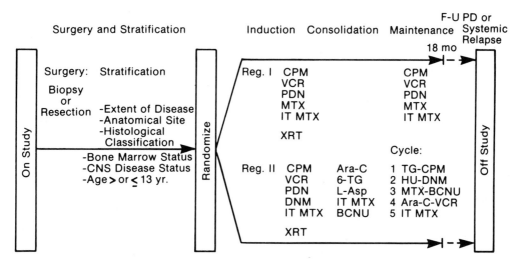

Fig. 13. CCG-551: Non-Hodgkin's lymphoma

Preliminary data from this study and its earlier pilot already demonstrate the need for systemic treatment in the approximately one-third of patients who present with localized or regional disease. Thus, 51 consecutive cases in this category (but excluding localized mediastinal disease) have not yet suffered a first relapse with followup intervals ranging from one to 30 months. There was one toxic death in complete remission in this group.

Multivariate analysis of the patients in this study will for the first time allow a comprehensive assessment of some of the biological variables.

Concurrent with this study, SWOG-7615, a single-arm study, is assessing a modified LSA_2-L_2 regimen in all children except those with Burkitt's lymphoma.

SUMMARY

This review shows clear evidence of major contributions by the Cooperative Groups to our understanding of both Hodgkin's disease and non-Hodgkin's lymphoma. The Cooperative Groups have established the activity of virtually all single agents in advanced Hodgkin's disease. They have confirmed the value of MOPP in advanced Hodgkin's disease with survival curves that are equivalent to those shown in the original trials at the National Cancer Institute. The Cooperative Groups have systematically explored the addition of various drugs to MOPP in an attempt to improve on the standard MOPP regimen (bleomycin, adriamycin), and examined alternative regimens, with less toxicity, in direct comparison with MOPP (BCVPP).

The Cooperative Groups have systematically explored the role of maintenance therapy in advanced Hodgkin's disease, confirming the studies which have failed to show it to be of significant benefit. They have established the cost of treatment of Hodgkin's disease in terms of complications. Both benign and malignant complications have been thoroughly documented.

The Cooperative Groups were the first to compare cytoxan, oncovin and prednisone with single agents in advanced non-Hodgkin's lymphoma. They have extensively explored the use of nitrosoureas in a similar setting. Less intensive treatment of nodular non-Hodgkin's lymphoma has been studied by Cooperative Groups. They have documented the value of adriamycin alone and in combination in the management of non-Hodgkin's lymphoma.

Most importantly, by their example the Cooperative Groups have made a significant impact on improving the standard of care of patients in the community setting.   Patients referred to cooperative group members have been returned to the community with excellent regimens and high quality care. This has now become, in fact, a detriment to further cooperative group research efforts, because the translation of research tools into clinical practice has allowed the community physicians to apply these tools to their patients without referral to research programs.

The Cooperative Groups are currently involved in studying the role of alternating, noncross resistant, combination chemotherapeutic regimens in advanced Hodgkin's disease and non-Hodgkin's lymphoma. The role of low-dose radiotherapy in the prevention of relapse in Hodgkin's disease is being explored in an attempt to define the minimal dose of combined modality treatment necessary in the mangement of poor prognosis Hodgkin's disease. The role of chemotherapy in the management of localized Hodgkin's disease is also under study. A number of protocols have examined the role of immunotherapy in the management of non-Hodgkin's lymphoma and the impact of this on nodular histologies is being documented. Other studies include the testing of active new agents in all kinds of lymphoma. Finally, ongoing registries have been developed for the identification and followup of malignant and nonmalignant complications of the management of lymphoma.

REFERENCES

1. Jones SE, Butler JJ, Byrne G, Coltman CA, Moon TE: Histopathologic review of lymphoma cases from the Southwest Oncology Group. Cancer 39:1071-1076, 1977.
2. Ward JA, Coltman CA, Maloney TR, Butler JJ: A retrospective review of the SWOG experience with patients with immunoblastic lymphadenopathy and Lennert's lymphoma treated with combination chemotherapy. Manuscript in preparation.
3. Chiuten DF, Creech RH, Glick J, Falkson G, Bennet JM, Begg CB, Muggia FM, and Carbone PP: The treatment of malignant lymphoma with VM-26. (American Society of Hematology Abstract), Blood 50 (5) Supplement 1, Nov. 1977.
4. Coltman CA, Fuller LM: Patterns of relapse in localized (Stage I and II) Hodgkin's disease (HD) following extended field radiotherapy (EFXRT) vs. involved field radiothearpy (IFXRT) plus MOPP. Blood 50:188, 1977.
5. Coltman CA, Montague E, Moon TE: Chemotherapy and total nodal radiotherapy in pathological Stage IIB, IIIA, and IIIB Hodgkin's disease. In Adjuvant Therapy of Cancer, SE Salmon and SE Jones, eds. Elsevier/North Holland, Amsterdam, pp.529-536, 1977.
6. Coltman CA, Montague E, Haskins C, and Moon TE: Chemotherapy (MOPP) and total nodal radiotherapy (TNRT) in pathological Stage IIB, IIIA and B Hodgkin's disease (HD). AACR 18:216, 1977.
7. Coltman CA, Frei E, Moon TE: MOPP maintenance (MM) vs. unmaintained remission (UMR) for MOPP induced complete remission (CR) of advanced Hodgkin's disease (HD): 7.2 year followup. Southwest Oncology Group. ASCO 17:289, 1976.
8. Coltman CA, Jones SE, Grozea PN, De Persio E, Moon TE: Bleomycin in combination with MOPP for the treatment of Hodgkin's disease: SWOG experience. In Bleomycin: Current Status and New Developments. SK Carter, ST Crooke, H Umezawa, eds. New York: Academic Press pp.227-242, 1978.
9. Durant JR, Brascho D, Green L: Accuracy of retroperitoneal ultrasonography in Hodgkin's disease and non-Hodgkin's lymphomas: A comparison with lymphangiography and gallium scanning. Radiology 125:485-487, 1977.
10. Jones SE, Tobias DA, Waldman RS: Computed tomographic scanning in patients with lymphoma. Cancer 41:480-486, 1978.
11. Panettiere F, and Coltman CA: Splenectomy effects on chemotherapy in Hodgkin's disease. Arch Intern Med 131:362-366, 1973.
12. Panettiere FJ, Coltman CA, Delaney FC: Splenectomy, chemotherapy and survival in Hodgkin's disease. Arch Intern Med 137:341-343, 1977.
13. Hermon TS, Jones SE: Systematic restaging in patients with Hodgkin's disease. Cancer 42:1976-1982, 1978.
14. Jain JK, Ratanatharathorn V, Bergsman K, et al: Practical approach to staging laparotomy in the management of lymphomas. Blood 50:194, 1977.
15. Gold GL, Slavin LG, Schnider BI: A comparative study with three alkylating agents: Mechlorethamine, cyclophosphamide, and uracil mustard. Cancer Chemother Rep 16:417-419, 1962.
16. Brindley CO, Slavin LG, Potee KG, Lipowska B, Shnider BI, Regelson W, Colsky J: The Eastern Cooperative Group in solid tumor chemotherapy. J Chron Dis 17:19-30, 1964.
17. Jacobs EM, Peters FC, Luce JK: Mechlorethamine HCl and cyclophosphamide in the treatment of Hodgkin's disease and the lymphomas. JAMA 203:104-110, 1968.
18. Carbone PP, Spur C, Schneiderman M, Scotto J, Holland JF, Schnider B: Management of patients with malignant lymphoma: A comparative study with cyclophosphamide and vinca alkaloids. Cancer Research 28:811-822, 1968.
19. Soloman J, Jacobs EM, Bateman JR, Lukes RJ, Weiner JM, Donohue DM: Chemotherapy of lymphoma with mechlorethamine and vinblastine. Arch Intern Med 131:407-417, 1973.
20. Stolinsky DC, Solomon J, Pugh RP, Stevens AR, Jacobs EM, Irwin LE, Wood DA, Steinfeld JL, Bateman JR: Clinical experience with procarbazine in Hodgkin's disease, reticulum cell sarcoma and lymphosarcoma. Cancer 26:984-990, 1970.
21. Nissen NI, Stutzman L, Holland JF, Glidewell OJ: Chemotherapy of Hodgkin's disease in studies by Acute Leukemia Group B. Arch Intern Med 131:396-401, 1973.
22. Luce JK, Gamble JF, Wilson HE, Monto RW, Isaacs B, Palmer RL, Coltman CA, Hewlett JS, Gehan EA, Frei E: Combined cyclophosphamide, vincristine, and prednisone therapy of malignant lymphoma. Cancer 28:306-317, 1971.
23. Lenhard RE: Eastern Cooperative Oncology Group studies. Arch Intern Med 131:418-420, 1973.
24. Luce JK, Frei E, Gehan EA, Coltman CA, Talley R, Monto RW: Chemotherapy of Hodgkin's disease. Arch Intern Med 131:391-395, 1973.
25. Frei E, Luce JK, Gamble JE, et al: Combination chemotherapy in advanced Hodgkin's disease, induction and maintenance of remission. Ann Intern Med 79:376-382, 1973.
26. Huguley CM, Durant JR, Moores RR, Chan YK, Dorfman RF, Johnson L: A comparison of nitrogen mustard, vincristine, procarbazine and prednisone (MOPP) vs. nitrogen mustard in advanced Hodgkin's disease. Cancer 36:1227-1240, 1975.
27. Stutzman L, Glidewell O: Multiple chemotherapeutic agents for Hodgkin's disease. JAMA 225:1202-1211, 1973.
28. Coltman CA, Frei E, Delaney FC: Effectiveness of actinomycin (A), methotrexate (MTX) and vinblastine (V) in prolonging the duration of combination chemotherapy (MOPP) -induced remission in advanced Hodgkin's disease (HD). A Southwest Oncology Group study. ASCO, 1973.
29. Coltman CA, Delaney FC: Five-drug combination chemotherapy for advanced Hodgkin's disease (HD). Clinical Research 21:876, 1973.

30. Coltman CA: MOPP plus low-dose bleomycin (MOPP+LDB) for advanced Hodgkin's disease - a five-year followup. Bleomycin meeting XII International Cancer Congress, Buenos Aires, 1978.

31. Jones SE, Coltman CA, Fisher R: Comparison of 3 combination drug programs for advanced Hodgkin's disease (HD): A preliminary report of the Southwest Oncology Group (SWOG) MOPP #5 study. ASCO 19:333, 1978.

32. Lessner HE, for the Southeastern Cancer Chemotherapy Cooperative Study Group: BCNU (1,3,Bisβ - chloroethyl)-1 nitrosourea) effects on advanced Hodgkin's disease and other neoplasia. Cancer 22:451-456, 1968.

33. Hoogstraten B, Luce JK: CCNU(1-(2-chloroethyl)-3-cyclohexyl-1-nitrosourea) and bleomycin in the treatment of solid tumors and lymphoma. AACR 14:3, 1973.

34. Tranum BL, Haut A, Rivkin S, Weber E: Methyl CCNU in Hodgkin's disease and other tumors. Southwest Oncology Group. ASCO 15:171, 1974.

35. Rege VB, Owens AH: BCNU in the treatment of advanced Hodgkin's disease, lymphosarcoma, and reticulum cell sarcoma. Cancer Chemother Rep 58:383-392, 1974.

36. Cooper MR, Spurr CL, Glidewell O, Holland JF: The superiority of a nitrosourea (CCNU) containing four-drug combination over MOPP in the treatment of Stage III and IV Hodgkin's disease. Leukemia Group B. AACR 16:111, 1975.

37. Durant JR, Bartolucci A, Gams RA, Dorfman RF, Velez-Garcia E: Southeastern Cancer Study Group trials with nitrosoureas in Hodgkin's disease. Cancer Treat Rep 60:781-787, 1976.

38. Durant JR, Gams RA, Velez-Garcia E, et al: BCNU, Velban, cyclophosphamide, procarbazine, and prednisone (BVCPP) in advanced Hodgkin's disease. Cancer 42:2101-2110, 1978.

39. Durant JR, Gams RA, Velez-Garcia E, Dorfman R: Advantage of 12 monthly cycles of BVCPP for complete remission (CR) in advanced Hodgkin's disease (AHD). Southeastern Cancer Study Group. ASCO 17:258, 1976.

40. Durant JR, Gams RA, Bartolucci AA, Velez-Garcia E, Dorfman RF: Treatment of Hodgkin's disease with a five-drug regimen. ASCO 16:245, 1975.

41. Bakemeier RF, DeVita VT, Horton J: Chemotherapy and immunotherapy of Hodgkin's disease (HD). ASCO 17:293, 1976.

42. Vinciguerra VP, Coleman M, Pajek TF, Rafla S, Stutzman L, Nissen NI: MER immunotherapy for advanced, recurrent Hodgkin's disease. A Cancer and Leukemia Group study. Accepted in Cancer Clinical Trials, 4/80.

43. Holland JF, Regelson W, Selawry OS, Costa G: Methylglyoxal-bisguanylhydrazone -- An active agent against Hodgkin's disease and acute myeloblastic leukemia. Acta, Un int Cancer 20:352-353, 1964.

44. Frei E, Luce JK, Talley RW, Vaitkevicius VK, Wilson HE: 5-(3,3-Dimethyl-1-triazeno) imidazole-4-carboxamide in the treatment of lymphoma. Cancer Chemother Rep 56:667-670, 1972.

45. Jones SE, Tucker WJ, Haut A, Tranum BL, Vaughn C, Chase EM, Durie BGM: Phase II trial of piperazinedione in Hodgkin's disease, non-Hodgkin's lymphoma, and multiple myeloma: A Southwest Oncology Group study. Cancer Treat Rep 61:1617-1621, 1977.

46. Bennett JM, Bakemeier RF, Ezdinli EZ, Horton J, Isreal L, Pocock S: The evaluation of new chemotherapeutic agents: Hexamethylmelamine (HXM) and bleomycin (Bleo) in malignant lymphomas. Proceedings of XI International Cancer Congress 4:780, 1974.

47. Frei E, Spurr CL, Brindley CO, Selawry O, Holland JR, Rall DP, Wasserman LR, Hoogstraten B, Shnider BI, McIntyre OR, Mathews LB, Miller SP: Clinical studies of dichloromethotrexate. Clinical Pharmacology and Therapeutics 6:160-170, 1964.

48. Cecil JW, Quagliana JM, Coltman CA, Al-Sarraf M, Thigpen T, Groppe CW: Evaluation of VP-16-213 in malignant lymphoma and melanoma. Cancer Treat Rep 62:801-803, 1978.

49. Chiuten DF, Creech RH, Glick J, Falkson G, Brodovsky H, Bennett JM, Begg CB, Muggia FM, Carbone PP: 4'-Demethl-epipodophyllotoxin-β-D-thenylidene Glucoside (VM-26). A new anticancer drug with effectiveness in lymphoma. Cancer Treat Rep 63:7-11, 1979.

50. O'Connell MJ, Silverstein MN, Kiely JM, White WL: Pilot study of two adriamycin-based regimens in patients with advanced malignant lymphomas. Cancer Treat Rep 61:65-68, 1977.

51. Rossof AH, Kerr RO, Braine HG, Coltman CA: A kinetically designed chemotherapeutic regimen for advanced refractory lym phoma patients. Med and Ped Oncology 4:133-139, 1978.

52. Wirtschafter DD, Scalise M, Cort H, Henke C, Gams RA: Clinical algorithms in a cooperative multiinstitutional clinical trial. Presented Society for Advanced Medical Systems, November 1977.

53. Wirtschafter D, Carpenter JT, Mesel E: A consultant-extender system for breast cancer adjuvant chemotherapy. Ann Intern Med 90:396-401, 1979.

54. A Collaborative Study: Survival and complications of radiotherapy following involved and extended field therapy of Hodgkin's disease, Stages I and II. Cancer 38:288-305, 1976.

55. Hoogstraten B, Holland JF, Kramer S, Glidewell OJ: Combination chemotherapy-radiotherapy for Stage III Hodgkin's disease. Arch Intern Med 131:424-428, 1973.

56. Hoogstraten B, Glidewell O, Holland JF, Blom J, Stutzman L, Nissen NI, Perlberg HJ, Kramer S: Long-term followup of combination chemotherapy-radiotherapy of Stage III Hodgkin's disease. A Cancer and Acute Leukemia Group B study. Cancer 43:1234-1244, 1979.

57. Grozea PN, Coltman CA, Montague E, DePersio EJ, Fisher R, Haskins C, Jones J: Results of two studies from the Southwest Oncology Group (SWOG), in the treatment of Stages IIIA and IIIB Hodgkin's disease (HD). Presented XVII Congress of the International Society of Hematology.

58. Toland DM, Coltman CA, Moon TE: Second malignancies complicating Hodgkin's disease: The Southwest Oncology Group experience. Cancer Clinical Trials 1:27-33, 1978.

59. Durant JR, Norgard MJ, Murad TM, Bartolucci AA, Langford KH: Pulmonary toxicity associated with BCNU. Ann Int Med 90:191-194, 1979.

60. Chilcote RR, Baehner RL, Hammond D, and the investigators and special studies committee of the Children's Cancer Study Group: Septicemia and meningitis in children splenectomized for Hodgkin's disease. N Eng J Med 295:798-800, 1976.

61. Ezdinli E, Wasser LP, Lenhard RE, Costello W, Berard CW, Hartsock R, Bennett JM, Carbone PP: Eastern Cooperative Oncology Group experience with the Rappaport classification of non-Hodgkin's lymphoma. Cancer 43:544-550, 1979.

62. Durant JR, Gams RA, Bartolucci AA, Dorfman RF: BCNU with and without cyclophosphamide, vincristine and prednisone (COP) and cyclo-active therapy in non-Hodgkin's lymphoma. Cancer Treat Rep 61:1085-1096, 1977.

63. Miller TP, Jones SE: Chemotherapy in the management of localized histiocytic lymphoma. Lancet 1:358-360, 1979.

64. Bartolucci A, Durant JR, Gams RA: Prognostic factors in non-Hodgkin's lymphoma: A multivariate analysis of over 300 cases. ASCO 18:304, 1977.

65. Herman TS, Hammond N, Jones SE, Butler JJ, Byrne GE, McKelvey EM: Involvement of the central nervous system by non-Hodgkin's lymphoma: The Southwest Oncology Group experience. Cancer 43:390-397, 1979.

66. Herman TS, Jones SE: Systematic restaging in the managment of non-Hodgkin's lymphomas. Cancer Treat Rep 61:1009-1015, 1977.

67. Gold G, Slavin LG, Schnider BI: A comparative study with three alkylating agents: mechlorethamine, cyclophosphamide, and uracil mustard. Cancer Chemother Rep 16:417-419, 1962.

68. Coltman CA, Luce JK, McKelvey EM, Jones SE, Moon TE: Chemotherapy of non-Hodgkin's lymphoma: 10 years' experience in the Southwest Oncology Group. Cancer Treat Rep 61:1067-1078, 1977.

69. Bennett JM, Lenhard RE Jr, Ezdinli E, Johnson GJ, Carbone PP, Pocock SJ: Chemotherapy of non-Hodgkin's lymphomas: Eastern Cooperative Oncology Group experience. Cancer Treat Rep 61:1079-1083, 1977.

70. Nissen NI, Pajak T, Glidewell O, Blom H, Flaherty M, Hayes D, McIntyre R, Holland JF: Overview of four clinical studies of chemotherapy for Stage III and IV non-Hodgkin's lymphomas by the Cancer and Leukemia Group B. Cancer Treat Rep 61:1097-1107, 1977.

71. Hoogstraten B, Owens AH, Lenhard RE, Glidewell OJ, Leone LA, Olson KB, Harley JB, Townsend SR, Miller SP, Spurr CL: Combination chemotherapy in lymphosarcoma and reticulum cell sarcoma. Blood 33:370-378, 1969.

72. Lenhard RE, Prentice RL, Owens AH, Bakemeier R, Horton JH, Shnider BI, Stolbach L, Berard CW, Carbone PP: Combination chemotherapy of the malignant lymphomas. Cancer 38:1052-1059, 1976.

73. Ezdinli E, Pocock S, Berard CW, Aungst CW, Silverstein M, Horton J, Bennett J, Bakemeier R, Stolback L, Perlia C, Brunk SF, Lenhard RE, Klaassen DJ, Richter P, Carbone P: Comparison of intensive versus moderate chemotherapy of lymphocytic lymphomas. Cancer 38:1060-1068, 1976.

74. Ezdinli EZ, Costello W, Lenhard RE, Bakemeier R, Bennett JM, Berard CW, Carbone PP: Survival of nodular versus diffuse pattern lymphocytic poorly differentiated lymphoma. Cancer 41:1990-1996, 1978.

75. Lenhard RE, Ezdinli EZ, Costello W, Bennett JM, Horton J, Amorisi EL, Stolbach L, Wolter J: Treatment of histiocytic and mixed lymphomas: A comparison of two, three and four-drug chemotherapy. Cancer 42:41-52, 1978.

76. Ezdinli E, Costello WG, Silverstein MN: Chemotherapy of prognostically favorable non-Hodgkin's lymphoma. An Eastern Cooperative Oncology Group study.

77. Coltman CA: Adriamycin in the therapy of lymphomas: Southwest Oncology Group studies. Cancer Chemother Rep 6:375-380, 1975.

78. McKelvey EM, Gutterman HU, Coltman CA Jr: Hydroxyldaunomycin (adriamycin) combination chemotherapy for advanced non-Hodgkin's lymphoma. ASH, 1973.

79. McKelvey EM, Gottlieb JA, Wilson HE, Haut A, Talley RW, Stephens R, Lane M, Gamble JF, Jones SE, Grozea PN, Gutterman J, Coltman CA, Moon TE: Hydroxyldaunomycin (adriamycin) combination chemotherapy in malignant lymphoma. Cancer 38:1484-1493, 1976.

80. Jones SE, Grozea PN, Metz EN, Haut A, Stephens RL, Morrison FS, Butler JJ, et al: Superiority of adriamycin-containing combination chemotherapy in the treatment of diffuse lymphoma. A Southwest Oncology Group study. Cancer 43:417-425, 1979.

81. Johnson GJ, Oken MM, Sponzo RW, Bennett J, Silverstein M, Glick J, Carbone PP: Cyclophosphamide (C), vincristine (V), and prednisone (P) plus adriamycin (A), bleomycin (B) or BCNU: A prospective clinical trial in an unfavorable diffuse non-Hodgkin's lymphoma (NHL). ASCO 19:395, 1978.

82. McKelvey EM, Moon TE: Curability of non-Hodgkin's lymphomas. Cancer Treat Rep 61:1185-1190, 1977.

83. Durant JR, Loeb V, Dorfman R, Chan YK: 1,3-Bis (2-Chloroethyl)-1-nitrosourea (BCNU), cyclophosphamide, vincristine and prednisone (BCOP), a new therapeutic regimen for diffuse histiocytic lymphoma. Cancer 36:1936-1944, 1975.

84. Meadows AT, Jenkin RDT, Chilcote R, Coccia P, Exelby P, Kushner J, Siegel S, Wilson J, Leikin S, Hammond D, for the Children's Cancer Study Group (CCSG). Remission induction in childhood non-Hodgkin's lymphoma (NHL) with cyclophosphamide (CPM), vincristine (VCR), prednisone and intravenous methotrexate (MTX). ASCO 19:365, 1978.

4

Multiple myeloma, chronic leukemia, and polycythemia vera

O. Ross McIntyre, Raymond Alexanian, Harvey Jay Cohen, and Stephen A. Landaw

INTRODUCTION

Since their development twenty years ago, Cooperative Groups have made major contributions to the improved understanding and treatment of a variety of hematologic malignancies. The development of research studies on multiple myeloma, the chronic leukemias, and polycythemia vera represented the first attempt by Cooperative Groups to study diseases of a chronic nature in a systematic manner. Such diseases must be approached differently from disorders with a very short life span, with a greater emphasis being placed on long-term treatments, accurate disease staging, survival time measurements, and an awareness of the late complications of treatment. In addition to securing an adequate number of patients for study, there are other important advantages from Cooperative Group efforts against these diseases. Individuals with a variety of professional interests are linked in a structure with sufficient administrative stability to conduct studies that may require several years to complete. Standard and quantitative definitions for the diagnosis, patient eligibility, evaluation of response, etc., help to eliminate the possible bias that may be introduced by individual investigators. Furthermore, the availability of a biostatistical group with expertise in the illnesses under investigation and specialized laboratories for the analysis of patient specimens facilitates the conduct of the clinical trials.

MULTIPLE MYELOMA

BACKGROUND

This malignant disorder of plasma cells results in the death of 8,000 patients each year in the United States. It represents 10 percent of all hematologic malignancies and causes the death of about one percent of the individuals who die from cancer. While the incidence of the disease is 4 per 100,000 annually, the incidence is nearly twice this in black males and is as common as all lymphomas in this population subgroup.

Because the disease is associated with a tumor marker in almost all patients (i.e., myeloma protein) and because of the accessibility of tumor samples from the bone marrow, the study of multiple myeloma has provided important insights on human tumor kinetics, as well as on improved methods for the measurement of tumor response. These advances have extended into closely linked disorders, such as Waldenstrom's macroglobulinemia, chronic lymphocytic leukemia, and amyloidosis. In 1964, the Chronic Leukemia-Multiple Myeloma task force, consisting of representatives from the different cooperative groups, described standard criteria for the diagnosis and for the evaluation of the effects of treatment on this disease.[1] These criteria of tumor response were based on myeloma protein reductions, as well as on changes in other disease manifestations, and have been widely used in documenting the effects of myeloma treatments. Recently, a more sophisticated method for the measurement of changing tumor burden has been developed and used in some Group studies.[2] This assessment is based upon considerations of the serum myeloma protein concentration, the changing catabolic rate with changing IgG concentration and the measured or assumed plasma volume. Simple computer programs have been developed that permit a rapid calculation of tumor reduction or relapse in each patient. Thus, unlike most other human cancers, myeloma represents a disease where a quantitative assessment of tumor mass change can be made with reasonable precision.

EARLY STUDIES

When Group activity in myeloma began, urethane was considered the treatment of choice. Concern for the efficacy of this agent led to a study initiated in 1958 which failed to show improved survival for urethane-treated patients versus patients randomized to a placebo.[3] In those with azotemia, survival was worse with urethane than in similar patients receiving the placebo. This experience emphasized the value of concurrently-treated control patients in subsequent investigations.

A number of clinical trials were then conducted with new agents that showed promise in animal studies; all failed to confirm useful activity in humans and, at times, produced toxicity in the absence of survival benefits.

Included in these studies, however, was melphalan (L-phenylalanine mustard, L-PAM) which produced a significant number of both subjective and objective responses.[4] At about this same time cooperative group studies also showed that cyclophosphamide was able to produce a similar frequency of responses.[5] Following these demonstrations, Cooperative Groups conducted a series of studies which defined the response rate for melphalan and demonstrated an improved survival over untreated patients (Table 1). In addition, patients responding to treatment had a significantly longer survival time than those not responding, and this prolongation was accounted for by the length of remission. Response rates were defined from several different regimens of melphalan, including a loading dose followed by daily therapy[6] and a higher dose intermittent regimen.[7] Subsequently, different regimens were tested with or without the addition of prednisone, and significantly higher response rates and longer survival times resulted from the melphalan-prednisone combinations.[8] Analysis of one of these studies provided evidence that prednisone at a dose of 1.2 mg/kg for ten weeks was detrimental to high-risk patients but not to low-risk patients.[9] Lower doses (0.6 mg/kg) or shorter durations of prednisone used in subsequent experiments were beneficial to high-risk patients.[10]

Two regimens producing similar response rates and survival times evolved from these experiments. A loading dose of melphalan 0.15 mg/kg followed by daily melphalan 0.05 mg/kg, with an 8-10 week course of prednisone tapering from 0.6 mg/kg has been frequently used. An intermittent regimen utilizing melphalan at a dose of 0.25 mg/kg with prednisone 60 mg/M^2 for 4 days every 6 weeks has advantages in

TABLE 1
Response Rates and Survival in Multiple Myeloma

Therapy	Period	Response Rate (%)	Median Survival (mos)
Before Melphalan	Prior to 1960	<10	<12
Melphalan alone	1960-1968	30	18
Melphalan-Prednisone	1968-1974	45	24
Combination CT	1974-present	60	30-35

$\geq$ 75% reduction in myeloma protein synthesis

terms of convenience of followup and is the more common regimen used at this time.

TESTING OF COMBINATIONS

Because several studies described therapeutic activity from cyclophos-phamide and carmustine (BCNU) in some myeloma patients resistant to melphalan, there was the possibility that cross-resistance to these alkylating agents was not inevitable.   Studies in the mouse myeloma model also demonstrated noncross-resistance in some instances.   Also, there were possible advantages to be gained from a combination of agents with different toxicities.   For this reason, combinations of different alkylating agents were then studied by several Cooperative Groups, always with added prednisone in view of the results described previously.   Although the studies are still ongoing, no major advantage has yet resulted when more than one alkylating agent was used in a combination regimen, such as with melphalan-cyclophosphamide-prednisone or melphalan-cyclophosphamide-prednisone-BCNU.   In one study, the use of intravenous L-PAM, cyclophosphamide, and BCNU with prednisone resulted in an improved survival time for patients at increased risk but failed to benefit other patients.[11]   This observation suggests that treatment designed specifically for patients in different prognostic groups may be more rational.

The role of alkylating agents, when given in combination with other drugs, has also been explored.   When vincristine was given at three-week intervals in combination with melphalan-cyclophosphamide-prednisone or cyclophosphamide-doxorubicin-prednisone, the response rate was about 15 percent higher (60 percent) and the median survival time about four months longer than the comparable control groups without vincristine.[12]   These observations suggested that, as with prednisone, vincristine had some useful role in the chemotherapy in myeloma patients.   The median survival time for all patients receiving a combination of vincristine-cyclophosphamide-doxorubicin-prednisone was 35 months (Table 1).   No improvement was observed in the frequency of remission or in the survival time when doxorubicin was added to combinations of melphalan-prednisone or cyclophosphamide-prednisone as part of the initial treatment.

Preliminary studies in one Cooperative Group now suggest improved results from a program that alternates intermittent courses of a vincristine-melphalan-cyclophosphamide-prednisone   combination (VMCP) with a vincristine-cyclophosphamide-doxorubicin-prednisone combination (VCAP).[13]   Sixty-five percent of patients are achieving 75 percent tumor reductions, in contrast to 45 percent of patients randomized concurrently to melphalan-prednisone (p < .05). Median survival is 29 and 22 months respectively.

Through the studies described above, a slow but steady improvement in myeloma patient response and survival has occurred. While superior responses and survival results have been reported in some instances from smaller, single institution studies, these are often affected by patient selection and/or criteria for response which are difficult to compare with other studies.

RELAPSE

Since about 40 percent of myeloma patients given standard therapy fail to have an adequate response, and since responding patients will eventually relapse, Cooperative Groups have also been involved in efforts to find agents or combinations which will be effective for resistant myeloma. In this way, doxorubicin, BCNU, CCNU, cyclophosphamide, and vincristine were tested both alone and in combination.[14,15] While patients failing on initial treatment have usually proven refractory to subsequent therapy, initially responding patients are more successfully treated. In one Cooperative Group, the combination of vincristine-BCNU-doxorubicin-prednisone achieved second remissions in about one-fourth of relapsing patients.[16] Recently, hexamethylmelamine has been effective in achieving response in some patients refractory to alkylating agent therapy.[17]

SECOND MALIGNANCIES

The large number of patients enrolled in Group studies has provided definition of the risk of leukemia after long-term alkylating agent treatments. In several patients the diagnoses of leukemia and myeloma are made simultaneously, suggesting a biologic susceptibility to both diseases.[18] On the other hand, 2 to 6 percent of all myeloma patients responding and treated for at least 2 years have developed acute leukemia, an incidence about 100 times higher than that of comparable individuals of similar age. Only through the collation of data obtained from a large series of patients could such an assessment of risk be made. The apparently increasing risk with longer duration of therapy has raised the question of how long treatment should be continued in these patients, as well as in other cancer patients receiving adjuvant therapy. For this and other reasons, studies to determine the need for indefinite remission maintenance treatment have been undertaken.

MAINTENANCE TREATMENT

In one study, indefinite maintenance therapy after one year of treatment in patients achieving a 75 percent or greater tumor reduction did not confer any advantage in comparison with patients followed without treatment until relapse.[19]   When such patients relapse, retreatment with the same regimen has produced an 80 percent likelihood of response and survival time equivalent to maintained patients.   Long remission durations were noted mainly in those responding patients with a low residual number of plasma cells, such as in patients with disappearance of serum and urine myeloma globulins or those who presented initially with a low tumor mass.   To further define the need for maintenance and the best type of maintenance, other randomized studies are currently underway.   The definition of groups of patients who require different induction or maintenance treatments on the basis of clinical staging or specific prognostic variables has assumed a new importance.   The Cooperative Groups are in the best position to define the criteria for the selection of specific treatment programs for subgroups of patients at different phases of their disease.

SUPPORTIVE THERAPY

In addition to conducting chemotherapy studies, the Groups have determined the effectiveness of different ancillary and supportive treatments for patients with multiple myeloma.   Most patients have severe depressions of normal immunoglobulin levels and infection is a major cause of morbidity.   A randomized trial determined that gamma globulin prophylaxis for infection was unsuccessful.[20]   Nonrandom trials and a single institution randomized trial have suggested a role for fluoride in the prevention of bone dissolution and pathologic fractures which are frequent in this disease.   In a large Group study, there was no difference in the survival between experimental and placebo-treated patients despite laboratory and x-ray evidence that the treatment caused flurosis of bone.[21]   In fact, patients who developed fluorosis complained of more bone pain.   Another Group study has demonstrated no obvious benefit from fluoride treatment when given with calcium, vitamin D and androgens.[22]

RISK FACTORS AND PROGNOSIS IN MYELOMA

Attempts to classify myeloma by stage or extent of disease are based on lessons gained in the treatment of solid tumors and lymphomas where histology and stage determine the best possible treatment.   Early analyses of patients entered on protocol identified several important risk factors.   Of these, renal function, hemoglobin, serum calcium and performance status were the most important.[23]   Multiple regression analyses performed subsequently have confirmed and extended these early observations.

Patients in some early studies were identified as good or poor risk from a combination of factors found to be associated with different survival times. Thus, poor-risk patients were those with moderate degrees of azotemia, hypercalcemia, and pancytopenia, while good-risk patients had values for these parameters that were within the normal range. In one study where both types of patients received intravenous melphalan, the median survival for poor-risk patients was 7 months and was 66 months for good-risk patients.[24]   Further progress in assignment of prognosis resulted from the application to Group studies of new methods which quantitate the body burden of myeloma cells at the onset of treatment.[2]   Tumor cell mass was calculated on the basis of knowledge of in vitro M-protein production per cell and the known in vivo turnover rate of M-protein at the observed M-protein concentration. A higher number of plasma cells was calculated for patients with severe anemia, hypercalcemia and extensive bone lesions. Other studies indicated a quantitative relationship between the severity of anemia, hypercalcemia or azotemia and a shortening of the survival time. Criteria were then developed by which patients were assigned to a "high", "intermediate", or "low" tumor mass grade, depending on simple laboratory measurements.

When this approach was applied, the response rate (i.e., 75 percent reduction of myeloma protein production) for groups of patients in each tumor mass category was similar (Table 2).[25]   Thus, the proportion of cells killed with a standard program of chemotherapy was similar for

TABLE 2
Correlations of Tumor Mass Grade with Prognosis

	High	Intermediate	Low
Frequency distribution (%)	44	41	23
Response Rate (% evaluable)	50	55	54
Survival (median months)	17	27	42

Median Survial Time (months)

Percent Reduction of Tumor Load

	High	Intermediate	Low
50-100	9	13	27
25-49	14	22	34
10-24	17	25	40
<10	33	34	46

patients with different loads. This finding confirmed, in a human tumor model, numerous previous observations by Skipper in rodent malignancies of a constant, fractional cell kill of cancer cells from a standard drug dose.

Patients with a high pretreatment tumor mass had a higher incidence of early death, a shorter survival and a shorter remission duration for responsive patients, in comparison with other patients demonstrating less extensive tumor. Patients presenting with a low pretreatment tumor mass achieved longer survival times and remission durations. These observations were attributed to the higher residual numbers of plasma cells remaining during "remission" in patients with a high tumor mass, a conclusion again consistent with numerous studies in animal models. When one combines the information on the pretreatment tumor mass and the degree of tumor reduction calculated from the myeloma protein change, a more precise index of prognosis is developed (Table 2).

Several attempts have been made to relate the myeloma protein type to prognosis.[26] While studies attempting to relate light chain type to prognosis in patients with only Bence Jones protein have produced conflicting results, the systematic study of M-proteins in Group studies has produced other benefits. The identification of the second case of myeloma producing IgE M-protein was an early result of Group studies, as was the survival analysis for infrequent subgroups of patients (i.e. those without evidence of serum or urine myeloma globulins). The median survival for patients producing IgA myeloma globulin was slightly less than those producing IgG or only light chain globulins. Patients producing IgA myeloma protein also had a higher frequency of renal failure and hypercalcemia than those with IgG peaks. While prognosis may be influenced in part by the specific protein produced, it is clear that prognosis depends more on the presence of those disease complications associated with a short survival (anemia, hypercalcemia, azotemia, high tumor mass) rather than on a specific myeloma protein type per se.

CHRONIC LEUKEMIAS

CHRONIC MYELOGENOUS LEUKEMIA

Chronic myelogenous leukemia (CML) is a disorder characterized by an easily-controlled benign disease phase, usually followed by a more malignant phase resistant to most forms of chemotherapy. Most patients demonstrate a Ph^1 chromosome in granulocyte, platelet, and erythroid precursors, with additional chromosome changes frequently developing during the resistant phase or "blast crisis". The annual incidence of CML is about 2/100,000 population. Most investigators feel that there has been little improvement in the median survival time of about 3 years despite 50 years of study. Recently, there have been advances in our understanding of the pathophysiology of the blast crisis. This has led to improved treatment concepts which will be discussed in the chapter on acute myelogenous leukemia.

One of the first achievements in chronic myelogenous leukemia by Cooperative Groups was to distinguish more clearly the diagnostic features of the benign phase from the resistant or myeloblastic phase.[27] Thus, the resistant phase was confirmed when the sum of myeloblasts and promyelocytes exceeded 30 percent of the cells on a bone marrow smear.

Cooperative Groups were the first to emphasize the utility of busulfan for the benign stage of CML. A greater inhibitory activity for busulfan was found on myeloid tissues in comparison with lymphoid tissues with about 85 percent of patients with CML responding well to this treatment.[28] Cooperative Groups have also demonstrated significant therapeutic activity with other alkylating agents such as cyclophosphamide and melphalan.

Drugs other than alkylating agents have also been active against CML. 6-Mercaptopurine was capable of reducing elevated granulocyte and platelet counts, but the frequency and duration of this effect was less than with busulfan.[29,30] Neither drug delayed the later myeloblastic transformation and neither prolonged the survival time in comparison with untreated patients. After many trials with other agents, no treatment has yet been identified that can forestall the development of the resistant, blastic phase of disease. In one study, 10 patients with CML and a Ph[1] positive marrow received an adequate trial of a combination of cytosine arabinoside and thioguanine; in 2 patients, the bone marrow was converted to a Ph[1] negative state, although severe nausea and vomiting were also induced.[31]

Treatment regimens for patients in the resistant or myeloblastic phase of CML have also been evaluated. Thus, a combination of hydroxyurea, 6-Mercaptopurine and dexamethasone achieved complete or partial control in about one-third of the patients.[32] A higher frequency of response was associated with a high percentage of marrow blasts, a high platelet count, females, and an age below 40 years.

CHRONIC LYMPHOCYTIC LEUKEMIA

This disease occurs in about 5/100,000 persons each year and is characterized by a widely variable survival. The initial phases of

Cooperative Group studies emphasized the evaluation of new agents (primarily alkylating agents) that might control the marked lymphocytosis and lymphadenopathy that were usually present. Chlorambucil was found to control these disease manifestations in about two-thirds of the patients.[33] Other alkylating agents, such as cyclophosphamide, were also shown to have clinical activity, although not superior to those found with chlorambucil. Simultaneously, corticosteroids were found to have a major antitumor effect, as well as being useful in the control of autoimmune hemolytic anemia and thrombocytopenia.

A clinical staging system (Table 3) has proved advantageous in the design of group studies.[34] This system, which predicts those patients with a poor prognosis (median survival 19 months), allows studies of comparable groups of patients with benign or advanced disease. In one study, patients with Stages III and IV disease were randomized to treatments with prednisone alone, daily chlorambucil with prednisone, or intermittent chlorambucil with prednisone.[35] Both the frequency of response and the survival time were longer when previously untreated patients received an intermittent chlorambucil-prednisone combination. The frequency of major complications, such as serious infection, was less. In addition, a clear survival advantage was recognized for responsive, in comparison with unresponsive, patients. Such superiority

TABLE 3
Clinical Staging of Chronic Lymphocytic Leukemia

Clinical Stage	Findings	Median Survival (mo)
0	lymphocytosis in blood and bone marrow	> 150
I	lymphocytosis in blood and bone marrow plus enlarged lymph nodes	101
II	lymphocytosis in blood and bone marrow plus enlarged lymph nodes, liver and/or spleen	71
III	lymphocytosis of blood and bone marrow with anemia, nodes; liver, spleen may or may not be enlarged	19
IV	lymphocytosis of blood and bone marrow with thrombocytopenia; nodes, liver, spleen may or may not be enlarged	19

was evident particularly in patients who achieved complete control of their disease.   When remissions had been achieved in patients with advanced disease, sustained control was more likely when chlorambucil-prednisone treatments were continued rather than when a cycle-active combination, such as cyclophosphamide-cytosine arabinoside, was substituted.[36] These conclusions are similar to those found previously with melphalan-prednisone treatment for multiple myeloma.

POLYCYTHEMIA VERA

BACKGROUND

Polycythemia vera is a rare and slowly progressive myeloproliferative disease usually occurring in older individuals and characterized by an excessive production of hematopoietic cells, especially of red blood cells.   The annual incidence is about 0.5 per 100,000 population.   The effectiveness of a Cooperative Group approach for the study of relatively uncommon illnesses is perhaps best demonstrated by the studies involving polycythemia vera.   At the time Group studies were initiated, it had been shown that the median survival of untreated patients was about two years and that the survival of P32-treated patients was greater than ten years.   However, the scientific community was polarized as to the relative advantages and risks of treatment with phlebotomy, alkylating agents or P32.[37]   One of the initial tasks was to establish criteria for the diagnosis of polycythemia vera and to separate this entity from the other causes of polycythemia.   Several institutions within the Group piloted studies aimed at elucidating the mechanisms responsible for the production of various secondary polycythemic states.

The efforts devoted to standardization of diagnostic criteria,[38] laboratory tests,[39] and histopathological examination[40] were followed by the collection of data on patients entered into the experimental studies. Through this mechanism, virtually all of the new information acquired about the pathogenesis, natural history, and treatment of polycythemia vera in the past ten years have eminated from studies by or associated with the Polycythemia Vera Study Group (PVSG).

CLINICAL TRIALS

In the first study performed by PVSG, patients were randomized to receive treatment with phlebotomy alone, chlorambucil, or P32.   Analysis of the patients entered revealed no significant bias in patient selection in the randomization. Accrual to this study was terminated in 1973, at which time 432 evaluable patients had been entered.

As the study progressed, it became evident that thrombotic complications were more common in patients treated with phlebotomy and this difference is now statistically significant.[41] Further analyses revealed that a prior history of thrombosis or an age > 70 were significant risk factors.

A number of patients with conversion to myeloid metaplasia or "spent" polycythemia have now appeared.[42] Myelofibrosis has occurred more frequently in patients randomized to phlebotomy. The degree of myelofibrosis correlates significantly with increased marrow cellularity at the time of diagnosis of polycythemia vera. Since patients treated with phlebotomy had not received hematosuppressive therapy, the finding of increased myelofibrosis suggested that the fibrosis might be due to failure to control the hyperproliferation.

Patients randomized to receive chlorambucil or P32 were noted to have an increased frequency of acute leukemia conversions, so that the risk of a second malignancy is now significantly higher for patients receiving myelosuppressive treatment.[41] One case of leukemia has occurred among the patients treated with phlebotomy, confirming earlier anecdotal reports that this complication occurs in patients who have not received myelosuppressive treatment. Table 4 indicates the frequency of these various complications. Despite the difference in complications noted above, no significant differences in survival are yet apparent among the three treatments (Fig. 1). In March, 1979 the 75 percentiles

TABLE 4
Polycythemia Vera: Specified Endpoints by Treatment Group

Endpoint	Treatment Group			
	Phlebotomy (135) %	Chlorambucil (141) %	^{32}P (156) %	Total (432) %
Death on study	20.9	31.9	23.1	25.3
Thrombosis	29.9	17.0	21.8	22.7
All Cancer	3.7	20.6	12.2	12.3
Solid Tumor	3.0	9.9	8.3	7.1
Leukemia	.7	10.6	3.8	5.1

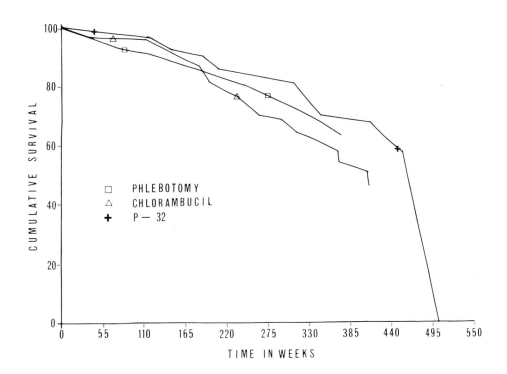

Fig. 1. Survival from date of randomization by treatment group

were 298 weeks, 239 weeks and 334 weeks respectively for phlebotomy, chlorambucil and P32.

The results indicate that for survival specific subsets exist which are at risk for death or complication. To further pursue a form of treatment which attempts to maximize survival and minimize the complications, a second major protocol was initiated in 1977. This trial compares the "best" myelosuppressive arm (P32) from the earlier protocol with the phlebotomy arm now supplemented with antiplatelet agents. The end point of the study is a thrombotic complication. The design should be able to answer the questions initially posed concerning the complex interrelationships between disease, treatment, and its complications.

EFFICACY STUDIES

While the major protocol was continuing, other patients were treated with agents which might have utility in this disease. One such study was a comparison of chlorambucil and melphalan in previously-treated patients.[43] Each patient received both drugs, and the time to relapse was measured. This study indicated that both drugs were equally effective in producing remission. Remission was longer in the melphalan arm, but this effect appeared to be related to the greater degree of myelosuppression caused by the doses chosen for melphalan relative to those for chlorambucil.

OTHER STUDIES

Detailed studies of marrow histology and cytogenetics at various stages of the illness have been included in the clinical trials. From this effort has come an improved understanding of the importance of bone marrow histology, especially in regard to cellularity, iron stores, megakaryocyte number and the extent of myelofibrosis as the disease is treated.

Cytogenetic studies have revealed that about 25 percent of previously untreated patients have an abnormal cytogenetic status.[44] Both structural and numerical abnormalities have been encountered. The numerical abnormalities predominate and are best explained by nondisjunction in the dividing marrow cells.[45] This provides a clue to the intracellular conditions which prevail in the polycythemic clone. Involvement of the C group chromosomes in this abnormality is common. A variety of structural abnormalities also occurs in the presence or absence of numerical abnormalities. Preliminary evidence suggests a higher incidence of second malignancies of all types in those with an initially abnormal cytogenetic status. While no cytogenetic lesion has been found to predict the transition to leukemia, an insufficient number of leukemia transformations have been studied so far to detect a relationship.

Because of the large number of polycythemia vera patients available for study, it was possible for randomized patients to be identified who would be of unique value in experiments which proved the clonal origin of the disease. These studies, performed in two black female patients, could probably not have been performed without the help of the Cooperative Groups, since females have polycythemia vera less commonly than males, and blacks constitute only about 5 percent of all patients with polycythemia vera.[46] These studies confirmed that there is a clonal abnormality in the stem cell which is responsible for the generation of erythrocytes, granulocytes, and platelets, but not for the cells leading to the production of fibroblasts or lymphocytes. Further studies on the pathophysiology of the disease have utilized PVSG patients to demonstrate autonomous erythroid colony formation by bone marrow cells independent of erythiopoietin stimulation.

STUDIES OF MYELOPROLIFERATIVE DISEASE

The success of this approach to the study of polycythemia vera has now resulted in the extension of studies to the other, more poorly defined myeloproliferative disorders. Definitions of major categories of myeloproliferative syndromes have been developed and protocols have been designed for these myeloproliferative disorders, some of which develop complications of polycythemia vera.

Patients identified in the different diagnostic categories are being assigned to one of two or more therapies that are most likely to control specific complications, such as anemia, hemolysis, splenomegaly or thrombocytosis. The decision to follow specific disease-related problems, rather than survival, is a major departure from usual treatment protocols. Such studies are required for these chronic disorders with uncertain etiology and treatment, and are best approached by Cooperative Groups. While it is too early to draw conclusions from these recently activated studies, one initial finding is that the dose of 32P found effective in polycythemia vera is not adequate for control of a platelet count in excess of 1×10 /cmm in primary thrombocytosis. Raising the initial and subsequent doses of 32P by 25 percent resulted in a response rate similar to that noted with melphalan without significant toxicity.[47]

REFERENCES

1. Committee of the Chronic Leukemia-Myeloma Task Force (NCI): Proposed guidelines for protocol studies: II. Plasma cell myeloma. Cancer Chemother Rep 4:145-158, 1973.
2. Durie BGM, Salmon SE: A clinical staging system for multiple myeloma. Cancer 36:842-854, 1975.
3. Holland JF, Hosley H, Scharlau C, Carbone PP, Frei E, Brindley CO, Hall TC, et al: A controlled trial of urethane treatment in multiple myeloma. Blood 27(3):328-342, 1966.
4. Bergsagel DE, Sprague CC, Austin C, et al: Evaluation of new chemotherapeutic agents in the treatment of multiple myeloma. L-phenylalanine mustard. Cancer Chemother Rep 21:87-99, 1962.
5. Korst DR, Clifford GO, Fowler WM, et al: Multiple Myeloma: II. Analysis of cyclophosphamide therapy in 165 patients. JAMA 189:758-762, 1964.
6. Hoogstraten B, Sheehe PR, Cuttner J, Cooper I, Kyle RA, Oberfield RA, Townsend SR, Harley JB, Hayes DM, Costa G, Holland JF: Melphalan in multiple myeloma. Blood 30:74-83, 1967.
7. Alexanian R, Haut A, Khan AU, Lane M, McKelvey EM, Migliore PU, Stuckey WJ, Wilson HE: Treatment for multiple myeloma: Combination chemotherapy with different melphalan dose regimens. JAMA 208:1680-1685, 1969.
8. Hoogstraten B: Steroid therapy of multiple myeloma and macroglobulinemia. Med Clin N Am 57:1321-1330, 1973.
9. Costa G, Engle RL, Schilling A, et al: Melphalan and prednisone: An effective combination for the treatment of multiple myeloma. Am J Med 54:589-599, 1973.
10. Cuttner J, Wasserman LR, Martz G, Roland W, Sonntag RW, Kyle RA, Silver RT, Spurr C, et al: The use of low-dose prednisone and melphalan in the treatment of poor-risk patients with multiple myeloma. Med Pediatr Oncol 1:207-216, 1975.
11. Harley J, McIntyre OR, Pajak TF: Improved survival of poor-risk myeloma patients receiving combination alkylating agent therapy, abstracted. Blood 50:192, 1977.
12. Alexanian R, Salmon S, Bonnet J, Gehan E, Haut A, Weick J: Combination therapy for multiple myeloma. Cancer 40:2765-2771, 1977.
13. Minutes, Southwest Oncology Group, March 1980.
14. Presant CA, Klahr C: Adriamycin, 1,3-bis(2-chloroethyl)-1-nitrosourea (BCNU), cyclophosphamide plus prednisone (ABC-P) in melphalan-resistant multiple myeloma. Cancer 42:1222-1227, 1978.
15. Bennett JM, Silber R, Ezdinli E, Levitt M, Oken M, Bakemeier RF, Bailar JC, Carbone PP: Phase II study of adriamycin and bleomycin in patients with multiple myeloma: An Eastern Cooperative Oncology Group Study. Cancer Treat Rep 62:1367-1369, 1978.
16. Bonnet JD, Alexanian R, Salmon S: Vincristine-BCNU-adriamycin-prednisone combination for treatment of melphalan-and cytoxan-resistant multiple myeloma. ASH 206:12, 1976.
17. Cohen HJ: Hexamethylmelamine (HMM): A new agent effective in the treatment of refractory multiple myeloma. Blood 50, Supplement 1:187, 1977.
18. Rosner F, Grunwald H: Multiple myeloma terminating in acute leukemia: Report of 12 cases and review of the literature. Am J Med 57:927-939, 1974.
19. Alexanian R, Gehan E, Haut A, Saiki J, Weick J: Unmaintained remissions in multiple myeloma. Blood 51:1005-1011, 1978.
20. Salmon SE, Samal BA, Hayes DM, Hosley H, Miller SP, Schilling A: Role of gamma globulin for immunoprophylaxis in multiple myeloma. N Eng J Med 277:1336-1340, 1967.
21. Acute Leukemia Group B and Eastern Cooperative Oncology Group: Ineffectiveness of fluoride therapy in multiple myeloma. N Eng J Med 286:1283-1288, 1972.
22. Cohen HJ, Abramson N, Bartolucci A, Bailar J: BCNU, cyclophosphamide and prednisone vs. melphalan and prednisone in multiple myeloma. ASCO 17:280, 1976.
23. Costa G, Engle RL, Taliente P: Criteria for defining risk groups and response to chemotherapy in multiple myeloma. AACR 10:15, 1969.
24. McIntyre OR, Leone L, Pajak TF: The use of intravenous melphalan (L-PAM) in the treatment of multiple myeloma. Blood 52:(ASH) Supplement I, 274, 1978.
25. Alexanian R, Balcerzak S, Bonnet JD, Gehan EA, Haut A, Hewlett JS, Monto RW: Prognostic factors in multiple myeloma. Cancer 36:1192-1201, 1975.
26. Acute Leukemia Group B: Correlation of abnormal immunoglobulin with clinical features of myeloma. Arch Intern Med 135:46-52, 1975.
27. Hayes DM, Ellison RR, Glidewell O, Holland JF, Silver RT: Chemotherapy for the terminal phase of chronic myelocytic leukemia. Cancer Chemother Rep 4:233-247, 1974.
28. Rundles RW, Grizzle J, Bell WN, Corley CC, Frommeyer WB, Greenberg BG, Huguley M, et al: Comparison of chlorambucil and myleran in chronic lymphocytic and granulocytic leukemia. Am J Med 27:424-432, 1959.
29. Shullenberger CC: Evaluation of the comparative effectiveness of myleran and 6-MP in the management of patients with chronic myelocytic leukemia. Cancer Chemother Rep 16:203-207, 1962.
30. Southeastern Cancer Chemotherapy Cooperative Study Group: Comparison of 6-Mercaptopurine and busulfan in chronic granulocytic leukemia. Blood 21:89-101, 1968.
31. Smalley RV, Vogel J, Huguley CM, Miller DS: Chronic granulocytic leukemia: Cytogenetic conversion of the bone marrow with cycle-specific chemotherapy. Blood 50:107-114, 1977.
32. Coleman M, Silver RT: Combination chemotherapy for aggressive chronic granulocytic leukemia: Prediction of response. ASCO 16:229, 1975.
33. Huguley CM: Treatment of chronic lymphocytic leukemia. Cancer Treat Rev 4:261-273, 1977.

34. Rai KR, Sawitsky A, Cronkite EP, Chanana AD, Levy RN, Pasternack BS: Clinical staging of chronic lymphocytic leukemia. Blood 46:219-234, 1975.
35. Sawitsky A, Rai KR, Glidewell O, Silver T: Comparison of daily versus intermittent chlorambucil and prednisone therapy in the treatment of patients with chronic lymphocytic leukemia. Blood 50:1049-1059, 1977.
36. Keller JW, Knospe WH, Huguley CM, Johnson L: Cyclophosphamide (CTX) and cytosine arabinoside (ARA-C) to consolidate remission in chronic lymphocytic leukemia (CLL)? ASCO 18:339, 1977.
37. Wasserman LR: The treatment of polycythemia vera. Sem Hemat 13:57-78, 1976.
38. Berlin NI: Diagnosis and classification of the polycythemias. Sem Hemat 12:339-351, 1975.
39. Smith JR, Kay NE: Polycythemia-1973. Laboratory and Clinical Evaluation. 54:141-147, 1973.
40. Ellis JT, Silver RT, Coleman M, Geller SA: The bone marrow in polycythemia vera. Sem Hemat 12:433-444, 1975.
41. Polycythemia Vera Study Group, manuscript in preparation.
42. Silverstein MN: The evolution into and the treatment of late stage polycythemia vera. Sem Hemat 13:79-84, 1976.
43. Minutes, Polycythemia Vera Study Group, November 1976.
44. Wurster-Hill D, Whang-Peng J, McIntyre OR, Hsu LX, Hirschhorn K, Modan B, et al: Cytogenetic studies in polycythemia vera. Sem Hemat 13:13-32, 1976.
45. McIntyre OR, Wurster-Hill D: Mechanisms responsible for the cytogenetic abnormalities encountered in patients with untreated polycythemia vera. Excerpta Medical International Congress Series No. 415, Sixteenth International Congress of Hematology, Kyoto, Japan, 652, 1976.
46. Adamson JW, Fialkow PJ, Murphy S, Prchal JF, Steinmann L: Polycythemia Vera: Stem-cell and probably clonal origin of the disease. N Engl J Med 295:913-916, 1976.
47. Polycythemia Vera Study Group, manuscript in preparation.

5

Central nervous system tumors

John B. Horton, Chu H. Chang, and Audrey E. Evans

INTRODUCTION

Tumor involvement of the central nervous system is a major cause of cancer morbidity and mortality in this country. Primary tumors of the brain are the most common solid tumors of children and, while brain tumors are not in the front rank in terms of producing mortality in adults, metastatic tumor to the brain is the cause of death in many types of cancer.

This review deals with the activity and accomplishments of the Clinical Cooperative Groups and is divided into three major areas; primary tumors of the brain in adults, pediatric brain tumors, and tumor metastases to the brain. The considerable activity of the cooperative groups relating to meningeal involvement in leukemia and lymphoma will not be reviewed since this is discussed elsewhere.

ADULT PRIMARY TUMORS

It is generally accepted that the median survival from the time of operation in patients with malignant glioma is approximately 5.5 months. Twenty percent of patients are alive at the end of one year, less than 10 percent at the end of two years, and only a few at five years. The extent of involvement of the brain by tumor is difficult to evaluate, either objectively or subjectively, so survival is currently the principal method used for demonstrating improvement in the treatment of a malignant brain tumor. Since survival is short, this parameter is effective.

PROGNOSTIC FACTORS

Cooperative Group studies using large patient numbers have defined several significant prognostic factors. Knowledge of these factors now enables stratification procedures to be used to allow better evaluation of therapeutic effect. Excluding treatment as a prognostic factor, characteristics that influence survival include age, varying extent of tumor removal, the presence of seizures and cranial nerve symptoms, and location of the primary tumor in either the parietal or other areas.[1] Another cooperative study not only confirms the favorable effect of young age but also shows that those patients with the best initial performance and mental status grade and least initial neurologic deficit have the best survival.[2]

PATHOLOGY

The number of well-studied patients entered into the several prospectively randomized, well-controlled treatment trials facilitates effective central pathology review. For example, one review of 718 patients[3] demonstrated that there were some instances of progression of histologic anaplasia. Of particular interest in the autopsied cases were several instances of excessive necrosis in white matter distant from persistent glioma in the patients who had received chemotherapy and radiotherapy. This observation suggests the presence of structural and/or metabolic alteration in the disease hemisphere that perhaps makes it more susceptible to further alterations secondary to the adjunctive therapy. Another ongoing pathology review found the limitations of the Kernohan method of classification of primary brain tumors and is stimulating nationally the more widespread adoption of the Rubenstein or WHO classification. Evaluation of one large ongoing study indicates that patients with Kernohan Grade III and Grade IV have

TABLE 1
Correlation of Survival with Histologic Type of
Malignant Brain Glioma

Histologic Type	Number	Deaths	Median Survival
Astrocytoma with foci of anaplasia	24	7	26.4 months
Glioblastoma multiforme	77	62	8.4 months

similar median survivals (9.8 and 8.2 months respectively). In contrast, categorization of patients by the Rubenstein classification gives a much better discrimination of prognosis (Table 1). Treatment effects also vary with histologic type. Hydroxyurea plus radiation, for example, is more effective than radiation alone in anaplastic astrocytoma (42 versus 10 months median survival). This benefit was less marked in the other histologic types.[4]

EVALUATION OF RESPONSE

The difficulty of evaluation of antitumor effect has already been mentioned. While it is possible to document symptomatic change in primary brain tumors, accurate and objective tests that reflect the status of the tumor and the surrounding normal brain are not now available. Current studies include radionuclide brain scanning and computerized tomography. The latter seems to be of greater promise and is now being incorporated into group protocols. The evaluation of brain tumor recurrence is particularly difficult and the subtle differences in symptoms and presentation between recurrence and brain necrosis are currently being defined.

TREATMENT

The major role of the cooperative groups has been in determination of optimal methods for treatment by study of sufficient patient numbers to allow proper statistical evaluation. Largely because of these groups, multimodal therapy is currently considered "standard" practice by many physicians. Much of the development of the individual treatment modalities has taken place with the Cooperative Group mechanism.

Extirpative surgery has been shown to be better than biopsy alone.[1] It is now established for the first time by prospective randomized studies that radiation, using conventional methods of fractionation and dosimetry, significantly increases the median survival over that of patients who do not receive postoperative radiotherapy.[5] There is a linear dose response relationship with evidence of beneficial results being greater at 6,000 rads over 7 weeks than at lower doses at 5,000 rads in 5 to 6 weeks, etc.[6] A higher dose of 7,000 rads in 9 weeks is currently under study.[2]

The Cooperative Groups have evaluated several chemotherapeutic agents. Initial studies have usually been in patients with recurrent tumors. It is now evident that effective drugs are usually those that are lipid soluble. Early studies included evaluation of the lipid soluble, rapidly acting bisepoxide, alkylating agent Epodyl,[7] and the nitrosourea

TABLE 2
Schema of Joint Study of Malignant Gliomas

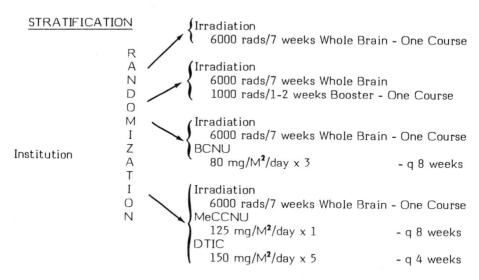

BCNU.[8]   The antitumor antibiotic Mithramycin was shown to be ineffective[9] but other nitrosoureas such as CCNU[10] and methyl CCNU[11] were shown to have effects, both alone and with radiation therapy.[12] Other agents that have been shown to have activity include DTIC,[13] procarbazine,[14] and podophyllin toxoids such as VM 26[12] and hydroxyurea.[4]

Based on the data that surgery, radiation therapy and several types of chemotherapy each had the capability of providing benefit, several prospectively randomized multimodal studies have been activated, each with appropriate controls and pathology and clinical review. The first such study initiated by the Brain Tumor Study Group compared the efficacy of BCNU 80 mg/M^2 per day for 3 days every 6-8 weeks, irradiation at 6,000 rads to the whole brain in 6 to 8 weeks, the combination of both and an untreated control group. All patients received conventional neurosurgical care, including tumor resection with adequate decompression. This study demonstrated that the maximum benefit occurred from those patients who received BCNU plus irradiation.[15]

Another study of malignant glioma, jointly conducted by two large Cooperative Groups, is comparing the effectiveness of whole brain irradiation alone, whole brain radiation plus a booster dose to the tumor, and whole brain irradiation plus a combination of methyl CCNU plus DTIC (Table 2). The "standard arm" is purposely designed to be identical to the previously described "best arm" of the BTSG study, i.e. radiation plus BCNU. This study is still in progress and median survivals in the range of one year are being obtained.[15] Another study group is comparing radiation therapy and CCNU with and without procarbazine.[14] As previously discussed, there is now sufficient data to suggest that the addition of hydroxyurea to radiation is of benefit, at least in patients with anaplastic astrocytoma.[4]

These treatment studies have demonstrated considerable prolongation of survival and, although this is more difficult to document, have allowed evaluation of the duration of useful life that has occurred. The programs have had an impact on patient care in that it is now generally accepted in this country that optimal therapy for malignant primary brain tumors constitutes a multimodal approach using surgical resection, radiation therapy and/or systemic chemotherapy.

TOXICITY

Considerable attention is currently placed on evaluating the toxicity of the treatment programs in progress. It is obvious that the presence of a brain tumor or the complication of this having been resected increases the likelihood of side effects on the normal brain tissue from the addition of radiation, either alone or in combination with chemotherapy. The use of higher doses of radiation therapy will allow the evaluation as to whether or not this gives an increased incidence and severity of toxic effects and will define the limit of brain tissue tolerance. Similarly, further evaluation of the interaction of radiation and chemotherapy will also be made. Well done autopsy pathologic studies, correlated with initial diagnostic material, are critical for this effort. It is essential to determine the therapeutic ratio of any mode of therapy in terms of the extent of tumor sterilization vs. the extent of nominal brain tissue damage.

FUTURE STUDIES

The development of future studies in the treatment of primary brain tumors will likely be concentrated in two areas: more effective radiotherapy and more effective chemotherapeutic agents. For radiotherapy, this includes the evaluation of different dose rate and fractionation schedules, high LET (Linear Energy Transfer) radiation and the use of radiation sensitizers. Initial studies of the hypoxic cell sensitizer of metronidazole have been instituted.[16] Misonidazole is now being studied in Phase II protocols and will shortly be incorporated into prospective studies. The effectiveness of hyperthermia, hyperbaric oxygen, or radionuclide implantation therapy are all capable of being tested of the pilot studies that are now being performed suggest effectiveness.

The future direction for chemotherapy is less clear. Definition of the true effectiveness of hydroxyureas as part of the multimodality approach is indicated. More Phase I and II studies on new chemotherapeutic agents are needed as well as investigation of new pharmacologic techniques for drug delivery, uptake and metabolism in the brain.

PEDIATRIC PRIMARY TUMORS

MEDULLOBLASTOMA AND OTHER TUMORS

Cooperative Group studies of childhood brain tumors have centered primarily on medulloblastoma. The history of these studies indicates a rather logical progression of effort. First, various institutional studies and reviews were undertaken to determine the basis for a study of adjuvant chemotherapy and the results of irradiation. One such study reported that intrathecal methotrexate caused alleviation of neurological signs in 15/18 patients lasting from six weeks to five months.[17] In another study, vincristine was given as a single agent weekly to 17 children with recurrent brain tumors and objective responses lasting from two months to four years were seen in half; 2/4 medulloblastomas had complete regression of symptoms and signs lasting 17 and 24 months.[18] The response to vincristine led to its inclusion in the multidrug chemotherapy of a randomized trial comparing surgical resection, CNS axis irradiation with and without VCR, CCNU and prednisone for patients with medulloblastoma and infratentorial ependymomas.

Other studies were conducted to determine the best methods for delivering a uniform dose of irradiation over the entire CNS axis while maintaining a low dose to other tissues. In a report by Van Dyke et al,[20] the technique was described in detail and the computed dose calculations were verified experimentally with thermoluminescent dosimetry in both a rectangular polystrene phantom as well as a human phantom. It was estimated that the overall dosage variation to the craniospinal axis by means of this technique was within 10 percent of the prescribed tumor dose for the average adult and better than 5 percent for the average child.

Currently three Phase III studies are being conducted for children with newly diagnosed brain tumors, including medulloblastoma and infratentorial ependymoma, Grade III and IV astrocytoma and brain stem glioma. These are randomized studies and the chemotherapy arm, consisting of vincristine, CCNU and prednisone for one year, is the same in each.

The largest entry has been in patients with medulloblastoma/ ependymoma. One hundred and sixty patients had been randomized by the fall of 1978. To date, the survival rate is the same on both study arms and no benefit from chemotherapy has emerged. However, only 20 percent of the patients have been on study 24 months or longer and the life table curves are unstable at this point, particularly in the case of a tumor which has a tendency to recur late. A similar medullo- blastoma study is being conducted in Europe in collaboration with members of the International Society of Pediatric Oncology (SIOP), the only difference being the absence of prednisone in the chemotherapy arm. Results reported at the SIOP annual meeting in September 1978, showed a tendency for the two arms to diverge at 18 months with the patients receiving chemotherapy having a better survival experience. Again, the number of patients on study longer than 24 months is small. The U.S. and European studies have a common arm of patients who receive surgery and neuraxis irradiation alone. There is a striking difference in the survival rate between the U.S. and European patients with better survival in the SIOP study. Efforts are underway to determine the possible causes of this difference.

The toxicity of the chemotherapy regimen is considerable, particularly during the first three months when combined with CNS axis irradiation. Opportunistic infections with pneumocystis carinii and severe varicella were seen.

At the time of this writing, there are insufficient study entries to determine the effect of chemotherapy in Grade III and IV astrocytomas and brain stem gliomas, and relapses are occurring on both arms at roughly the same rate.

Plans are underway to develop a second study for patients with medulloblastoma and consideration is being given to determine the correct dose of irradiation to the spine in particular, since the price of large field irradiation in a child is high and the chance of spinal seeding in the absence of local primary recurrence is low.

A Phase II study was reported[21] in which 24 children with recurrent brain tumors of various histologies received MOPP. Ten had prior chemotherapy. The diagnosis was medulloblastoma in ten and glioma in ten. The combination of drugs were given for 14 days of each four- week period if the WBC was at least 4,000/mm^3. The responses were classified as unequivocal or partial, and the combined responses were 18/24 or 75 percent. Nine of the responses were unequivocal. Although the report does not describe the duration of response, there was a striking difference in the median survival between the 18 responders and the 6 nonresponders i.e. 9.4 months versus 2 months. The authors concluded that MOPP chemotherapy was effective in the treatment of recurrent brain tumors and that prior failure on chemotherapy should not preclude trials with other agents.

PINEAL AND SUPRASELLAR TUMORS

To determine the need for and feasibility of a therapeutic study of tumors in the pineal and suprasellar region, the Groups surveyed member institutions to determine the results of treatment and assess the methods used to date.[22] The years covered were 1960 to 1975 and 118/140 patients were evaluable, having adequate treatment records. The median age was in the second decade with 93/118 occurring under the age of 20. There were 79 males and 39 females.

The primary focuses of the study were to determine the histology of the tumors in this region, the treatment employed and the survival rate. Until recently, most tumors were not biopsied because surgical intervention in this site led to a high operative mortality, but more recently, neurosurgical advances have justified biopsy. Thirty-six of 57 patients, where a tissue diagnosis was available, were found to have germinomas. The next most frequent diagnoses were teratomas and pineal parenchymal tumors of which there were seven each.

Treatment was with radiation therapy in all cases. Sixty received local treatment with a generous margin, 49 cranial and 9 craniospinal. Most were treated with a tumor dose of 5,000 rads in 5-6 weeks but 21 received 4,500 rads or less. None received adjuvant chemotherapy. Overall survival was 65 percent with survival being better for the younger age group, 66 of 101 and 7 of 17 below and above 30 years of diagnosis. Histology influenced survival in that the germinoma group had a 72 percent survival compared to 21 percent for pineal parenchymal tumors and malignant teratomas.

It was not possible from this review to determine any effects of the variation in treatment. The recurrence rate was not different for the patients receiving 5,000 rads or more and 4,500 rads or less. Spinal cord metastases occurred in 9 of 108 patients who had not received craniospinal axis irradiation and 0 of 9 of those who had been so treated. However, the authors did not conclude that an 8 percent spinal recurrence rate warranted total CNS irradiation.

Two questions remained unanswered by this review: 1) can the dose of irradiation for pineal and suprasellar germinomas be safely reduced, and 2) will the increase of surgical intervention give rise to any increase in spinal cord metastases (14 percent biopsied versus 1 to 7 percent unbiopsied). Since the recurrence rate was not different in the patients receiving more than 5,000 rads and less than 4,500 rads, the group has embarked upon a study comparing two doses of irradiation to determine if the disease control is the same and the side effects such as pituitary dysfunction are less in the patients receiving the lower dose. Multi-agent chemotherapy will be employed for patients with recurrent disease.

LONG-TERM TOXICITY

A major concern and current focus of the cooperative groups is in the evaluation of both acute and long-term toxicity to the CNS as a result of the intervention modalities used and the longer survivals that have occurred as a result of these intervention methods. Prospective studies involving psychometric analysis, performance of neurologic examinations, CT scans, etc. are underway to determine the long-term hazard and to attempt to determine whether modification of curative treatment methods should be instituted.

METASTATIC TUMORS TO THE BRAIN

Metastatic tumors to the brain are a major cause of fatality from various common types of primary carcinoma, particularly carcinomas of lung, breast and melanoma. Instances where it is feasible for surgical removal of apparently isolated metastases are uncommon and the majority of patients are treated with various combinations of cortico-steroids, radiation therapy and, in some instances, chemotherapy.

EVALUATION

Once again, evaluation of the effectiveness of treatment is not easy. Various scales of symptomatic change have been developed by cooperative groups and these have been of value in monitoring the clinical benefit of treatment. A simple, workable scale for quantitating the extent of symptomatic deficit is summarized in Table 3.[23] In contrast to the use of survival in evaluation of treatment in patients with primary malignant brain tumors, there are difficulties with using the parameter in metastatic tumors since, although survival is short, death is not necessarily related only to the intracerebral aspects of the disease.

TREATMENT

One of the early cooperative group studies confirmed the value of corticosteroids in the management of this disease.[24] Another group evaluated over 2,000 patients using five different radiation treatment

TABLE 3
Classification of Symptomatic Status of Patients
With Tumor Metastasis to the Brain

A.   General Performance Status

Class	Description
1	Normal
2	Symptoms, but ambulatory
3	In bed, up to 50% of the time
4	In bed, more than 50% of the time
5	100% bedridden

B.   Neurological Function

Class	Description
1	Able to work, neurological findings minor or absent.
2	Able to be at home, although nursing care may be required. Neurological findings present, but not serious.
3	Requires hospitalization and medical care with major neurological findings.
4	Requires hospitalization and is in serious physical or neurological state, including coma.

schedules of whole brain irradiation ranging from 4,000 rad/4 weeks to 2,000 rad/1 week in two sequential Phase III randomized studies to determine palliative effectiveness in patients with metastatic brain disease.[23] The initial neurologic function status and general performance status have been used as prognosticators of response.

These latter studies have shown that whole brain irradiation improved neurologic function in approximately 50 percent of patients. Improvement of specific neurologic symptoms is as high as 90 percent. Patients who present with initial neurologic function 3 have a higher response rate (65 percent) than those presenting with neurologic function 2 (37 percent). Within each neurologic function class, ambulatory patients show a higher response rate than nonambulatory patients. Treatment schedule and primary site had no influence on response in these studies. Administration of corticosteroids during irradiation favored more rapid improvement but did not appear to influence the overall frequency of improvement. Since all treatment schedules were comparable with respect to frequency of improvement, duration of improvement, time of progression, survival and palliative index, it is concluded that a short time-dose fractionation scheme, such as 3,000 rad/2 week be recommended, thus resulting in less expense and inconvenience.

Those patients with a controlled primary lesion and brain as the only site of metastases constitute a prognostically favorable group and may benefit from whole brain irradiation to higher doses (such as 5,000 rad/4 weeks). This selected population is currently under investigation in a Phase III, randomized study by the same group.

The radiation treatment schedules are generally well tolerated and the direction of future research will likely center on the evaluation of various radiation sensitizers. A Phase II study of radiation plus the hypoxic cell sensitizer misonidazole has already been started.

PROPHYLAXIS

It is recognized that the results of treatment of overt metastasis to the brain are poor with average survivals approximating 15 weeks. Prophylactic treatment of microscopic brain metastases may lead to a better quality of survival and improved survival rate.

Some tumors, for example small (oat) cell carcinoma of the lung, have a particularly high incidence of developing brain metastasis. Cooperative group studies in this tumor have shown that combination chemotherapies that include nitrosoureas or other drugs that cross the blood-brain barrier may reduce the incidence of expression of intracerebral metastasis. Prophylactic radiation to the brain (PBI) is well tolerated when used in multimodal treatment studies. It significantly reduces the incidence of expression of brain metastases, although survival is not influenced.[24] These significant discoveries by the Cooperative Groups are currently being actively refined and further explored.

CONCLUSION

Some of the accomplishments of the Cooperative Groups regarding the treatment of CNS tumors include:

A. Primary brain tumors in adults

   1. Methods for detection, diagnosis and followup of brain tumors have been refined.

2.   The clinically relevant prognostic factors have been described for primary brain tumors in adults.

3.   Methods of pathologic classification have been evaluated, refined and promoted.

4.   The optimal roles of surgery and radiation therapy have been defined.

5.   Many chemotherapeutic compounds have been tested for effectiveness.

6.   The value of multimodal treatment has been demonstrated with significant numbers of studied patients.

B.   Pediatric brain tumors

1.   Several studies of the natural history of brain tumors in childhood have been conducted to serve as a basis for therapeutic studies.

2.   Phase II studies of single agents have helped to define which chemotherapeutic agents are effective preparatory to Phase III studies.

3.   Phase III studies have been initiated which include all the common brain tumors in childhood.

C.   Metastatic tumors

1.   Simple scales for quantitating symptomatic changes have been developed.

2.   The role of corticosteroids has been established.

3.   The optimal methods for radiation have been established.

4.   Active studies for prophylaxis are in progress.

Future improvements will likely be associated with a gain in the therapeutic ratio from radiation therapy. This can come from an increase in the effectiveness of tumor treatment or a reduction in normal tissue injury. Most radiation sensitizers sensitize both normal and malignant cells. A notable exception is the newly discovered class of drugs which selectively sensitize hypoxic cells with no effect on well-oxygenated normal tissue. The cooperative groups have conducted Phase I and II studies on a new hypoxic cell sensitizer, misonidazole, in malignant glioma and a number of Phase III studies are being initiated. The use of heavy radiation particles, such as neutrons, heavy ions, and pi-mesons in radiotherapy could lead to a selective increase in tumor injury, i.e. and improvement in therapeutic ratio. Quality control, consistency and uniformity of treatment techniques, and treatment planning are ensured by specific mechanisms, and the accrual of patients onto group studies has been very gratifying. This kind of accrual is not possible on the basis of patients seen in any one institution.

The Cooperative Groups have greatly improved the communication between the neurosurgeon, the radiation therapist and the chemo-therapist, leading to improved care. Also, the cooperative groups have expanded their communication with other cooperative groups outside the United States and parallel studies are being conducted.

REFERENCES

1. Gehan E, Walker M: Prognostic factors for patients with brain tumors. Natl Cancer Inst Monogr 46:189-195, 1977.
2. Horton J, Chang CH, Schoenfeld D: Combined modality approaches in malignant brain glioma. AACR 18:212, 1977.
3. Mahaley MS Jr, Vogel FS, Burger P, Ghatak NR: Neuropathology of tissues from patients treated by the Brain Tumor Study Group. Natl Cancer Monogr 46:77-82, 1977.
4. Irwin L: Western Cooperative Oncology Group Studies 807,808. Natl Cancer Inst Monogr 46:235-236, 1977.
5. Walker MD, Gehan EA: An evaluation of 1-3 Bis (2-Chloroethyl)-1-nitrosourea (BCNU) and irradiation alone and in combination for the treatment of malignant glioma. AACR 13:67, 1972.
6. Walker MD, Strike TA, Sheline G: The dose-effect relationship of radiotherapy in the treatment of malignant glioma. American Radium Society, 4:22, 1978.
7. Horton J, Olson KB, Cunningham TJ, Sullivan JM: Epodyl (AY 62013) in advanced cancer involving the brain and other organs. Cancer, 20:1837-1840, 1967.
8. Lerner H, Carbone P, Colsky J, Lurie P: BCNU effect in primary and secondary brain cancer -- EST 0669. AACR 19:123, 1978.
9. Walker MD, Alexander E, Hunt WE, Leventhal CM, Mahaley MS, Mealey J, Norrell HA, Owens G, Ransohoff J, Wilson CB, Gehan EA: Evaluation of mithramycin in the treatment of anaplastic gliomas. J Neurosurgery, Vol. 44, June 1976.
10. Hildebrand J: EORTC brain tumor studies 26741 and 26742. Natl Cancer Inst Monogr 46:231-232, 1977.
11. Walker MD: Nitrosoureas in central nervous system tumors. Cancer Chemother Rep, 4:21-26. 1973.
12. Gutin PH, Walker MD: Methyl CCNU, VM-26, and cranial irradiation in therapy for malignant brain tumors. Cancer Treatment Rep 61:1715-1717, 1977.
13. Taylor SG, Nelson L, Baxter D, Rosenbaum C, Sponzo RW, Cunningham TJ, Olson KB, Horton J: Treatment of Grade III and IV astrocytoma with dimethyl triazeno imadazole carboxamide (DTIC) alone and in combination with CCNU or methyl CCNU (MeCCNU). Cancer 36:1269-1276, 1975.
14. Quagliana J, Eltringham J, Kushner J, Hoogstraten B: Radiation therapy and CCNU ± procarbazine in patients with grade III and IV astrocytomas of the brain. Natl Cancer Inst Monogr 46:229, 1977.
15. Walker MD: Chemotherapy: Adjuvant to surgery and radiation therapy. Seminars in Oncology, 2:69-72, 1975.
16. Urtasun R, Band P, Chapman DJ, Feldstein ML, Mielke B, Fryer C: Radiation and high-dose metronidazole in supratentorial glioblastomas. N Eng J Med 294:1364-1367, 1976.
17. Newton WA, Sayers MP, Samuels LD: Intrathecal methotrexate therapy for brain tumors in children. Cancer Chemother Rep 52:257-261, 1968.
18. Rosenstock JG, Evans AE, Schut L: Response to vincristine of recurrent brain tumors in children. J Neurosurgery 45:135-140, 1976.
19. Jenkin RDT: Medulloblastoma in childhood: Radiation therapy. Canad Med Assoc Journal 100:51-53, 1969.
20. Van Dyke J, Jenkin RD, Leung PMK, Cunningham JR: Medulloblastoma: Treatment technique and radiation dosimetry. J Rad Oncol Biol Phys 2:993-1005, 1977.
21. Cangir AL, van Eys J, Berry DH, Hvizdala E, Morgan SK: Combination chemotherapy with MOPP in children with recurrent brain tumors. J Med and Pediatr Oncol 4:253-261, 1978.
22. Wara WM, Jenkin RD, Evans A, Ertel I, Hittle R, Ortega J, Wilson CB, Anderson J, Hammond D: Tumors of the pineal and suprasellar region: Childrens Cancer Study Group treatment results 1960-1975. Cancer 43:698-701, 1979.
23. Borgelt B, Gelber R, Kramer S, et al: The palliation of brain metastases: Final results of the first two studies by the Radiation Therapy Oncology Group. Intl J Radiation Oncol, Biol and Physics 6:1-9, 1980.
24. Horton J, Baxter DH, Olson KB, The Eastern Cooperative Oncology Group: The management of metastases to the brain by irradiation and corticosteroids. Am J Roentgenology, Radium Therapy and Nuclear Med 3:334-336, 1971.

6

Head and neck tumors

Harvey J. Lerner, Robert C. Donaldson, and Lawrence W. Davis

GENERAL CONSIDERATIONS FOR HEAD AND NECK TUMORS

Cancer of the head and neck is a term that encompasses a large variety of tumors, although most of these are squamous cell carcinoma. The natural history and the proportion of patients presenting with regional lymphatic metastases, as well as those eventually developing distant metastases, vary greatly according to the site of the primary tumor. Ultimate survival is related to the proportion of patients developing local and regional control of the tumor, although distant metastases will undoubtedly become a more significant problem as a higher proportion of patients have control of their local disease.

Some general points can be made concerning head and neck tumors. In the past, a relatively high incidence of local and regional failure led to the observation that head and neck tumors rarely metastasize systemically. However, since local and regional control has become much more common following management by combined surgery and radiation therapy, distant failure has become much more frequent. For example, in patients with nasopharynx and oropharynx primaries presenting with cervical lymph node metastases, distant metastases have ultimately been documented in more than 30 percent of patients dying of their disease.

Even though head and neck neoplasms account for only six percent of invasive cancers in the United States, the obvious defects of speech or swallowing function by the radical surgical management of these cancers has emphasized the importance of these tumors beyond their incidence. Severe impairment of quality of life for survivors remains a

117

management problem in these patients. While high cure rates and preserved function can be achieved in very early lesions using radiation therapy, combinations of surgery and radiation therapy appear to give the best local control for locally advanced tumors. The optimum combination of radiation therapy and surgery as well as the extensiveness of both procedures remain unanswered questions. In addition, the role of systemic chemotherapy in contributing both to local control and control of distant metastatic disease remain questions to study.

Additional problems do exist, though, in the study and management of these patients. Many patients who present with massive tumors are in poor general condition with a poor nutritional status. Almost all are heavy drinkers and smokers, and their prognosis is poor even if the presenting tumor is controlled. Many develop second and third malignancies of the upper air and food passages, while others die of intercurrent infections or malnutrition. There are many challenges for investigation of these tumors.

Results of 17 Cooperative Group protocols for treatment of head and neck cancer have been reviewed. The majority of the patients have squamous cell carcinoma originating in the mucous membrane lining the nasopharynx, mouth, pharynx and larynx. Discussion will be limited to this cell type since the number of patients with other cell types is too small even to suggest trends in response to treatment. The protocols are divided into two major groups - first, those that have large enough patient populations for statistically valid conclusions to be drawn, and second, those with small numbers of patients, but important from the standpoint of being pilot projects.

The purpose of a large methotrexate study was to determine whether methotrexate given prior to irradiation was more effective in local control and survival in patients with locally advanced untreated, squamous carcinoma of the oral cavity, oropharynx, hypopharynx, and supraglottic larynx than radiation therapy given alone. The primary endpoints of the study were survival and control of cancer within the irradiated field. Patients with primary lesions, stage T-3 or T-4 with nodes N-0 - N-3, or with primary tumors T-1 or T-2, but with nodes N-2 or N-3 were eligible for the study. Patient accession was closed in October of 1972.

Seven hundred and nine patients were randomized into this study, and 631 (89 percent) were eligible for analysis. The preliminary findings indicated that:

1. Heavy smokers and drinkers of alcohol had a significantly poorer survival than nonsmokers and nondrinkers.

2. Tumor status at 90 days following the initiation of therapy is a clear predictor of outcome since it correlated with tumor clearance and survival.

3. Those patients having surgery as a part of initial management, although not controlled in the study, had a significantly superior survival than those patients not having surgery. The majority of surgical procedures were planned-radical-neck dissections.

4. There was no significant difference in local control or survival between the two treatment arms although there is a slight but non-statistical survival benefit in the patients with oral cavity and hypopharyngeal lesions receiving methotrexate.

5. Methotrexate combined with irradiation offers no statistical advantage over irradiation alone.[1,2]

In 1971 a study began to evaluate the role of oxygen. Patients were randomized to receive radiotherapy either alone or while breathing adjuvant oxygen consisting of 95 percent oxygen and 5 percent carbon dioxide at atmospheric pressure. The rationale for this study was based on the experimental evidence that tumors contain necrotic cores and that there are areas in which tumor cells are hypoxic. Response to radiation therapy is less with hypoxic cells than with well-oxygenated ones, and radiotherapy while breathing carbogen might result in dilatation of the blood vessels from the carbon dioxide and greater perfusion of the anoxic areas with oxygen-rich blood. There were several pilot studies conducted which support this premise. Patients with untreated T-2, 3 and 4 squamous cell carcinomas of the oral cavity, oropharynx, nasopharynx, hypopharynx and larynx as well as patients with any stage untreated carcinoma of the esophagus were eligible for this study. Patients with distant metastases were excluded. Case accession was closed in October of 1976 at which time 328 cases had been randomized onto this study including 77 patients with carcinoma of the esophagus. Analysis of the data indicates no treatment advantage for patients breathing adjuvant carbogen during radiation therapy as judged either by local control or survival. Breathing a mixture of 95 percent oxygen and 5 percent carbon dioxide during irradiation offers no advantage over irradiation alone.[3]

Radiation therapy in the treatment of malignancies of the head and neck region is typically delivered five days a week for six to seven weeks. Some treatment schemas use a high daily increment of radiation with a planned interruption of the treatment.

A protocol was designed to determine if split-course irradiation has better treatment tolerance, tumor control, and curability than the standard, uninterrupted radiation therapy course. The primary endpoints of the study are tumor control, patient tolerance to treatment, and immediate and late normal tissue reactions, and survival. Eligible patients include those with untreated carcinoma of the nasopharynx, tonsillar fossae and base of the tongue. This study also includes patients with carcinoma of the uterine cervix and urinary bladder.

Case accession for patients with base of tongue lesions closed in July of 1976. Cases are being accessed to the other head and neck sites. There are currently more than 400 cases on study. Preliminary analysis of the data has shown no differences in local tumor control or treatment tolerance between the two radiation therapy courses. Therefore, split course irradiation offers no statistical advantage over continuous course therapy.[4] Acute reactions were also similar. The overall median survival differs for the three regions, 15 months for the tongue, 19 months for the tonsil and 31 months for the nasopharynx.

Preliminary data analysis of the methotrexate study had an interesting observation that when surgery was added radiation therapy patients had improved survival as compared to those not undergoing surgery. However, surgery was not subject to randomization in that study, and it was impossible to determine whether this improvement was due to selection or represented a therapeutic gain. Because of that, and because of the body of information indicating that radiation therapy combined preoperatively with surgery resulted in better local control of tumor than either modality alone, and because very little information was available on the effectiveness of surgery combined with postoperative irradiation therapy, a study was designed to determine the value of radiation therapy alone or in combination with surgery for squamous cell carcinoma of the oral cavity, pharynx, and larynx. Radiation therapy was given either pre- or postoperative in definitive doses and surgery reserved for persistent or recurrent tumor was also included in lesions to the oral cavity and oropharynx since this was judged to be a valid treatment option. Furthermore, this study represents again, the close cooperation of radiation oncologists and surgical oncologists in study design and in the systematic development of randomized studies.

Patients with T-2, T-3 or T-4 untreated squamous carcinomas of the oral cavity, oropharynx, supraglottic larynx and hypopharynx, except those with N-3A, fixed nodes, are eligible for the study as long as considered operable.

The endpoints of the study are local control, complications, functional status post therapy, and survival time.

Three hundred forty-six patients were entered into the study, and preliminary analysis of the data indicates the following:

1. There are fewer radiotherapy complications in patients receiving radiotherapy preoperatively as compared to postoperatively. The rates of surgical complications are similar for all three treatment groups.

2. Primary tumor control for patients treated with a combination of radiation and surgery (in either treatment arm) is excellent.

3. At 18 months the disease-free survival is 46 percent for pre- and 52 percent for postoperative radiation. Preoperative irradiation offers no statistical advantage over postoperative radiation in the control of supraglottic cancer. [5]

A study comparing a) Methotrexate alone (M); b) Methotrexate plus leucovorin rescue (LM); and c) Methotrexate plus leucovorin plus cyclophosphamide plus cytosine arabinoside (MLCC) in patients with advanced disease showed significantly different response durations. Methotrexate alone had a median response duration of 120 days as compared to 47 and 61 days of ML and MLCC respectively. There were also major differences in survival by treatment. Methotrexate alone had a median survival of 5.1 months as compared to 4.4 for Methotrexate with leucovorin and 3.2 for MLCC. This trial indicated that Methotrexate alone was the best treatment. It had the best response rate, the most complete responders, the longest duration of response, and the best survival. The latter two of these differences were statistically significant. [6]

Protocols classified as pilot studies because of the small number of evaluable patients are summarized as follows: [7]

1) 5-Fluorouracil, Methotrexate, Vincristine and Cyclophosphamide

2) 5-Fluorouracil, Methotrexate, Vincristine and Cyclophosphamide plus Prednisone.

3)   1-(2-chloroethyl)-3-cyclohexyl-1-nitrosourea (CCNU) alone.

4)   Adriamycin alone.

5)   Dimethyl triazeno imidazole carboxamide (DTIC) alone.

6)   Cytosine arabinoside alone.

The best results occurred with protocol #2 above with 6/12 squamous cell carcinomas showing 50 percent or greater reduction in tumor volume with an average duration of 3 to 7 months.

A Phase I study treated 15 patients with irradiation plus a multidrug combination consisting of cyclophosphamide, vincristine and bleomycin during irradiation therapy and followed with a maintenance schedule substituting methotrexate for vincristine.[8] Six of 15 patients are alive without gross evidence of disease 4 to 12 months from onset of treatment. This is a remarkable response considering that 14 of the 15 were classified as having Stage IV disease.

The lone immunotherapy protocol compares methotrexate alone with methotrexate plus methanol extract residue of BCG (MER) and offers a third crossover arm whereby patients failing after six weeks of methotrexate alone then receive MER added to methotrexate.[9] Although the number of patients is too small for statistical evaluation, the trend is for methotrexate and methotrexate plus MER to be equally effective, producing a 50 percent decrease in cancer volume in 40 percent of the patients. Of more significance may be that 4/7 crossover patients responded with 50 percent regression of tumor. These results suggest that six weeks of methotrexate prior to MER may have improved the stage for MER by first depressing serum blocking factors enabling MER to selectively stimulate cell-mediated immunity.

An outpatient therapy schedule has been developed for Cis-diamminedichloride Platinum consisting of two 50 mg/M^2 doses one week apart repeated at 4-10 week intervals.[10] This schedule proved to be minimally toxic. Sixteen out of 65 evaluable patients had > 50 percent reduction in tumor volume. The duration of regression ranged from 36 to 476 days, median 138 days.

Intraarterial infusion was the subject of only one cooperative group study - 258 patients with squamous cell carcinoma of the head and neck were infused with ten different chemotherapy drugs and schedules with an overall 50 percent response rate with 50 percent reduction in gross tumor volume.[11] There is no breakdown as to which treatment schedule was best. In only 12 percent of the responding patients did the regression last longer than six months. The low percentage of six month responders probably is a reflection of the fact that head and neck cancer is more often than not a systemic disease requiring more treatment than simple local intraarterial infusion for long-term arrest.

CONCLUSIONS AND RECOMMENDATION FOR FUTURE

Future control of squamous cell carcinoma of the head and neck lies in exploration of combination therapies in order to define proper patient selection, the correct dose, frequency and sequence of administration of surgery, irradiation, chemotherapy and immunotherapy.

Head and neck cancer lends itself well as a "relatively" ideal study model, i.e.:

1) It remains a local-regional disease for a long period of time prior to distant metastases.

2) It can be measured with direct vision, and often with calipers, and does not require indirect measurement such as scans, x-rays, or palpation through other tissues.

3) The effect of therapy on advanced disease can be readily seen and objectively measured and photographed.

4) It can be primarily treated by a single modality or multiple modalities, i.e., surgery, radiation therapy, immunotherapy, and chemotherapy.

5) Since local-regional failure often occurs prior to distant metastases, it is also a very good system to evaluate adjuvant therapy (of any modality).

6) The primary tumor or lymph node metastases can be treated by the direct injection of therapeutic agents.

7) In addition, head and neck cancers can be sampled at various times during therapy.

The Cooperative Cancer Study Groups are now sufficiently organized and have indepth multimodal ability to provide the patient volume for the scientific, biologic and therapeutic study of head and neck cancer.

124   REFERENCES

1. Fazekas JT, Davis L, Concannon J, Bogardus C, Sommer C, Borgelt B, Lindberg R, Kramer S, Jesse R (Radiation Therapy Oncology Group): The value of intravenous methotrexate as an adjuvant to definitive radiotherapy in advanced cancers of the oral cavity, oropharynx, hypopharynx and supraglottic larynx.
2. Kramer S (Radiation Therapy Oncology Group): Methotrexate and radiation therapy in the treatment of advanced squamous cell carcinoma of the oral cavity, oropharynx, supraglottic larynx and hypopharynx. Canadian J of Otolaryngology 4: 213-218, 1975.
3. Rubin P, Marcial V, Hanley J, Mann S, Brady L (Radiation Therapy Oncology Group): The national study on adjunctive oxygen breathing in the radiation treatment of head and neck and esophageal cancer.
4. Marcial VA, Hanley J, Davis L, Hendrickson F, Ortiz H (Radiation Therapy Oncology Group): Split-course radiation therapy of carcinoma of the base of the tongue: Results of a prospective national collaborative clinical trial of the Radiation Therapy Oncology Group.
5. Snow JB, Gelber RD, Kramer S, Davis LW, Marcial VA, Lowry LD (Radiation Therapy Oncology Group): Evaluation of randomized preoperative and postoperative radiation therapy for supraglottic carcinoma: Preliminary report. Submitted to Annals of Otology, Rhinology, Laryngology.
6. DeConti RC (Eastern Cooperative Oncology Group): Phase III comparison of methotrexate with leucovorin vs. methotrexate alone vs. a combination of methotrexate plus leucovorin, cyclophosphamide and cytosine arabinoside in head and neck cancer. ASCO 17:248, 1976.
7. Dowell KE, Armstrong DM, Aust JB, Cruz AB: Systemic chemotherapy of advanced head and neck malignancies. Cancer 35: 1116-1120, 1975.
8. Silverberg IJ, Phillips TL, Friedman MA, Fu KK (Radiation Therapy Oncology Group): A Phase I study of radiotherapy and multidrug chemotherapy in advanced head and neck cancer. (Abstract)
9. Donaldson RC, Banda F, Keehn R (VA Surgical Adjuvant Cancer Chemotherapy Group): Methotrexate plus MER for head and neck cancer. In Neoplasm Immunity: Solid Tumor Therapy, RG Crispen, ed. Philadelphia: Franklin Institute Press, pp. 243-248, 1977.
10. Panettiere FJ, Lehane D, Fletcher WS, Stephens R, Rivkin S, McCracken JD, (Southwest Oncology Group): Chemotherapy of Head and Neck cancer with cis-platinum. Med and Ped Oncol, In Press.
11. Conn JH, Fain WR, Chavez CM, Rogers LS (Infustion Study Group of VA Surgical Adjuvant Cancer Chemotherapy Group): Cancer chemotherapy by continuous intraarterial infusion. Bull de la Societe Internationale de Chirurgie 27:588-599, 1968.

7

Breast cancer

Douglass C. Tormey, Bernard Fisher, Bill L. Tranum,
and Ruheri Perez-Tamayo

INTRODUCTION

Over the past two decades the Cooperative Groups have been involved in determining the relative value of various treatment modalities for the management of both primary and metastatic breast cancer. Moreover, they have directed their efforts toward answering significant biological questions concerning the disease. Relative to the latter, they have defined a great many factors which affect the natural history of breast cancer, especially from the time of diagnosis. The observations contained in this area alone have enabled a clearer description of the disease process, and thereby have allowed sharper insights to the development of future approaches. This report is limited to reviewing the more important findings in the areas of natural history and treatment. It is in no way intended to be a detailed, complete and all inclusive narrative, but is more an outline which emphasizes and demonstrates the accomplishments of the Cooperative Group approach.

OBSERVATIONS RELATIVE TO THE NATURAL HISTORY AND STAGING OF BREAST CANCER

RELATION OF NUMBER OF INVOLVED AXILLARY NODES TO PROGNOSIS

A finding of singular importance was noted from 1968 to 1970.[1,2,3] Previously it had been generally accepted that the prognosis of cancer of the breast was related to the presence or absence of axillary nodal involvement without regard for the number of nodes demonstrating tumor.   When sufficient data had accumulated, a plot of numbers of nodes containing tumor in a surgical specimen versus the 24-month postoperative recurrence rate was carried out.   In this preliminary examination it was observed that while a progressive increase in recurrence rate accompanied the presence of more positive nodes, a sharp rise occurred with the involvement of approximately four nodes. Consequently, patients with lymph nodes were grouped into those with 1 to 3 or 4 plus involvement in subsequent analyses of data. The validity of such grouping was confirmed by the observance of a 25 percent difference in 5-year survival of patients in the two groups.[1]   At that time the following comment was made: These findings afford a possible explanation for differences in recurrence and survival rates in different reported retrospective nonrandomized series. The positive node patient population in one study may differ from that of another with respect to the number of involved nodes.   Consequently, interpretation of data without such information may be difficult.[1]

Subsequently, it has been observed that the 10-year treatment failure rate and survival rate are also dependent upon the number of axillary nodes involved.[4] When all nodes are free of tumor the treatment failure rate at ten years was 24 percent and the survival rate 65 percent.   In patients with 1 to 3 involved axillary nodes these rates were 64 percent and 38 percent, respectively, while in those with >4 involved nodes the figures were 86 percent and 13 percent, respectively (Table 1).

LOCATION OF TUMOR AND PROGNOSIS

Over the next few years a number of manuscripts were addressed to

TABLE 1
Breast Cancer Results At 10 Years

Histopathologic Axillary Nodal Status	Treatment Failure Rates	Survival Rates
Negative	24%	65%
Positive	76%	25%
1-3	64%	38%
>4	86%	13%
All Patients	50%	46%

answering a series of questions which related to factors that could influence prognosis. In one such study a detailed evaluation was carried out to determine how tumor location affected prognosis[2] This data, collected from more than 1,000 patients across 45 institutions, afforded an opportunity to reassess the long-established principle that the location of a primary breast carcinoma influences prognosis. It was observed that of 1,063 breast carcinomas, 56 percent were in the outer half of the breast, and four-fifths of these were found in the upper outer quadrant. Inner half lesions comprised 17 percent of the total, and in only 5 percent of all patients were tumors found in the lower inner quadrant. Twelve percent were considered as diffuse in that such lesions were either not discrete, extended from the center of the breast to involve more than one quadrant, or were multifocal in origin.

Examination of the relationship between tumor location and axillary nodal involvement revealed that upper inner quadrant lesions and interquadrant lesions of the upper half of the breast were significantly less often associated with positive axillary nodes (34 percent), than were tumors at other sites (52 percent). With upper inner quadrant lesions the number of nodes involved was more frequently 1 to 3 rather than 4 plus. Subareolar tumors likewise demonstrated a lower incidence of nodal involvement than did outer quadrant lesions, but when they were involved, there was a greater tendency for four or more nodes to contain tumor.

When the five-year recurrence rate of patients was related to tumor location, without regard to nodal status, it was noted that inner quadrant lesions resulted in a slightly lower incidence of recurrence than did those tumors which occurred elsewhere. The highest recurrence rate (62 percent) occurred in patients with diffuse tumors. When tumors were grouped as inner half, outer half, middle vertical or upper half, lower half and middle horizontal no significant difference in the recurrence rate between groups was noted.

In 497 patients with negative axillary nodes, no significant difference in recurrence occurred when tumors were at any site or were considered diffuse. Similarly, the 508 patients with positive axillary nodes demonstrated no significant difference in recurrence when their tumors were located at any particular site or combination of sites. Only those patients with diffuse tumors and four or more positive axillary nodes had a significantly higher recurrence rate.

When survival rates were related to tumor location without regard for nodal status, no tumor location provided a significant advantage over any other. Only those tumors classified as diffuse resulted in a significantly greater mortality.

In patients with negative nodes, for the most part, no tumor location - not even subareolar or diffuse tumors - was associated with a significantly different survival rate. Only when a comparison was made between upper half lesions and those in the lower half and middle horizontal segments combined was a significant difference in favor of the former lesions found.

Survival of patients with positive axillary nodes was not significantly different when tumors occurred in inner or outer, upper or lower halves of the breast. Only when tumors were subareolar, in the middle vertical segment of the breast, or diffuse, was the survival rate found to be worse, and this was primarily the result of patients having 4 plus positive nodes rather than 1 to 3 positive nodes. Table 2 summarizes these findings relative to survival and tumor location.

Failure to observe a significant increase in the recurrence rate in patients treated by conventional radical mastectomy when their lesions were in the inner half or central portions of the breast, in spite of the acknowledged greater incidence of internal mammary nodal metastases

TABLE 2
Five-Year Survival Rate According
To Location Of Tumor And Number Of Positive Nodes

TUMOR LOCATION	1 TO 3 POSITIVE NODES		4 PLUS POSITIVE NODES	
	NO. OF PATIENTS	PERCENT SURVIVAL	NO. OF PATIENTS	PERCENT SURVIVAL
Quadrant				
Upper Outer	131	64	110	39
Upper Inner	24	63	16	38
Lower Outer	24	54	21	33
Lower Inner	16	56	8	50
Overall for all Quadrants	195	62	155	38
Interquadrant				
Upper Outer and Inner	10	30	16	25
Lower Outer and Inner	6	83	6	33
Upper and Lower Inner	3	67	2	50
Upper and Lower Outer	9	89	12	33
Overall for all Interquadrants	28	64	36	31
Subareolar	11	73	16	13
Diffuse	22	50	56	14
TOTAL	256		263	
Outer Half	164	65	143	38
Inner Half	43	61	26	43
Middle Vertical	27	59	38	21
Upper Half	165	62	142	37
Lower Half	46	59	35	37
Middle Horizontal	23	78	30	23

with such tumors, provoked certain conclusions. The findings confirmed a previous suggestion made in 1967 that positive lymph nodes merely denote that disseminated tumor cells, which produced such growths as a result of intrinsic cell properties or host factors or both, are capable of developing metastases elsewhere throughout the body as well and that the absence of lymph node involvement does not mean that tumor cell dissemination has not taken place. Negative nodes may reflect conditions which, in addition to preventing nodal growth of tumor, also inhibit metastases from occurring in other places in the body. Moreover, the presence of positive internal mammary nodes in addition to axillary node involvement may be of no more biologic or prognostic significance, as is seemingly demonstrated in this study, than if axillary nodes alone are involved. The findings led to the conclusion that there is no reason to anticipate from these data that the utilization of a specific surgical approach for the therapy of breast carcinoma, based on location of the tumor, will be more rewarding than will be any other.[2]

PRIMARY TUMOR SIZE AND AXILLARY NODE INVOLVEMENT

To elucidate the validity of the concept that the size of breast neoplasms influences prognosis, an analysis was carried out in 1969 utilizing information obtained from 2,578 patients entered into Cooperative Group trials. When all patients were distributed according to tumor size at the time of surgery without regard for their nodal status, it was of interest to note that only 5 percent had tumors smaller than 1.0 cm. The greatest proportion of tumors, 50 percent, ranged from 1.0 to 3.0 cm. Seventeen percent of all patients came to surgery with tumors 3.1 to 4.0 cm in size, and in 28 percent, tumors were greater than 4.0 cm.

To determine the relationship between primary tumor size and axillary node involvement, the distribution of the former within each nodal status category was evaluated (Fig. 1). Because of the very large number of patients, each of the distributions was found to be statistically different (p < 0.01) from the other. Negative node patients tended to have smaller tumors than did those with 1 to 3 positive nodes. They, in turn, had smaller tumors than did patients with 4 or more positive lymph nodes. However, despite the statistical significance of the differences in distributions, the clinical significance of the differences was less impressive. For example, the median tumor size for negative node patients was 2.7 cm; for patients with 1 to 3 positive nodes 2.9 cm; and for those with 4 plus nodal involvement 3.7 cm. The median size of all positive node patients combined was 3.3 cm.

The relationship between the size of the primary tumor and axillary nodal involvement was also examined another way. The percentage of patients within each tumor size grouping having positive or negative

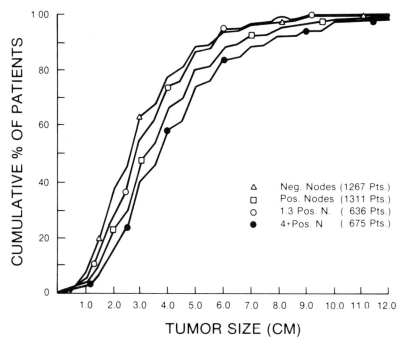

Fig. 1. Tumor size of 2,578 patients with regard for nodal status

nodes was determined. It was thus observed that fewer patients with small tumors had positive nodes than did those whose tumors were large. Of interest, however, were the findings that as many as 22 percent of patients having the smallest tumors (<1.0 cm) did have positive lymph nodes, and that those with the largest tumors (6.0+ cm) demonstrated only a 63 percent involvement. There was a good correlation between increasing tumor size and greater percentage of positive lymph nodes, but the differences were smaller than might have been anticipated.

It was of interest to determine whether in those patients who have positive nodes the number of nodes involved was related to tumor size. Results of such a comparison demonstrated (Fig. 2) that the proportion of patients with 4 plus positive nodes increased with increasing tumor size. In those whose tumors were between 1.0 and 1.9 cm, 56 percent had 1 to 3 positive nodes and 44 percent had 4 or more nodes involved. The opposite prevailed when tumors were 6.0+ cm. Then, 35 percent had 1 to 3 nodes containing tumor and 65 percent had 4 or more nodes involved. However, from a point of view of clinical significance, it was of interest that only 10 percent more patients having positive lymph nodes with 5.0-5.9 cm tumors had 4 plus positive nodes than did similar patients with 1.0-1.9 cm tumors (44 percent vs 54 percent).

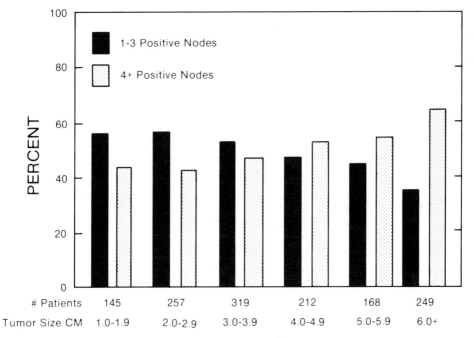

Fig. 2. Percent of patients with auxillary metastases having 1 to 3 or 4+ nodes involved

EFFECT OF PRIMARY TUMOR SIZE AND NODAL STATUS ON FIVE-YEAR MORTALITY RATE

The 5-year mortality rate was derived from 1,105 patients. Without regard for nodal status, it can categorically be stated that the larger tumors resulted in a greater mortality rate than did those which were smaller. Tumors from 3.0 to 6.0+ cm in size differed little in 5-year mortality (43 percent to 55 percent); those < 3.0 cm had a mortality rate ranging from 18 percent for < 1.0 cm to 28 percent for 2.0-2.9 cm. Thus the largest increase occurs when tumors are 3.0 cm or greater in size.

Consideration of survival by tumor size within nodal status categories resulted in findings consistent with those relative to recurrence. Survival of the patients with the largest tumor (> 6.0 cm) and negative axillary nodes was only 10 percent different than that observed for patients with the same nodal status and the smallest tumors (< 1.0 cm.), 75 percent and 85 percent, respectively. Similarly, in patients with 1 to 3 positive axillary nodes, no strong trend in survival in favor of those with smaller tumors was encountered. Only in those patients with 4 plus positive nodes was it evident that the larger the tumor the poorer the survival (i.e., 65 percent in those with 1.0-1.9 cm tumors versus 15 percent when tumors were 6.0+ cm).   Just as with the recurrence rate, consideration of tumor size alone could not foretell survival. For the largest tumors ($\geq$ 6.0 cm) with negative nodes, the survival rate was 75 percent.   However, the rate decreased to 55 percent when 1 to 3 nodes were involved with metastases and to 15 percent when 4 or more nodes were positive.

NUMBER OF LYMPH NODES EXAMINED AND PROGNOSIS

In a trial conducted in 43 institutions, it was possible to correlate the recurrence and survival rates of 2,768 patients with breast carcinoma with the number of lymph nodes obtained and examined in surgical specimens.[5] The range of the number of nodes examined per specimen was remarkably great from institution to institution.   The median number varied from a low of eight at one institution to a high of 28 at another.   Analysis of data to determine whether or not the number of nodes per specimen differed relative to the nodal status, revealed that the distribution of the number of nodes examined in specimens containing all negative nodes was similar to that obtained when 1 to 3 were tumor-positive. In both, the mean number examined was 17. Patients with 4 or more axillary nodes containing tumor averaged 21 nodes examined per specimen.

It is suggested that the great range in the number of nodes per specimen is related to a combination of anatomic differences, errors in identification of all nodes by the pathologist, and variation in the extent of surgical dissection.   A comparison of methods used for identification of nodes in resected specimens revealed that diligence of search was more important than techniques used. However, the failure to observe any nodes in some specimens despite exhaustive efforts to identify them suggests that sometimes the presence of only a few regional nodes is a true finding.

The results obtained failed to demonstrate that the discovery and examination of a greater number of nodes in a specimen were more meaningful in determining prognosis than if only a few were recovered. It was observed that patients having five to ten nodes reported as negative had essentially the same recurrence and survival rates as did those with 25 or 30 nodes free of tumor. The concept that the latter represents a purer negative node group was not substantiated. Likewise, when specimens from patients with positive nodes contained one to five or more than 30 nodes, recurrence and survival rates were similar. The patient with two positive nodes out of five examined was not found to be at greater risk than another having two with tumor out of 30 recovered.

These findings have evoked certain considerations relative to their significance and have prompted conclusions which, while contrary to current thought, cannot be dismissed without further evaluation. Since recurrence and survival rates were found to be independent of the number of lymph nodes found, it could be concluded that it mattered little if all regional nodes were surgically removed. Moreover, the findings tend to minimize the importance of the conclusions of those who have uncritically claimed better results for their surgical efforts because more nodes have been recorded in their resected surgical specimens.

INCIDENCE OF NONSIMULTANEOUS BILATERAL PRIMARY BREAST CANCER

The risk of carcinoma developing in the second breast has been a subject which has received considerable attention. Unfortunately, much of the information presented has been difficult to evaluate. Consequently, in 1973 a Cooperative Group reported its experience in that regard. [6]

A total of 52 second primary tumors were diagnosed from one to 67 months after removal of the first breast in a series of 2,734 patients entered in clinical trials, 1.9 percent. Survival of the patients with bilateral primary carcinoma, within stage, calculated from time of diagnosis of the first primary tumor, was similar to survival of those with unilateral primary tumors. The incidence of second primary lesions on the basis of patient years at risk was 4.3 per 1,000 patients per year, which was similar to the first six years of several other series reported in the literature. Patients under 40 years of age at the time of initial diagnosis have a risk of second primary breast carcinoma relative to that of a first primary tumor of 25.0 compared with a risk of 2 to 5 for other age groups. Patients with large first primary tumors, 6.0 centimeters or more in diameter, also had a much greater incidence of second primary carcinoma than those with smaller tumors. The incidence was determined for three nodal status groups on the premise that if the incidence was greatest for groups with a poor prognosis, second primary tumors might really be metastases. The results are not clear. While the high incidence for younger patients appeared to be limited to those with positive nodes, in the older patients those with negative nodes had a higher incidence. It was estimated that in the first five years only 2 percent of the patients would benefit from a bilateral mastectomy. If a bilateral procedure was routinely used for prophylaxis against second primary tumors, this would result in a maximum gain in five years of only 0.8 percent in the relative survival rate. The additional incidence of second primary carcinoma after five years was not thought to be great enough to justify routine bilateral mastectomy.

ADDITIONAL PATHOLOGIC FINDINGS OF SPECIAL IMPORTANCE

A)   Observations Concerning Multicentricity: Knowledge concerning the multicentricity of breast cancer is of extreme importance not only for its biologic importance but also for its relationship to treatment procedures.   In one study[7] microscopic foci of multicentric cancer were detected in 121 of 904 breasts surgically removed for a clinically overt, invasive cancer.   This incidence rate of 13.4 percent is regarded as a conservative estimate since lesions occurring in the same quadrant as the dominant mass were excluded from the analysis.   Only one randomly selected block of the quadrants was examined and in several cases only one or two were available for study.   When all quadrants were examined multicentric cancers were found in the same breast in 21.9 percent of the cases.   In 9.3 percent of the cases the multicentric cancers were designated as noninvasive (lobular in situ and/or intraductal) and in 4.1 percent invasive.   The occurrence of multicentric cancers was significantly (p <.05) associated with grossly nonencapsulated primary cancers with maximum diameters greater than 5 cm, the presence of a moderate or marked intraductal component, noninvasive cancer in its vicinity, and tumor involvement of the nipple. Lymphatic tumor emboli were observed in quadrants in 18 or 2.0 percent of the cases.   A positive association of such emboli was noted with primary tumors in the left breast or beneath the nipple, noncircumscribed primaries, a nuclear grade of 1, intralymphatic and blood vessel invasion, calcium, involvement of the overlying skin as well as nipple and four or more lymph nodes with metastases.   The relationship of these findings is under extensive consideration in the design of future clinical trials.

B)   Significance of Regional Node Histology Other Than Sinus Histiocytosis: The morphologic appearances of regional lymph nodes in radical mastectomy specimens obtained from 303 women entered into a prospective study of invasive breast cancer were analyzed with relation to 31 other histologic and 8 clinical features, including short-term treatment failure (3 months to 4 years, average 24 months).[8] A lymphocyte predominance pattern was significantly associated with a stellate tumor border, absent cell reaction within the dominant tumor, absent sinus histiocytosis of lymph nodes, combination tumor types and a patient age of 55 years or more.   A similar relationship between age of patient and sinus histiocytosis was found with the germinal center predominance pattern.   In addition, this histologic appearance was associated with circumscribed tumors, severe cell reaction and the infiltrating ductal carcinoma NOS and medullary types.   Nodes with an unstimulated appearance were also found to be related to an absent cell reaction but marked sinus histiocytosis and a patient age of 45-54 years. However, this study failed to indicate any value of such histologic nodal assessments as prognostic discriminants for breast cancer.

C)   Significance of Extranodal Extension of Axillary Metastases: One hundred fifty-eight patients with axillary nodal metastases were divided into those with only one node involved and those in whom one or more nodes manifested extranodal extension. The relationships of these patterns to 33 pathologic and seven clinical features of these cases were investigated by contingency table analysis.[9] Statistically significant associations (p < .05) were found between extranodal extension of such metastases and short-term treatment failure, as well as the presence of four or more involved nodes, infiltrating ductal NOS histologic tumor type, stellate tumor border and nipple involvement. When the metastases were confined to the nodes, there was a greater likelihood that the cancers were either medullary or tubular histologic types. Associations with severe cell reaction and a nuclear grade of 1 were also found, but appeared to reflect the high frequency of medullary carcinomas in this group. The results suggest that evaluation of extranodal extension of axillary nodal metastases in patients with breast cancer may represent an important prognostic discriminant.

D)   Significance of Axillary Nodal Micro- and Macrometastases: Two hundred seventy-eight of 565 patients in a prospective randomized clinical trial exhibited axillary nodal metastases. Patients in whom the largest nodal metastasis measured < 2 mm in its greatest diameter were regarded as having micrometastases and those in whom the lesions were ≥ 2 mm as having macrometastases.[10] Micrometastases were encountered in only 8 percent of the cases. Contingency table analysis disclosed that the group with macrometastases had a greater likelihood of being clinically assessed as Stage II; their primary tumor would be ≥ 2 cm; they would have 4 or more positive nodes; extension of the metastasis through the nodal capsule would have occurred; and uninvolved nodes would exhibit a germinal center predominance pattern. Life table analyses revealed that the disease-free survival of patients with negative nodes is markedly better than patients with micrometastases (p = .001), and cases with macrometastases (p = .0005). Multivariate analysis revealed that the apparent effects on survival and treatment failure rates in patients with micro- and macrometastases were more directly related to the number of nodes involved with metastases than to the size of the latter.

E)   Detection and Significance of Occult Axillary Nodal Metastases: Blocks of axillary lymph nodes from 78 patients with invasive breast cancer, which after "routine" pathological examination

TABLE 3
Consistent Associations with Pathologic Nodal Status

Negative

Clinically negative axilla
Gross and histologic circumscription
Nuclear Grade 3
Sinus histiocytosis moderate, marked
Histologic Grades 1 and 2
Elastica absent
Lymphatic invasion absent
Size less than 4.1 cm

4 Plus Positive

Clinically positive axilla
Nipple involvement
Blood vessel invasion
Perineural extension
Nuclear Grade 1
Sinus histiocytosis absent
Histologic Grade 3
Elastica moderate
Lymphatic invasion
Cancer in vicinity of main tumor
Size 4.1 + cm

were regarded as negative for metastases, were step-sectioned at 20 μ intervals.[11] Occult metastases were detected in 19 (24 percent) of the cases. A significant association between such metastases and a lack of or slight degree of an intraductal component of the dominant cancer was noted. There was no relationship between occult metastases and 15 other histopathological and 3 clinical features investigated. It is of interest that none of ten patients with only tumor emboli died of their disease whereas four of nine cases in whom the occult lesion appeared as a "true" metastatic deposit died of their cancer and a fifth already has recurrence.

F)   Pathologic Interrelationships: The National Surgical Adjuvant Breast Project has conducted an extensive indepth analysis of the pathology of breast cancer from a cooperative group study patient cohort.[12] Space prohibits more than a cursory review of the findings. The interrelationships of 32 pathologic and seven clinical parameters encountered in this study of 1,000 examples of invasive breast carcinoma were determined. In some instances the biological significance of these associations is at present unclear, while in others there is no information as to the rank of their significance. Nevertheless, the associations that were encountered not only help further characterize the various forms of breast cancer but also provide information regarding the possible biological significance of some of their features.

From the previous pages it is evident that the absence or presence of axillary lymph node metastases plays a very important role in the prognosis of breast cancer. The consistent associations with pathologic nodal status are summarized in Table 3.

Several of the guidelines used in the examination of the specimens in this study and conclusions of the study represent at least minimum requirements necessary for a meaningful pathologic evaluation of breast carcinoma. These are presented in a condensed version.

1. Simple descriptive terminology is the most practical as well as inclusive. This allows for the consideration of cancers with complicated histologic appearances, not clearly encompassed by existing classifications.

2. The distribution of histologic types was as follows: a) infiltrating ductal without special features or NOS (52.6 percent); b) medullary (6.2 percent); c) lobular invasive (4.9 percent); d) mucinous (2.4 percent); e) tubular (1.2 percent); f) adenocystic (0.4 percent); g) papillary (0.3 percent); h) carcinosarcoma (0.1 percent); i) Paget's disease (2.3 percent); j) combinations with NOS (28.0 percent); and k) combinations of the above without an NOS component (1.6 percent).

3. Oxyphilic or apocrine change and squamous metaplasia are features of tumor types rather than distinct entities.

4. Carcinomas totally or in part comprised of small or multinucleated giant or basaloid cells are arbitrarily classified according to their basic growth pattern, i.e., NOS, lobular invasive, etc., rather than as distinct entities.

5. Atypical medullary tumors exhibited some but not all of the features of medullary cancer, lacking either: a) histologic circumscription, b) marked lymphoid infiltrate, or c) Grade 1 nuclear forms. Significant associations with this tumor type, were distinctly different from those of the classical medullary form. Since they were less strikingly different than those found with the NOS type they were for the time being included in the group of NOS lesions.

6. The value of segregating combination tumor types from their "pure" forms is apparent from the differences in significant associations between the two. This consideration also militates against the common practice of designating breast cancers only by their most malignant components. The true merit of this contention should also be determined by survival studies.

7. All 23 examples of Paget's disease were associated with a carcinoma of the underlying breast substance. Only 2 were regarded as being intraductal or noninvasive.

8. Cancers, exclusive of those with epidermal nipple involvement, that were regarded by light microscopy as being purely intraductal were deleted.

9. Adenocystic carcinoma is commonplace in breast cancers and represents a variation of tubule formation.

10. A simplified highly reproducible method of histologic grading of breast cancer based upon the presence of tubule formation and nuclear grade has been introduced. Approximately 70 percent of the cancers were considered as poorly differentiated (Grade 3) and only 2.5 percent as well differentiated or Grade 1.

11. Nuclear grade was associated with many of the same features noted with histologic grade. The reproducibility of nuclear grading was between 85 and 90 percent.

12. The nuclear as well as histologic grades appear to be predictable from an assessment of the type of intraductal component observed within the primary tumor.

13. The lack of microscopic circumscription was notably attendant with short-term treatment failure, as well as the presence of positive axillary nodes and lymphatic invasion.

14. The median size of 3.0 cm for tumors in this study is similar to that recorded for the period 1948-1968. Tumors 4.1 cm or larger were consistently associated with four or more positive axillary nodes, blood vessel and lymphatic invasion, multicentric cancers, and short-term treatment failures at all periods of observation.

15. A severe cell reaction to the tumor was associated with features suggesting a high degree of malignancy rather than "host resistance".

16.   No apparent biologically significant relationships with degree or type of stromal connective tissue response to the tumor were evident.

17.   Elastica content of breast cancers appears related to the degree of connective tissue, stromal response and age of the patients.

18.   Approximately half of the breast cancers contained some degree of mucin. The exclusive presence of PAS-positive mucin was observed in tumors with high histologic grade or malignancy, as well as the occurrence of a severe cell reaction and lymphatic invasion.

19.   Tumors containing calcium were significantly associated with glycogen, short-term treatment failure and elastica.

20.   Squamous metaplasia was apparently related to the occurrence of sinus histiocytosis of axillary nodes, as well as skin involvement and tumor necrosis.

21.   A marked intraductal component of the primary tumor was associated with features indicating the multifocal origin of breast cancer, particularly de novo remote multicentric cancers, as well as nipple involvement.

22.   Marked tumor necrosis was found to be associated with neoplasms of high histologic grade and short-term treatment failure.

23.   Noninvasive cancer in the vicinity of the primary tumor was associated with other features of multicentricity, as well as clinical and pathologic evidence of nodal metastases.

24.   Blood vessel invasion was encountered in only 4.7 percent of the cases, whereas lymphatic extension occurred in 33 percent and was regarded as questionable in another 22.7 percent.

25.   Perineural space invasion was associated with lymphatic invasion, positive nodes and short-term treatment failure.

26.   Undetected multicentric or de novo cancers were observed in quadrants of breast tissue remote from the dominant mass in 13.4 percent of the cases. In 9.1 percent they were of the noninvasive type (lobular carcinoma in situ and/or

Tormey, Fisher, Tranum and Perez-Tamayo

intraductal carcinoma) and in 4.3 percent they were of the invasive NOS type.

27. Approximately three-fourths of the cases exhibited some degree of sinus histiocytosis of axillary nodes, but this was marked in only 8.5 percent. Its absence was associated with the presence of four or more nodal metastases.

28. Axillae clinically assessed to be positive for nodal metas-tases failed to reveal such involvement pathologically in 24 percent of the patients. The incidence of positive nodal metastases in patients whose axillae were regarded as clinically negative was 39 percent. The overall error in clinical assessment of the axillary status was 32 percent.

29. Younger patients (20-44 years) were associated significantly with tumors of high-grade malignancy. This finding may have been influenced by the greater frequency of medullary cancers in this age group.

TABLE 4
Pathologic Associations with Short-Term Treatment Failure

Pathologically Positive Axillary Nodes

Location: Tumor In Subareolar Area

Tumor Size: 6.1+ CM / 5.1-6.0 / 4.1-5.0 / 3.1-4.0 / 2.1-3.0 / 1.1-2.0 / 0-1.0

Noncircumscribed Tumor (Macro And Microscopic)

Histologic Type: NOS; NOS + Lobular / NOS + Tubular; Medullary; Lobular Invasive; NOS + Mucinous / NOS + Papillary; NOS + Lobular + Tubular / Mucinous; Tubular

Nuclear Grade: 1 / 2 / 3

Histologic Grade: 3 / 2 / 1

Tumor Necrosis

Lymphatic Invasion

Blood Vessel Invasion

Cell Reaction To Tumor

Mucin: Absent/Slight / Moderate / Marked

Intraductal Component Of Cancer: COMEDO / Solid Or Papillary / Adenocystic Or Combinations

Microscopic Involvement Of Skin Overlying Tumor

Nipple Involvement

Capsulary Extension Of Nodal Metastases

Intralymphatic Extension In Quadrants Remote From Primary Tumor

30.   Patients of the black or other nonwhite races had a greater
      likelihood that their tumors were of the medullary type with
      its attendant features.

When 1,665 patients had entered the study and the average period of
followup was 3 years the relationship of pathologic discriminants to the
spread of breast cancer was further evaluated.[13] These are presented
in Table 4.

It is noteworthy some of the associations delineated in the earlier
analysis[12] are no longer present with the longer followup and that new
associations have been added.

RELATION OF DURATION OF SYMPTOM TO TREATMENT FAILURE

The conventional view regarding the natural history of breast cancer
implies that the primary tumor grows with time, subsequently spreads
to regional lymph nodes and then disseminates systemically. Yet all
previous studies have failed to disclose any consistent relationship
between the duration of symptoms and survival.

Of a Cooperative Group trial on 1,539 patients, durations of symptoms
exceeding nine months were not correlated with a greater average
monthly failure rate.[14] This is despite the relationship of duration of
symptoms with ominous prognostic indications such as tumor size,
nipple and skin involvement. This information reflects the heterogeneity of tumor characteristics and possibly the importance of host-
tumor relationships in the natural history of patients with breast
cancer. Interestingly, blacks had longer periods of symptoms than
whites.

FACTORS INFLUENCING PROGNOSIS AFTER RECURRENCE

In the patients with recurrent breast cancer there are several biological
characteristics of tumor involvement and host adaptability that influence the probability of success and thereby survival with subsequent
therapy. An extensive indepth analysis was conducted in 281 patients
entered in a Cooperative Group trial of chemotherapy for recurrent
disease.   The primary purpose of the analysis was to identify the
pretreatment characteristics ("prognostic factors" or "covariates") that
are most closely related to the initial response to chemotherapy. A
total of 22 covariates were considered and of these race was eliminated
because the very poor responses of blacks (12 of 39, 31 percent,
compared to 151 of 242, 62 percent for whites) could not be explained
by association with other covariates. Of the 21 remaining covariates,

TABLE 5
Covariates And Their Influence On Response

Not Significant	Inconsistent Effect	Consistent Effect
Menopausal Status	Duration of Metastatic	Disease-free Interval
Total Duration of Disease	Disease	Nodal Metastases
Oophorectomy Previously	Bone Involvement	Performance
Type of Mastectomy	Age	Number of Metastatic
Postoperative Radiation		Sites
Histology		Liver Involvement
Lung Involvement		SGOT Elevation
Pleural Involvement		
Skin Involvement		
Other Sites		
Hemoglobin		
Alkaline Phosphatase		

15 were not associated with response at a significance level of 0.05 or less. Six of the other nine covariates were consistent (Table 5). Longer disease-free intervals were associated with higher proportions of response as were node involvement (nonaxillary) and good performance status. Involvement of several sites, liver metastases and elevated SGOT levels led to poor results. Ambulatory patients with long disease-free intervals and no liver involvement had the best prognosis. The inconsistent influence of age was also found in another study,[16] but skin involvement did respond well to chemotherapy.

In a study of 60 patients the good initial performance status and long disease-free interval were also associated with longer survival.[17] Liver metastases had a poor prognosis, while no definitive influence was observed with the number of sites involved with metastatic disease.

MANAGEMENT OF STAGE I AND II DISEASE

From 1956 to the close of 1978 the management of breast cancer patients has been influenced significantly by the impact of clinical research performed by Cooperative Groups. Prior to the introduction of the multiinstitutional concept, trials in breast cancer were limited to institutional series of cases using historical controls or to relatively small trials of randomized cases. The large numbers of patients available for randomized controlled trials in the Group studies has enabled more definitive testing of therapeutic approaches as well as the demonstration of a multitude of variables which affect prognosis.

Cooperative Groups continue to search for early detection and recognition of appropriate clinical stages in patients with breast carcinoma which would benefit most from treatment by single or multiple modalities having the least morbidity and highest possible efficiency for the various patient subsets. Radical mastectomy had become the standard procedure indicated for a relatively small and select group of patients at an early clinical stage in the late 1800's and early 1900's. Unfortunately, this subset was not large enough to affect the overall survival of the group as a whole. Less-than-radical mastectomy plus radiation appeared to be "equivalent" to radical mastectomy. Super-radical or extended surgery appeared to be beneficial in a very small subset of patients. As such, it was difficult to justify due to its lack of impact on the overall group. Even with the introduction of new diagnostic methods such as mammography and radionuclide scans, the many accumulated statistical reports revealed no further improvement in survival into the 1970's. Accountable was the previously unrecognized

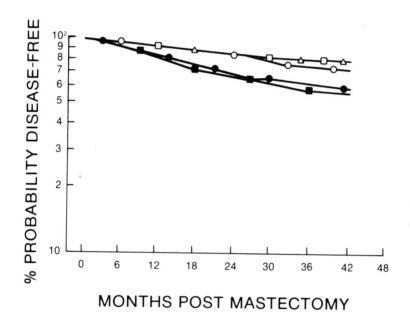

			No. Patients at Risk			
			Total	1 Yr	2 Yr	3 Yr
(A)	△	C NEG RADICAL MX	354	309	247	132
(B)	□	C NEG TOTAL MX + RAD	282	259	203	105
(C)	○	C NEG TOTAL MX	344	306	244	116
(D)	●	C POS RADICAL MX	277	230	167	83
(E)	■	C POS TOTAL MX + RAD	224	175	123	50

P-VALUE: A vs B vs C-NS
D vs E   -NS

NSABP PROTOCOL #4

Fig. 3. Probability (percent) of survival without disease

frequent dissemination of breast cancer and/or the inability of standard surgery or radiation to prevent distant metastases at significant rates in the breast cancer patient group at large.[18]

Following the demonstration that standard postoperative radiotherapy did not impart a major treatment benefit,[19] a randomized clinical trial began to compare the worth of alternative treatments with radical mastectomy. Radical mastectomy, total mastectomy combined with standard radiation and total mastectomy alone, produced equivalent results in breast cancer patients with clinically negative axillary nodes (Fig. 3).[20] When the axillary nodes were clinically positive (clinical Stage II), total mastectomy plus radiation, or radical mastectomy alone produced results equivalent to standard radical mastectomy. Published survivals were similar, and distant metastases developed at no different rate. With radiation therapy, regional and local recurrences were less frequent, but this factor did not lead to improved survivals. Again, this was taken as evidence of the disseminated nature of Stage II disease. This study led to the important discovery that leaving behind positive axillary nodes did not lead to a higher incidence of treatment failures or distant metastases during an average period of followup of 36 months. This provides reinforcement for the view that positive axillary lymphnodes are not the predecessor of distant tumor spread but are a manifestation of disseminated disease.

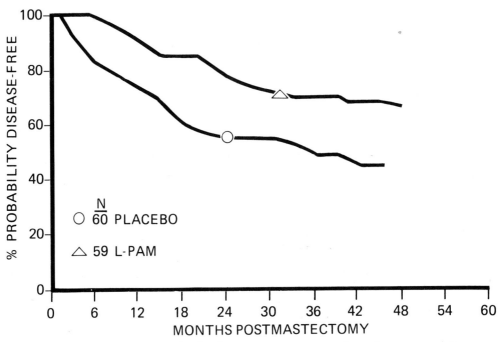

Fig. 4. Disease-free survival after mastectomy of patients age 49 or younger

A randomized study was simultaneously conducted for women with intact ovaries, who were less than 50 years of age.[21] The 5-year survival was 54 percent for patients who had a prophylactic oophorectomy for breast carcinoma, 57 percent for a group which received a placebo and 56 percent for patients who, beginning with the day of operation, received a total of 0.8 mg per kg triethylenethiophosphoramide (TSPA) over 3 days. Since the recurrence rates were also not statistically significantly different, this study failed to substantiate any worth of prophylactic oophorectomy.

An important new direction to the management of Stage II disease was given in 1972 when a large prospective, randomized, multiinstitutional, cooperative trial was begun to evaluate the efficacy of prolonged L-phenylalanine mustard (L-PAM) administration following operation in lengthening the disease-free interval. An update of the results of this study, when the duration on protocol ranged between 46 and 76 months, indicate a significant difference in disease-free survival in favor of patients receiving L-PAM.[22] This difference is limited to an important subset of patients 49 years or younger (Fig. 4) especially those with only 1 to 3 positive lymph nodes. Survival was 87 percent for L-PAM and 56 percent for placebo patients (p < .005). No such difference was found for the older patients.

The L-PAM has been compared with combinations of chemotherapeutic agents by three cooperative groups and all found the combinations to be superior. L-PAM + 5-Fluorouracil (5-FU) appears thus far to show

TABLE 6
Rates of Recurrence in Subsets of Patients With Stage II Breast Cancer

Comparisons		L-PAM	CMFVP
All Patients		70/189 = 37%	29/177 = 16%
Premenopausal		31/78 = 40%	11/68 = 16%
Postmenopausal		39/109 = 36%	18/106 = 17%
1-3	Lymph Nodes	17/71 = 24%	5/72 = 5%
$\geq$4	Lymph Nodes	53/118 = 45%	24/102 = 24%
1-3	Lymph Nodes		
	Premenopausal	7/28 = 25%	2/25 = 8%
	Postmenopausal	10/43 = 23%	3/47 = 6%
$\geq$4	Lymph Nodes		
	Premenopausal	24/50 = 48%	9/43 = 21%
	Postmenopausal	29/66 = 44%	15/58 = 26%

greater benefit for the patients 50 years and older.[23]   In a study comparing L-PAM with a combination of cyclophosphamide (C), metho-trexate (M), 5-FU and vincristine (V) the combination resulted in a superior disease-free interval (DFI) for patients 50 years or older.[24]

In another large study L-PAM was compared to CMF-V to which prednisone was added (CMFVP).[25]   The results thus far show marked superiority of the 5-drug combination over that of L-PAM (Table 6, Fig. 5).   Prior reports of adjuvant chemotherapy in Stage II breast cancer concluded that such chemotherapy was only beneficial for the younger or premenopausal women. The important finding in the L-PAM versus CMFVP study is that the menopausal status does not influence the rate of recurrence with L-PAM or with CMFVP overall. These observations are more in line with the studies which show that in Stage III disease the chemotherapeutic regimens do equally well in the younger as in the older patients. They also are of importance for the design of future studies.

Many other investigations continue combining several drugs, radiation, hormonal agents such as tamoxifen and immunostimulating agents such

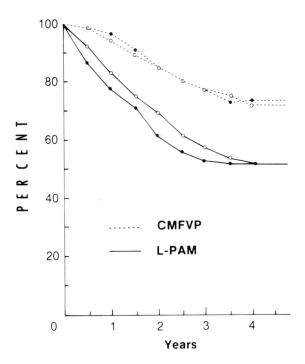

Closed Circles - Premenopausal
Open Circles   - Postmenopausal

Fig. 5. Disease-free survival with two adjuvant chemotherapies

as MER and C parvum.[26-30] Especially important is the search for the optimum number and best combination of chemotherapeutic agents, the comparisons of short-term versus long-term treatment and continuous versus cyclic courses. Since chemotherapy is often accompanied by acute or subacute toxicity, which could possibly lead to delayed effects, it is essential for Cooperative Groups to investigate many aspects of combined modality therapy. Thoughts along these lines were well expressed by Fisher in the form of eleven questions[31](Table 7).

Due to the impact of the success of multiinstitutional multimodality trials, there has been a resurgence of interest in the use of modern postoperative and preoperative radiation therapy for purposes of increasing local-regional control, disease-free interval, and survival, while preserving breast tissue. Radiosensitizers, particle radiation, dose fractionation, hyperthermia, and irradiation-chemotherapy combinations are being studied in all clinical stages, but in particular in Stage III breast cancer patients--and even Stage IV.

TABLE 7
Questions Raised by the Preliminary Results of Adjuvant
Therapy Trials

---

1.   Will there be sustained differences in disease-free rates?
2.   Will they be manifested in long-term survival rates?
3.   Will undesirable sequellae such as second neoplasms occur?
4.   Will there be a predilection for recurrences at certain sites?
5.   Will recurrences be more difficult to treat effectively?
6.   Does adjuvant therapy prolong the disease-free state following operation but shorten survival following recurrence so that there is little or no total survival benefit?
7.   How long should such therapy be given?
8.   Is the sequencing of drugs more meritorious than the repetitive use of the same agent(s)?
9.   Will immunostimulating agents lead to greater tolerance to chemotherapy by the host?
10.   Will such agents enhance host immune response and when employed with chemotherapy result in an additive or synergistic effect?
11.   How relevant is information obtained from patients with advanced disease to those with minimal disease after operation?
      a.   Response of overt mass predictive of sensitivity of cells in micrometastases?
      b.   Are drugs which are marginally or not effective in advanced cancers also ineffective following removal of a primary?

The days of standard radical mastectomy for breast cancer patients as the single method of treatment appear to be over. The impact of cooperative clinical research in all fields is changing the treatment of breast cancer. Survival has improved, as shown by group studies. The old plateau of previous decades appears to have been broken.

Research thought appears to be proceeding along the following lines of speculation at present:

1)   Substituting for radical mastectomy a less radical procedure that can be as little as excisional biopsy if supplemented by irradiation and/or chemotherapy in the earlier stages.

2)   In less early Stage I and Stage II patients, investigating the relative effectiveness of less-than-radical mastectomy (total mastectomy? segmental mastectomy?) plus radiation therapy with or without radiosensitizers, with or without chemotherapy, with or without immunostimulators.

3)   For Stages II, III, and IV, seeking increased effectiveness with radiation therapy and chemotherapy and/or hormone manipulation (with the assistance of hormone-dependence determination by estrogen receptor or similar tests) and/or immunostimulation.

Further progress in chemotherapy may produce a tolerable regime breaking the future plateau of success which might be anticipated in the absence of progress in radiation therapy or other fields of medicine. Radiosensitizers, particle radiation, and differing fractionation schedules appear promising. Disseminated disease, however, remains today the single most serious obstacle to the successful treatment of breast cancer patients in all clinical stages. Systemic therapy modalities must be further developed to control the dissemination of disease with safe and tolerable consequences before the value of radiation therapy--or of surgery, for that matter--is proportionately reduced. Early detection and prevention, when that becomes an ideal reality, will reduce the indication for all existing modalities.

TREATMENT OF ADVANCED BREAST CANCER

Of the 90,000 new cases of breast cancer that develop yearly, it is expected that 80 percent will ultimately die of their disease. The potential impact of successful systemic therapy is therefore immense. Presently, systemic therapy for advanced disease is looked on as palliative rather than curative. Nevertheless, treatment concepts

TABLE 8
Response Rates of the Most Effective Drugs

DRUG	RESPONSE %	DRUG	RESPONSE %
Adriamycin	38*	5-FU	22
	31	5-FUDR	22
Cyclophosphamide	27	Melphalan	19
Mitomycin-C	24	Thiotepa	17
Methotrexate	23	Vincristine	14

* Patients with no prior chemotherapy

derived for advanced disease are currently being employed in an attempt to provide cure of "operable" disease.

The development of Cooperative Groups engendered the fundamental concept of comparing one treatment with another in a prospective manner. This was made possible by multiple contributors pooling data under a uniform protocol within shortened time frames of patient accrual. Such studies not only identified schemes of administration and rates of response and toxicities that the practicing physician could expect when using these agents in the treatment of metastatic breast cancer, but also provided a firm basis for drug selection.

SINGLE DRUG THERAPY

Early studies of the Cooperative Groups involved hormone manipulation for the treatment of advanced breast cancer. The initial limited supply of single chemotherapeutic drugs has now increased considerably. Response rates of 15 to 35 percent are common but of relatively short duration[32-34](Table 8).

Due to the development of more successful combinations of chemo- therapeutic agents single drugs are used with less frequency for the initial treatment of advanced disease. New agents that showed promise in initial clinical trials are soon incorporated into combinations for treatment. Of the many newer agents that have been tested thus far, none have shown greater activity than that of drugs in current usage.

COMBINATION CHEMOTHERAPY

Following the introduction of combination chemotherapy, four questions arose in breast cancer: 1) Which are the critical constituents of each combination? 2) Are the combinations better than single drugs? 3) Is it better to give the drugs simultaneously or sequentially? 4) Are continuous courses of combinations better than intermittent courses?

The first popular combination of cyclophosphamide, methotrexate, 5-Fluorouracil, vincristine, and prednisone (CMFVP), led to clinical trials that suggested that each drug contributes to the rate or length of response.[35,36] In other combinations in which one or more drugs were added to a fixed dose of adriamycin, 40 mg/M^2, the rate and length of remission as well as the median survival were the same though there was an arithmetic advantage to the length of remission as more drugs were added[37](Table 9).

The strategy of drug administration appears to be critical to the success that has been achieved with chemotherapy in the hematologic malignancies. The same questions, of single versus combination therapy, and of simultaneous or sequential drug administration, have been approached in breast cancer.

Reports of comparison between CMFVP and adriamycin, and between CMF and melphalan, favor the multiple drug regimens in the rate and duration of remission (Table 10). One Cooperative Oncology Group selected the CMFVP regimen to test the relative value of simultaneous or sequential administration in advanced breast cancer.[40] The simultaneous combination had a higher rate of response, 46 percent versus 18 percent, and a longer median survival, 48 weeks versus 24 weeks.

TABLE 9
Adding Drugs to Fixed Dose of Adriamycin

REGIMEN	RESPONSE CR+PR %	MEDIAN RESPONSE DURATION (WKS)	MEDIAN SURVIVAL (WKS)
AF	42	22	61
AFC	43	33	66
AFCM	49	35	65

A = Adriamycin; F = 5-Fluorouracil; C = Cyclophosphamide; M = Methotrexate

TABLE 10
Single Drugs Versus Combination in Advanced Disease

REGIMEN	RESPONSE CR+PR %	MEDIAN DURATION OF RESPONSE	REFERENCE
CMFVP	54	9 months	38
Adriamycin	38	5 months	
CMF	53	6 months	39
Melphalan	20	3 months	

Because of the innumerable combinations and potential methods of applying individual drugs in sequence, it is difficult to conclude that combination treatment will always be superior to sequential use of drugs. Even so the concept of combination therapy has thus far proven to be superior in Cooperative Group trials.

Frequently used regimens and their response rates are shown in Table 11.

Selecting the best combination of drugs for the treatment of breast cancer is fraught with hazards. Variability in determining what constitutes a response in patients with primarily bone or pleural

TABLE 11
Combination Chemotherapy in Advanced Disease

REGIMEN	RESPONSE CR+PR %	MEDIAN DURATION OF RESPONSE (WKS)	MEDIAN DURATION OF SURVIVAL (WKS)	REFERENCE
AC	42	37	70*	37
AFC	45	42	70*	37
A + CMFVP	44	39	70*	37
CMFVP	59	43	60	38
CMFP	59	34	56*	41
AV	53	30	56*	41
CMF	49	21	56*	41

A = Adriamycin; C = Cyclophosphamide; F = 5-Fluorouracil;
M = Methotrexate; V = Vincristine; P = Prednisone
* = Median of entire study.

metastasis partially explains the wide difference in response rates even when comparing the same drugs. The initial studies recorded responses of 78 percent for adriamycin plus cyclophosphamide and adriamycin, 5-Fluorouracil and cyclophosphamide, whereas the same regimens tested in a groupwide study had response rates of 42 and 45 percent, respectively.[37] Survival was similar in both studies, suggesting similar benefits from chemotherapy but differences in evaluating response.

With the development of adriamycin Phase II studies promptly demonstrated its effectiveness in breast cancer.[42] However, response duration was relatively short, prompting the addition of conventional drugs to adriamycin in an attempt to increase the rate of response as well as prolong the duration.[37, 38, 43]

A regimen with adriamycin was designed to take advantage of adriamycin's known rapid onset of action plus using CMFVP in full doses. In this latter regimen it was observed that three cycles of adriamycin followed by CMFVP was not better than AFC or AC (Fig. 6).[37]

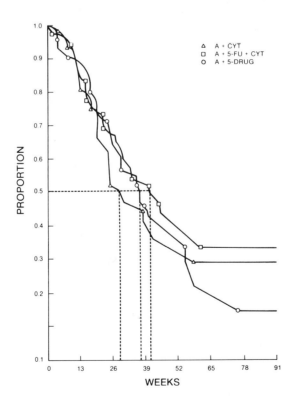

Fig. 6. Length of response by treatment

In a prospective trial of cyclophosphamide, adriamycin and 5-Fluorouracil (CAF) versus CMFVP on an intermittent schedule, the CAF combination was found to be superior in rate of response, 64 percent and 37 percent as well as duration of response, 32 weeks and 17 weeks, respectively. This important study showed the superiority of an intermittent combination containing adriamcyin over one which omitted it. However, the intermittent CMFVP regimen chosen for the above study may not be the most effective schema for using these five drugs.[38]

Presently, one can anticipate a response rate of approximately 50 percent or greater with a median duration of 37 weeks and a median survival of 70 weeks using either AC, CAF, CAFVP, or adriamycin followed by CMFVP. With the apparent plateau that has been reached in the treatment of advanced breast cancer, studies have been developed to test the value of adding immunotherapy to chemotherapy, using noncross-resistant combinations, and combining hormones with chemotherapy. Immunotherapy is presently being evaluated in organized trials after some favorable results with BCG and levamisole had been reported in nonrandomized studies. At present it is much too early to even assume that immunotherapy can have a beneficial effect.

HORMONAL MANAGEMENT

At one time in the history of the treatment of breast cancer, exogenous hormones and castration were primary treatments of advanced disease. Clinical studies repeatedly demonstrated that approximately one-fourth of premenopausal patients with metastatic disease would respond to castration and a lesser percent to androgens.[45] A similar number of postmenopausal patients would respond to estrogens or androgens. Combining hormone manipulation with cytotoxic chemotherapy appears to be additive in selected studies[46] but was indiscriminate in that there was no basis for selecting which patients should receive hormone treatment. With the discovery of estrogen binding properties of the tumors of patients with breast cancer there developed some predictive logic for selecting those patients to treat with hormone manipulation.

The presence of estrogen receptors in the cytoplasm of breast cancer cells and response to hormone manipulation correlate in 60 to 70 percent of patients so treated. An even better correlation (90+ percent) exists between the absence of estrogen receptors and failure to respond to hormone manipulation.[47] With the development of the family of antiestrogens, exogenous hormone therapy could be carried out without some of the unpleasant side effects of androgens and high dose estrogens. Tamoxifen,[47] has become the most popular anti-estrogen drug for clinical use.

With the high level of predictability of response to hormone therapy depending upon estrogen receptor (ER) status, it has been recommended that patients with breast cancer have their primary tumor charac-terized as ER+ or ER-. Approximately 60 percent of breast cancers will bind radioactive estradiol and 60 percent of the estrogen receptor positive tumors will improve with hormone therapy. Premenopausal patients with metastatic breast cancer comprise the group most likely to have their treatment altered depending upon estrogen receptor affinity. Castration, antiestrogen, androgens and adrenalectomy or hypophysectomy are all potential treatment modalities if the tumor is ER+, whereas none would be considered as a sole therapy if there were no estrogen binding activity. The quantitative level of estrogen binding activity also appears to correlate with the likelihood of responding to hormone manipulation.

Tamoxifen is well tolerated with minimal side effects. Hot flashes and occasional mild leukopenia and thrombocytopenia have been described but are tolerable and usually transient.[47] As with all exogenous hormone therapy hypercalcemia and generalized bone pain can be precipitated with tamoxifen. This requires careful attention and interruption of therapy. This hypercalcemic response may occur in ER positive tumors and there is evidence that the tumors will in some cases later respond to continued tamoxifen if the acute phase is successfully managed.

Future treatment will involve hormone manipulation, both surgical and exogenous hormone, added to cytotoxic chemotherapy primarily in estrogen receptor positive patients. Just as importantly, the time and morbidity of such treatment will be avoided in estrogen receptor negative patients with advanced disease.

SUMMARY AND PROSPECTUS

In the not too distant past a standard operation followed by standard radiotherapy was the uniform treatment for primary breast cancer. Recurrence in premenopausal patients was treated with castration and in the postmenopausal patients with hormones. Because of the ability of Cooperative Groups to compare one treatment against another, ask biological questions that can be tested, and follow-up on promising new leads with clinical trials, there is reason to expect that treatment should be tailored to fit the individual patient with breast cancer. Determining the type of surgery, choosing patients for a combined modality approach with systemic therapy, and selecting effective chemotherapeutic regimens is possible because of the prospective clinical trials that have been completed. Nevertheless, systemic therapy for both early and advanced disease will remain in a continuous state of flux until a method of cure is found.

The addition of multiple drugs in an aggressive manner has resulted in a higher rate of remission in advanced disease and a median survival of over one year. Cure for metastatic disease still eludes the oncologist. One of the most important results of the data coming from Cooperative Groups is that breast cancer is a treatable disease no matter what the stage at first diagnosis. Further investigation in an organized manner will continue to identify best treatments, and it is hoped that cure will be attainable.

Multiinstitutional Cooperative Group clinical trials have provided a critical vehicle for increasing our knowledge about breast cancer and simultaneously improving the quality of delivery of therapy. These trials have helped foster the development of experienced, critical investigators across the country who in turn pool their intellectual and clinical capabilities, thus providing the resources necessary to answer biologically relevant problems in breast cancer.

We can now divide the patient population into a wide variety of prognostic subsets. This in turn is permitting the development of lesser therapeutic procedures for good-risk patients and more intensive procedures for poor-risk patients. The capability to divide and treat the patient population in this manner has been facilitated by the orderly and efficient cooperation of groups from many institutions which dedicate their patient, laboratory, and clinical resources to clinical trials.

The advances achieved through the multiinstitutional clinical trials approach have formed a shifting baseline for the development of still newer biological concepts and therapies. The consequent development of combined modality approaches has been geared to increasing the number of patients with the best life-quality and survivorship characteristics possible.

As we approach the goal of cure with the fewest possible side effects, the answers become much more difficult to obtain. Ever increasing numbers of patients, time, and labor are required to detect smaller and smaller differences. As a result, the resources available to multiple institutions working cooperatively assume increasing critical importance for the detection of those differences, and for the achievement of our goals.

REFERENCES

1. Fisher B, Ravdin RG, Ausman RK, Slack NH, Moore GE, Noer RJ, and Cooperating Investigators: Surgical adjuvant chemotherapy in cancer of the breast: Results of a decade of cooperative investigation. Ann Surg 168:337-356, 1968.
2. Fisher B, Slack NH, Ausman RK, Bross IDJ: Location of breast carcinoma and prognosis. Surg Gynecol Obstet 129:705-716, 1969.
3. Fisher B, Slack NH, Bross IDJ, and Cooperating Investigators: Cancer of the breast: Size of neoplasm and prognosis. Cancer 24:1071-1080, 1969.
4. Fisher B, Slack N, Katrych D, Wolmark N: Ten-year follow-up results of patients with carcinoma of the breast in a cooperative clinical trial evaluating surgical adjuvant chemotherapy. Surg Gynecol Obstet 140:528-534, 1975.
5. Fisher B, Slack NH: Number of lymph nodes examined and the prognosis of breast carcinoma. Surg Gynecol Obstet 131:79-88, 1970.
6. Slack NH, Bross IDJ, Nemoto T, Fisher B: Experiences with bilateral primary carcinoma of the breast. Surg Gynecol Obstet 136:433-440, 1973.
7. Fisher ER, Gregorio R, Redmond C, Vellios F, Sommers SC, Fisher B: Pathologic findings from the National Surgical Adjuvant Breast Project (Protocol No. 4) I. Observations concerning the multicentricity of mammary cancer. Cancer 35:247-254, 1975.
8. Fisher ER, Gregorio R, Redmond C, Dekker A, Fisher B: Pathologic findings from the National Surgical Adjuvant Breast Project (Protocol No. 4) II. The significance of regional node histology other than sinus histiocytosis in invasive mammary cancer. Am J Clin Path 65:21-30, 1976.
9. Fisher ER, Gregorio RM, Redmond C, Kim WS, Fisher B: Pathologic findings from the National Surgical Adjuvant Breast Project (Protocol No. 4) III. The significance of extranodal extension of axillary metastases. Am J Clin Path 65:439-444, 1976.
10. Fisher ER, Palekar A, Rockette H, Redmond C, Fisher B: Pathologic findings from the National Surgical Adjuvant Breast Project (Protocol No. 4) V. Significance of axillary micro- and macrometastases. Cancer 42:2032-2038, 1978.
11. Fisher ER, Swamidoss S, Lee CH, Rockette H, Redmond C, Fisher B: Detection and significance of occult axillary node metastases in patients with invasive breast cancer. Cancer 42:2025-2031, 1978.
12. Fisher ER, Gregorio RM, Fisher B, and other cooperating investigators: The pathology of invasive breast cancer: A syllabus derived from findings of the National Surgical Adjuvant Breast Project (Protocol No. 4). Cancer 36:1-85, 1975.
13. Fisher ER, Fisher B: Relationship of pathologic and some clinical discriminants to the spread of breast cancer. Int J Rad Oncol Biol Phys 2:747-750, 1977.
14. Fisher ER, Redmond C, Fisher B: A perspective concerning the relation of duration of symptoms to treatment failure in patients with breast cancer. Cancer 40:3160-3167, 1977.
15. George SL, Hoogstraten B: Prognostic factors in the initial response to therapy by patients with advanced breast cancer. J Natl Cancer Inst 60:731-736, 1978.
16. Smalley RV: Prognostic factors indicating likelihood of response to combination chemotherapy (CT) in patients with metastatic breast carcinoma. ASCO, 17:285, 1976.
17. Taylor SG, Pocock SJ, Shnider BI, Colsky J, Hall TC: Clinical studies of 5-Fluorouracil + Premerin in the treatment of breast cancer. Med Ped Oncol 1:113-121, 1975.
18. Tormey DC, Carbone PP: Changing concepts in the therapy of breast cancer. Methods in Cancer Research 13:1-29, 1976.
19. Fisher B, Slack NH, Cavanaugh PJ, Gardner B, Ravdin RG: Postoperative radiotherapy in the treatment of breast cancer. Ann Surg 172:711-732, 1970.
20. Fisher B, Montague E, Redmond C, and other cooperating investigators: Comparison of radical mastectomy with alternative treatments for primary breast cancer. Cancer 39:2827-2839, 1977.
21. Ravdin RG, Lewison EF, Slack NH, Dao TL, Gardner B, State D, and Fisher B: Results of a clinical trial concerning the worth of prophylactic oophorectomy for breast carcinoma. Surg Gynecol Obstet 131:1055-1064, 1970.
22. Fisher B, Glass A, Redmond C, Fisher ER, and other cooperating investigators: L-Phenylalanine mustard (L-PAM) in the management of primary breast cancer. Cancer 39:2883-2903, 1977.
23. National Surgical Adjuvant Project for Breast and Bowel Cancers. Minutes, March, 1979.
24. Davis HL, Metter GE, Ramirez G, Grage TB, Cornell G, Fletcher W, Moss S, Multhauf P: An adjuvant trial of L-PAM versus CMF-V following mastectomy for operable breast cancer. ASCO 20:358, 1979.
25. Rivkin S, Glucksberg H, Rasmussen S: Adjuvant chemotherapy in Stage II breast cancer. ASCO 20:353, 1979.
26. Tormey D, Falkson G, Weiss R, Perloff M, Glidewell O, Holland JF: Postoperative chemotherapy with/without immunotherapy for mammary carcinoma. Adjuvant Therapy of Cancer II SE Jones and S Salmon, Eds. Grune and Stratton, Inc. pp.253-260, 1979.
27. Primary Breast Cancer Therapy Group: Comparison of chemotherapy with L-PAM/5-FU versus L-PAM/5-FU/MTX for breast cancer with one or more positive axillary nodes, Activated May, 1976.
28. Primary Breast Cancer Therapy Group: L-PAM/5-FU/tamoxifen chemotherapy for surgically "curable" breast carcinoma with one or more positive axillary nodes, Activated March, 1976.
29. Primary Breast Cancer Therapy Group: Chemotherapy with L-PAM/5-FU and immunotherapy with C parvum for new breast carcinoma with positive axillary nodes, Activated April, 1976.
30. Southeastern Oncology Group: Phase III randomized adjuvant chemotherapy with CTX/MTX/5-FU plus radiation versus short or long-term chemotherapy for breast carcinoma, Activated Sept., 1976.
31. Fisher B: Biological and clinical considerations regarding the use of surgery and chemotherapy in the treatment of primary breast cancer. Cancer 40:574-587, 1977.

32. Segaloff A: Investigations in breast carcinoma. National Cancer Institute Monograph No. 3:257-276, 1960.
33. Tormey D, Carbone P, Band P: Breast cancer survival in single and combination chemotherapy since 1968. AACR 18:64, 1977.
34. Hoogstraten B, Fabian C: A reappraisal of single drugs in advanced breast cancer. Cancer Clin Trials 2:101-109, 1979.
35. Ramirez G, Klotz J, Strawitz JG, Wilson WL, Cornell GN, Madden RE, Minton JP: Combination chemotherapy in breast cancer. Oncology 32:101-108, 1975.
36. Leone LA, Rege V: Treatment of metastatic, recurrent or inoperable carcinoma. AACR 14:125, 1973.
37. Tranum B, Hoogstraten B, Kennedy A, Vaughn C, Samal B, Thigpen T, Rivkin S, Smith F, Palmer RL, Costanzi J, Tucker W, Wilson H, Maloney TR: Adriamycin in combination for the treatment of breast cancer. Cancer 41:2078-2083, 1978.
38. Hoogstraten B, George SL, Samal B, Rivkin SE, Costanzi JJ, Bonnet JD, Thigpen T, Braine H: Combination chemotherapy and adriamycin in patients with advanced breast cancer. A Southwest Oncology Group study. Cancer 38:13-20, 1976.
39. Canellos GP, Pocock SJ, Taylor SG, Sears ME, Klassen DJ, Band PR: Combination chemotherapy for metastatic breast carcinoma: Prospective comparison of multiple drug therapy with L-phenylalanine mustard. Cancer 38:1882-1886, 1976.
40. Smalley RV, Murphy S, Huguley CM, Bartolucci AA: Combination versus sequential 5-drug chemotherapy in metastatic carcinoma of the breast. Cancer Research 36:3911-3916, 1976.
41. Carbone PP, Bauer M, Band P, Tormey D: Chemotherapy of disseminated breast cancer: Current status and prospects. Cancer 39:2916-2922, 1977.
42. Hoogstraten B: Adriamycin in the treatment of advanced breast cancer. Studies by the Southwest Oncology Group. Cancer Treat Rep 6:329-334, 1975.
43. Tormey D, Leone L, Perloff M, Bloomfield C: Evaluation of intermittent versus continuous and of adriamycin versus methotrexate 5-drug chemotherapy regimens for breast cancer. ASCO 19:320, 1978.
44. Smalley RV, Carpenter J, Bartolucci A, Vogel C, Krauss S: A comparison of cyclophosphamide, adriamycin, 5-Fluorouracil and cyclophosphamide, methotrexate, 5-Fluorouracil, vincristine, prednisone (CMFVP) in patients with metastatic breast cancer. Cancer 40:625-632, 1977.
45. Hall TC, Dederick MM, Nevinny HB, Muench H: Prognostic value of response of patients with breast cancer to therapeutic castration. Cancer Treat Rep 31:47-48, 1967.
46. Falkson G, Falkson HC, Leone L, Glidewell O, Weinberg V, Holland JF: Improved remission rates and durations in premenopausal women with metastatic breast cancer. ASCO 19:416, 1978.
47. Lerner HJ, Band PR, Israel L, Leung BS: Phase II study of tamoxifen: Report of 74 patients with Stage IV breast cancer. Cancer Treat Rep 60:1431-1435, 1976.

8

Lung cancer

Julius Wolf, Robert Livingston, Carlos A. Perez, and Leo L. Stolbach

INTRODUCTION

Significant contributions have been made in the treatment of patients with lung cancer by the Cooperative Groups over the past twenty years. In addition to the substantial improvement in survival of patients with small cell carcinoma, gains in survival and palliation have been accomplished in patients with the other cell types. The need for continued and increased efforts in adjuvant therapy of patients undergoing resection continues to be critical because the surgical cure rate has not improved, due in large measure to the failure to find better methods of early case finding.

This chapter will not detail the very large number of Phase I and II studies in patients with pulmonary cancer completed by the Cooperative Groups listed in Table 1. Without these studies, the current multiple drug regimens and multimodality therapies could not have been developed. Many of the agents, because of interesting or exciting laboratory results, had to be tested clinically. Without a mechanism for large scale controlled clinical trials, some would still be untested or studied under unfavorable circumstances, thus producing misleading results. Perhaps some of the drugs now being used -- nitrosoureas, adriamycin, vinca alkaloids -- would still be awaiting trials in cancer of the lung.

At the beginning of the cooperative trials in the therapy of lung cancer, it became obvious that evaluation of therapy was impossible without

TABLE 1
Cooperative Groups Studying Pulmonary Cancer

   Cancer and Acute Leukemia Group B (CALGB)

   Eastern Cooperative Oncology Group (ECOG)

   Radiotherapy Oncology Group (RTOG)

   Southeastern Cancer Study Group (SECSG)

   Southwest Oncology Group (SWOG)

   Veteran Administration Lung Group (VALG)

   Veteran Administration Surgical Adjuvant Group (VASAG)

   Western Oncology Group (WOG)

knowledge of the natural history and the elucidation of determinants of
survival and of response to therapy. It was almost impossible to
evaluate the data in the literature because of the retrospective nature
of most studies and of the lack of uniformity of the histologic
classification. The solid basis for the advances in therapy was built on
the foundations provided by the Groups and by the histologic studies of
Dr. Yesner and his colleagues of the VA Lung Group. Since it was still
ethically possible in the early 1960's to conduct controlled trials using
an inert compound, the data from these trials provided invaluable
knowledge of the natural history of lung cancer.

Ten years ago small cell carcinoma of the lung was a disease in which
relatively few investigators were interested. Radiation therapy to the
primary lesion and the mediastinum was the usual treatment for about
one-third of patients who presented with regional involvement, and
cyclophosphamide was commonly employed for patients with disseminated disease. In both instances the therapeutic goal was palliation, and the prevailing attitude was pessimistic: long-term survival,
except for the rare patient who presented with a peripheral resectable
coin lesion, was rare. Today combination chemotherapy is the core of
most treatment programs for both limited and extensive disease. The
role of radiation therapy has been questioned, and its scope is in the
process of redefinition. Most important, various therapeutic programs
have been developed that can produce long-term disease-free survival
in a small fraction of patients, including some who have widespread
disease at the outset. The prevailing attitude has become optimistic,
with a belief among most of the workers in the field that small cell
carcinoma is potentially curable. The initial evidence that chemotherapy could prolong survival of patients with extensive small cell
carcinoma came from a study, which showed significant improvement in
survival for patients receiving cyclophosphamide versus supportive care

only.[1]   Other studies have shown that response rates and survival can be further improved by the use of active drug combinations, and Cooperative Group trials have provided the most convincing evidence of the value of elective whole-brain irradiation.   They have shown that chemotherapy plus irradiation produces results in limited disease which are superior to those achieved by radiation therapy alone.   Studies now ongoing in the Groups should define the role (if any) of radiation therapy to the primary tumor in limited disease; the studies already completed have shown it to be of no survival benefit in extensive disease.

Cooperative Group studies in small cell carcinoma have had a significant impact on the attitute of referring physicians, surgical and medical house staff, medical students and, most importantly, the patients themselves toward this form of lung cancer. Such changes in attitude are necessary if important advances are ever to be made available to the average patients.

PATHOLOGY

In 1959, the World Health Organization agreed to establish a tentative classification for lung cancer which was immediately put into use by the Pathology Panel of the VA Lung Group having received an advanced copy of the classification.   The Panel consisted of Drs. Raymond Yesner, Oscar Auerbach, and Bruno Gerstl.

TABLE 2
World Health Organization Lung Cancer Classifications

    1.   Squamous cell carcinomas
       (a) with abundant keratin
       (b) with intercellular bridges
       (c) without keratin or bridges

    2.   Small cell undifferentiated carcinomas
       (a) with oat cell structure
       (b) with polygonal cell structure

    3.   Adenocarcinomas
       (a) acinar
       (b) papillary
       (c) poorly differentiated

    4.   Large cell undifferentiated carcinomas

    5.   Combined carcinomas

TABLE 3
Distribution of Cell Types

	I	II	III	IV	V
Squamous Cell	49.1%	34.5	60	40	12
Small Cell	19.2	23.2	0	10	2
Adenocarcinoma	15.8	25.6	15	15	58
Large Cell Undifferentiated	15.5	14.7	25	35	
Combined	0.4	2.0			

> I   VALG patients - Inoperable - Biopsy
> II   VALG patients - Inoperable - Autopsy
> III VASAG Five-year survivors
> IV   VASAG Nonfive-year survivors
> V   Solitary nodule study patients

It was soon established that a high degree of unanimity could be reached by these three pathologists reading slides independently using the modified criteria of the World Health Organization. The classification used by the VA Lung Group and subsequently adopted by most of the Cooperative Groups and others studying lung cancer therapy in this country is listed in Table 2. [2-5]

Distribution of cell types in over 10,000 specimens studied is shown in Table 3. Column I lists the cell type distribution found in the patients who were inoperable when first seen. Column II lists the distribution of the cell types as diagnosed from autopsy material in a subset of the same patients previously diagnosed by biopsy. There is a tendency to underread adenocarcinoma cell type in biopsies and diagnose the biopsy material as squamous cell. In operable patients, the predominant cell type is squamous cell, especially in those who survive five years. In the patients with solitary nodules, the predominant cell type is adeno-carcinoma.[6]

It soon became clear that there were major difficulties in the use of the classification because nearly all cancers showed varying degrees of differentiation from field to field and transitions from group to group did occur. Examination of 10,000 biopsies had yielded about 200 examples of combined tumors showing transitions between major categories, of which the commonest combination was differentiated squamous and mucin producing adenocarcinoma. Numerous examples also existed of transitions between small cell and squamous carcinoma, between small cell and adenocarcinoma, and even a few showing all three major categories in the same field. Careful examination also showed that tumor transitions commonly exist between small cell carcinoma of the oat cell type and of the polygonal type, between polygonal type and undifferentiated large cell carcinoma, between large cell and poorly differentiated squamous carcinoma, between undifferentiated large cell and poorly differentiated adenocarcinoma, and between greater differentiation in the squamous cell group and the adenocarcinoma group.[7]

These observations have led to the construction of the unified theory of lung cancer which is best demonstrated by a Y construct (Figure 1). Transitions occur between all designated categories and types -- chiefly between adjacent type and also between the extremities. At the base of the Y is small cell carcinoma, a homogenous neoplasm, traversed by delicate blood vessels about which the cells tend to palisade. The uniform small cell carcinoma undergoes transition to the polygonal small cell, but transitions to large cell carcinoma are subtle and may provide considerable difficulty in diagnosis. At this point there is a branching and transition may occur to either squamous cell carcinoma or adenocarcinoma. The WHO Expert Committee on Lung Cancer met in Geneva in October, 1977 and the revised nomenclature based on the studies of the VA Lung Group will be in harmony with the Y concept proposed by Dr. Yesner.

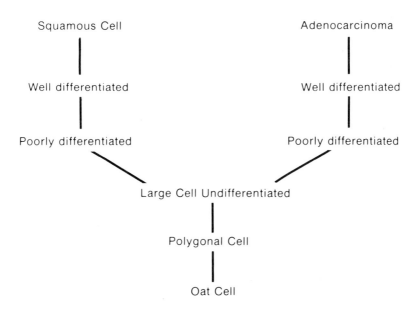

Fig. 1. Y concept of the unified theory of lung cancer

NATURAL HISTORY

CELL TYPE

Data from the control group in the early protocols in the VA Lung Group indicated that survival varied with cell type.[8],[9] Patients with adenocarcinoma had the longest median survival (13 weeks) followed by those with squamous cell carcinoma (9.5 weeks) after entry into study. Patients with large cell undifferentiated carcinoma or small cell undifferentiated carcinoma had a median survival of about six weeks (Figure 2). Other studies demonstrated that cyclophosphamide had a greater effect on small cell carcinoma than nitrogen mustard whereas nitrogen mustard appeared to have a better effect on squamous cell carcinoma than cyclophosphamide.[1]

TREATED SMALL CELL

The Cooperative Group studies have also contributed significantly to an understanding of the treated "natural history" of small cell lung cancer. In limited disease,[10],[11] the majority of patients relapsed in the chest,

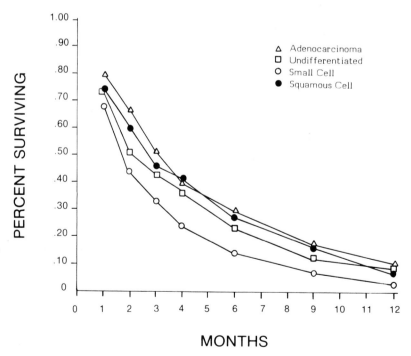

MONTHS

Fig. 2. Survival by cell type - inert compound

TABLE 4
Sites of Involvement at Presentation

104 LIMITED DISEASE
243 EXTENSIVE DISEASE

METASTATIC SITE	No. PTS.	PERCENT OF ALL PTS. WITH INVOLVEMENT		PERCENT OF EXTENSIVE DISEASE WITH INVOLVEMENT	
		ISOLATED	TOTAL	ISOLATED	TOTAL
Liver	84	12	24	16	35
Bone	74	10	22	15	30
Bone marrow	38	4	11	5	16
Brain	33	5	10	7	14
Pleura	32	5	9	7	13
Skin, nodes soft tissue	34	5	10	7	14
"Isolated"		36		50	

and at least half of this group appear to have developed recurrence in the radiated field. An analysis of the sites of involvement at presentation is shown in Table 4, and response and relapse patterns by site in extensive disease are shown in Table 5. An important point, not made in the tables, is that 10 percent of the responding patients with extensive disease relapsed initially in "nonbrain" CNS sites, suggesting the need for some type of elective or "prophylactic" treatment aimed at this area (e.g., intrathecal chemotherapy).

TABLE 5
Response and Relapse Patterns by Site in Extensive Disease

SITE	SMALL CELL		
	PERCENT INVOLVED	PERCENT RESPONDING	SINGLE SITE OF RELAPSE PREVIOUSLY INVOLVED (%)
Primary Tumor	> 50	> 50	10
Liver	35	52	10
Bone	30	56	3
Marrow	16	67	1
Brain	14	52	3
Nodes, Soft Tissue	14	60	6
Pleura	13	78	0

SURGICAL EXPERIENCE

The major factor influencing long-term survival in patients who have undergone a curative resection is the extent of the tumor at the time of the resection.[12]   If the tumor was confined to the lung, long-term survival was a much greater possibility than if the tumor had spread to adjacent lymph nodes or to contiguous structures. A second but less important factor was the age of the patient; this had an adverse effect especially in patients with tumor confined to the lung who were 60 years of age or older. The presence of mediastinal node involvement and the presence of other pulmonary disease also adversely affected long-term survival.

SOLITARY PULMONARY NODULE

The factors that influenced survival in 1,135 patients with a solitary pulmonary nodule who were studied were the size of lesions and age of the patient.[13]   Data indicated that five-year survival was better with patients whose lesions were less than 3.5 cm in diameter, and patients under 55 years of age fared better than those 65 or over. There was also evidence that survival in those patients with a normal chest x-ray less than one year prior to diagnosis was somewhat poorer than in those who had a positive x-ray a year or more before, indicative of the slower growing tumors.

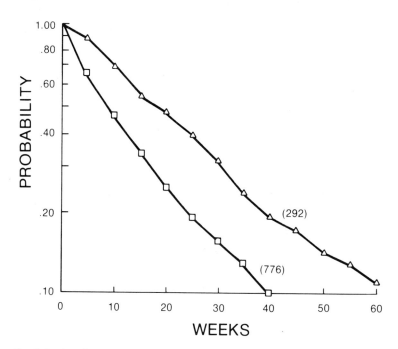

Fig. 3. Limited versus extensive disease - inert compound

EXTENT OF DISEASE

One of the first tasks in the early studies was to attempt to classify the patients according to extent of the disease.[1,8,9] Two classes were established -- limited or extensive. Subsequent survival experience indicated that these groups are in fact different. Limited disease patients are those in whom the nonresectable tumor was limited to one hemithorax and the apparent tumor mass was totally encompassed in every portal for possible x-ray therapy. There were no contralateral nodes nor cervical nodes or extrathoracic metastases. All other patients were classified as having extensive disease. Median survival of the limited disease group patients was 15 weeks while in the extensive disease group, median survival was 8 weeks (Figure 3).

PERFORMANCE STATUS

A third determinant of prognosis was the initial performance status using the Karnofsky Scale where a performance status of 100 indicated that the patient had no complaints and no symptomatic evidence of disease. There was easily demonstrated a difference in survival by performance status. Patients with a performance status of 90 percent on entrance into the study had a median survival of 22 weeks; those with 60 percent had a median survival of 9.5 weeks; and those with 40 percent had a median survival of 4.5 weeks (Figure 4).[8,9]

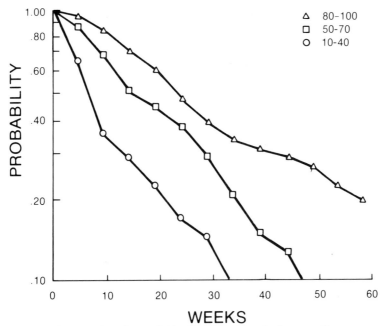

Fig. 4. Survival distribution of limited patients by performance status

SURGICAL ADJUVANT THERAPY

The Veterans Administration Surgical Adjuvant Group has conducted numerous trials to evaluate various regimens of adjuvant chemotherapy after resection. These included two doses of nitrogen mustard, cyclophosphamide, cyclophosphamide and methotrexate, and pre-operative radiotherapy. None of these demonstrated any benefit in survival. Failure to complete treatment was a common problem due to toxic reactions in some but in many it was a reluctance of well feeling patients to continue taking potent drugs. How much this contributed to treatment failure is not certain. The majority of patients dying succumbed as the result of the tumor. The five-year survival rate was about 25 percent in both control and treated groups. The three-year survival rate of those without metastatic lymph node involvement was 36 percent and for Stage I disease was 30.8 percent. It is important to note that thus far there has been no improvement in surgical five-year cure rate since 1960.[14,15]

"BIG ACTH"

In an attempt to discover a biological marker to assist in identifying patients with residual tumor and thus justify continuation of adjuvant therapy, Dr. R. Yalow working with both the VA Lung Group and VA Surgical Adjuvant Group explored further her finding that immuno-reactive "big" ACTH was produced by lung tumors. While ACTH was detectable in 47 of 49 patients with squamous cell and 15 of 19 patients with adenocarcinoma and not detectable in normal lung, abnormal levels in the plasma were found in only half of patients with squamous cell and in only one quarter of those with adenocarcinoma. The amounts produced by the tumors could not account for the elevated tumor levels found in the plasma. There was no significant fall after resection nor were high plasma levels associated with shorter survival. She proposed that the tumor per se was not the sole source of the circulating immunoreactive ACTH[16] and that it could not be used as a marker.

RADIATION THERAPY

ACCOMPLISHMENTS

Although there has been minimal improvement in the survival of patients with primary pulmonary carcinoma, the protocols developed by the Cooperative Groups involving radiation therapy have significantly contributed to a better understanding of the natural history of the disease, the response of the various histological types to irradiation and the optimal volume or doses of radiation to be employed in the treatment of these patients.

Radiation therapy is a potential cure in a small number of patients with pulmonary carcinoma limited to the thorax. In addition, irradiation has palliative indications in patients with extensive lung cancer who have hemoptysis, severe dyspnea because of large mediastinal or hilar masses or chest pain because of pleural or chest wall invasion. Significant palliation has been achieved in 75 to 80 percent of the patients.

Roswit et al[17] and Wolf et al[18] reported a study with a slightly better than one-year survival (22 percent) in a group of patients treated with 4,000 to 5,000 rads, in contrast to 16 percent survival in a control group given an inert compound. In patients with nonsmall cell carcinoma, there is a recently completed study in which preliminary analysis shows a 50 percent one-year survival and 25 percent two-year survival of patients with extensive intrathoracic disease without clinical evidence of distant metastasis. The study was designed to determine the optimal dose of irradiation to be given. The groups treated with 5,000 or 6,000 rads have a higher survival rate than those receiving 4,000 rads with either continuous or split course.[19]

The patients treated with the higher doses had an intrathoracic tumor control of about 60 percent, in contrast to only 40 percent for those in the 4,000 rads group. The study also demonstrated that if this type of radiation is properly delivered, the incidence of major complications are relatively low (less than one percent life-threatening and three percent major complications).

Three additional valuable observations in this study were the following:

A.   Patients with no evidence of hilar or mediastinal lymph nodes by radiographic evaluation have a two-year survival rate of 40 percent in contrast to only 20 percent for those with lymph nodes present. This correlation had been observed in surgical patients but not reported hitherto in clinically staged patients treated with irradiation. The finding is important because it points out the significance of clinical and radiographic staging of these patients.

B.   There was a definite correlation between the degree of tumor regression and the survival of patients; those showing complete response have a two-year survival of about 40 percent, as opposed to 20 percent with partial regression and 0 percent for the small group of patients with progression of disease after radiotherapy.

C.   Performance status of the patients correlated well with survival.

Another Group also reported higher survival rates with increasing doses of irradiation.[20]   The uncorrected median survival of patients receiving less than 1,400 rets was 20.4 weeks as compared to 43.1 weeks for those treated with more than 1,700 rets.   This group also demonstrated that performance status influenced survival and that patients with small cell undifferentiated carcinoma had an improved prognosis when irradiation was combined with chemotherapy (CCNU and hydroxyurea).   No significant prolongation of survival was noted in patients with nonsmall cell type when irradiation was combined with chemotherapy in comparison with a similar group of patients treated with radiotherapy alone.   It was also pointed out that the patients in the radiotherapy-chemotherapy group failed to show an increase in median survival with higher doses of irradiation, as was demonstrated in the radiotherapy alone group.

This study is of significance, not only because of the demonstration that the addition of chemotherapy did not result in prolongation of survival in the nonsmall cell carcinoma as opposed to the small cell type, but also because it showed that higher doses of radiotherapy correlate with better therapeutic results.

Other studies have been launched by the Cooperative Groups to evaluate the combination of radiation and chemotherapy in nonsmall cell carcinoma.   One studied the synergistic effect of 5-Fluorouracil (5-FU) with radiation in nonsmall cell carcinoma of the lung.[21]   It showed that 2,000 rads combined with 5-FU was as effective in shrinking tumor mass as 4,000 rads and was significantly more effective than 2,000 rads alone.   Recently pilot studies have been launched to evaluate, in patients with limited disease, standard radiation or hemibody radiation followed by cytoxan, adriamycin, methotrexate and procarbazine (CAMP), and to evaluate standard radiation followed by treatment with hexamethylmelamine, adriamycin and methotrexate (HAM).   One Group has activated a study to evaluate treatment with mitomycin-C, adriamycin, cytoxan and bleomycin followed by radiation to previous major areas of clinical involvement as well as "prophylactically" to the brain. No data is yet available regarding these studies.   However, as newer, more effective forms of therapy are identified that may be effective in advanced disease, these same forms of therapy will be evaluated as adjuvants to surgery and/or radiotherapy.

Aggressive combination of multiagent chemotherapy and irradiation to the intrathoracic disease as well as elective radiotherapy to the brain has been shown to control the intrathoracic tumor in about 80 percent of the patients in small cell carcinoma and the brain metastasis in 97 percent.[10] On a large scale, this study confirmed the findings reported by other investigators in pilot studies or in a small series of randomized patients.

UNRESOLVED PROBLEMS

It is apparent from the previous discussion that two major issues remain unresolved in the treatment of these patients. One is the local and regional (intrathoracic) tumor control, the other, the management of micrometastases.[22]

1.   Local-regional tumor control

Nonsmall cell tumors show a moderate response to irradiation, about 60 percent of the lesions demonstrating complete or partial regression with doses of 5,000 to 6,000 rads. For the large tumor, it is apparent that higher doses of irradiation are necessary. However, because of surrounding sensitive normal structures, such as the heart, esophagus, and spinal cord, it will be necessary to seek adjuvants that enhance the antitumor effects of irradiation without further damage to normal tissues. Possibilities that need to be explored are:

a.   Hypoxic sensitizers, such as misonidazole

b.   Hi-LET particles, such as neutrons or Pi mesons or

c.   Hyperthermia.

Small cell undifferentiated carcinoma exhibits an excellent response to irradiation, with about 90 percent of the tumors regressing after combinations of this modality with multi-agent chemotherapy (25 to 30 percent complete responders and 50 to 55 percent partial responders). Tumor regression seems to depend on the dose of radiation, as evidenced by the reports of persistent intrathoracic carcinoma or progression (40 to 50 percent of the patients treated with doses as high as 4,500 rads TD). Therefore, higher doses of irradiation or combination with aggressive cytoxic agent combinations are necessary.

With the advent of CT scanning it is possible to delineate the primary tumor and regional lymph nodes with greater accuracy. Also, the surrounding normal structures can be

readily identified. This information may be used in radiotherapy treatment planning, which could lead to dose optimization and increasing levels of irradiation to achieve
higher tumor control without increasing the complications.
Also, the quality of life may be enhanced in these patients.

2.   Treatment of distant metastases

Prophylactic irradiation of the brain has been demonstrated
to be extremely effective in preventing the clinical manifestation of intracranial metastasis.[23] It is possible that a
similar approach, irradiating pharmacological sanctuary
areas, may prove beneficial. Elective irradiation of high
risk metastatic sites, such as the liver, adrenal glands and
bones, deserves further investigation. The use of hemibody
irradiation in combination with chemotherapeutic agents
may be of value in the treatment of micrometastases.

SMALL CELL CARCINOMA

ACCOMPLISHMENTS

One of the best illustrations of how Cooperative Groups can build on
and extend the results of pilot efforts is in the field of small cell
carcinoma therapy. Following a pilot study consisting of cyclophosphamide, vincristine, and methotrexate with sequential radiation therapy to the primary tumor and whole brain, this regimen was compared
to high-dose cyclophosphamide alone, or to the combination with high-
dose methotrexate-citrovorum factor added. The results of this study
revealed the following: 1) the complete response rate in limited disease
was 30 to 40 percent, and did not differ by regimen; 2) median survivals
of almost a year, better than those which could be expected with
radiation alone, were achieved for patients with limited disease; and 3)
patients who received "prophylactic" whole brain irradiation had lower
rates of recurrence in the brain, although no significant survival benefit
could be demonstrated.[24]

Einhorn et al treated 29 patients, 25 of them with extensive disease,
with a combination of cyclophosphamide, vincristine, adriamycin and
bleomycin.[25] They observed an overall response rate of 76 percent, a
median survival of 8 months for the patients with extensive disease, and
2 of 4 patients with limited disease had prolonged, disease-free
survival. One Cooperative Group based their study on Einhorn's pilot,
but made several changes: 1) whole-brain irradiation was added, since 5
of 29 patients in the pilot relapsed in this site; 2) chest radiation

therapy was delivered, in "sandwiched" fashion, to patients with limited and extensive disease; and 3) bleomycin, a drug of no real activity as a single agent, was deleted.[10]   A complete response rate of 42 percent in limited and 14 percent in extensive disease, was achieved, with median survivals of one year and six months, respectively. More important, is the fact that 15 percent of the limited and 4 percent of the extensive disease patients survived beyond two years -- results better than those previously reported for radiation therapy alone.

Currently, an exciting lead in the treatment of small cell carcinoma is the pilot study of Cohen et al from the National Cancer Institute, who used intentional, early alternation of very aggressive, mutually noncross-resistant chemotherapy combinations.[11]   They reported complete response rates of 40 percent in extensive disease and 74 percent in limited disease, with a median survival in extensive disease projected at greater than one year. This concept of cycling combinations is used in a study design consisting of mutually noncross-resistant combinations plus whole-brain irradiation to prevent de novo relapse at this site.[26] This study should determine, quickly and efficiently with the statistical power of large numbers, whether Cohen's approach really represents a major step forward.

COMBINED MODALITY APPROACH

For many investigators working primarily in the solid tumor field, Group efforts in small cell carcinoma offered the first opportunity for medical oncologists and radiation therapists to work together in the design and analysis of studies.   Moore et al have described two important aspects of this interaction: 1) the observation that intentionally sequenced, "sandwich" radiation therapy to the chest and adriamycin-containing chemotherapy could be safely combined, without an undue rate of serious complications; and 2) the effectiveness of prophylactic whole-brain irradiation, in a multiinstitutional setting.[23,27] Salazar and his colleagues are actively piloting an innovative approach which involves the use of hemibody irradiation and combination chemotherapy in sequence.[28] Based on an analysis of the patterns of relapse in two completed, groupwide studies, radiation therapy is being redesigned for the primary tumor in patients with limited disease in an attempt to improve local control.

NONSMALL CELL CARCINOMA

The initial studies of the VA Lung Cancer Group reported in the early 1960's, represented a landmark in the carrying out of well designed control studies comparing chemotherapeutic agents, hormones, and radiotherapy, with a control treatment. The nontreated control groups were shown to be necessary since there was considerable variation in the survival of the group treated with an inert compound in the various studies. The major findings of these studies were that nitrogen mustard improved median survival by several weeks and that cortisone significantly shortened survival when compared to the inert compound.[29] Following this initial model, the Group continued to carry out both pilot studies looking at newer agents and Phase II and III studies evaluating the activity of single agents and combinations of chemotherapeutic agents in the treatment of this malignancy.[30-39]

Initially these studies did not separate patients with small cell carcinoma from those with nonsmall cell, but it soon became obvious that small cell carcinoma was much more responsive to a number of chemotherapeutic agents than was nonsmall cell carcinoma. In view of this finding, the small cell carcinoma patients were separated out in subsequent studies, and protocols tended to look at the response of patients with nonsmall cell cancer as a group. The study of nonsmall cell carcinoma of the lung has progressed in a logical fashion during the past 20 years. In a recent study, the combination of cytoxan and adriamycin was shown to be significantly better than cytoxan alone or cytoxan plus CCNU in squamous cell carcinoma of the lung. The median survival of patients with well differentiated squamous carcinoma and poorly differentiated squamous carcinoma were 23 and 26 weeks respectively for patients treated with adriamycin and cytoxan, compared to 10 and 13 weeks for patients treated with cytoxan alone. The combination of adriamycin and CCNU was also found to be better than cytoxan alone in patients with poorly differentiated squamous carcinoma.[38] However, the conclusion drawn from this study was that little meaningful improvement in performance status was obtained in these patients even though there was a statistically significant improvement in median survival.

The other Cooperative Groups have carried out studies evaluating a number of single agents, and in general, reported response rates in the range of 20 percent or less.[40-48] These studies included evaluation of hydroxyurea, adriamycin, methotrexate, hexamethylmelamine, dibromodulcitol, BCNU, cytoxan, CCNU, L-asparaginase, procarbazine, DTIC, streptozotocin, and bleomycin. Most of these studies did not result in any meaningful improvement in median survival.

Subsequently, the most promising single agents were incorporated into combination chemotherapy studies of the Cooperative Groups. The response rates obtained with the combination of an alkylating agent and a nitrosourea were not found to be better than that obtained with an alkylating agent alone.[47] The use of a nitrosourea in combination with an alkylating agent was in part based on the finding that this combination showed considerable synergistic activity in several experimental tumor systems, including the Lewis lung carcinoma. However, these combinations did not show significant increases in survival when evaluated in controlled studies.

The combination of an alkylating agent and nitrosourea with a vinca alkaloid and bleomycin known as "COMB", which was reported by two Groups, did not increase median survival significantly, and the toxicity from this combination was found to be considerable.[49],[50] This 4-drug combination, which combined a nitrosourea in the form of methyl CCNU with cytoxan with the addition of vincristine and bleomycin was based on the fact that vincristine can produce reversible mitotic arrest for 4 to 24 hours after its administration and the bleomycin is most effective at killing cells which are in the G_2 and M phases of the cell cycle. The overall result with this combination in pilot studies showed a reasonable response rate and represented an attempt to combine several agents which individually had minimal activity in carcinoma of the lung in order to develop a combination which might give significant activity when utilized in a controlled setting.[50] Unfortunately, the side effects outweighed the possible beneficial effects of the combination even though "COMB" produced some impressive tumor regressions. The administration of vincristine and bleomycin was associated with a debilitation syndrome consisting of anorexia, apathy and progressive weakness which was generally reversible upon discontinuation of these agents.

Another set of combination regimens has been developed utilizing adriamycin. This agent was reported in several reviews to have an overall response rate of 25 percent in squamous carcinoma, 17 percent in adenocarcinoma, and 13 percent in large cell carcinoma[51],[52] and was evaluated as a single agent by several Cooperative Groups.[41],[45],[53] It was shown that there was a significant improvement in survival for the combination of adriamycin and cytoxan over that obtained with cytoxan alone. Subsequently, in pilot studies, adriamycin was combined with CCNU, vincristine, bleomycin, and nitrogen mustard. These pilot studies carried out at the M. D. Anderson Hospital showed an initial response rate of 45 percent.[54] However, in a large follow-up study by a Cooperative Group comparing this 5-drug combination with a 3-drug combination of nitrogen mustard, adriamycin, and CCNU, the response rates were 21 percent and 16 percent respectively, with resulting median survivals of only 12 and 14 weeks respectively.[55] There was significant toxicity from this combination with fatal toxicities of approximately 4 percent in each group and life-threatening toxicities of 7 and 12 percent respectively. High response rates have been reported with other pilot combinations using adriamycin, including a combination of methotrexate, adriamycin, cytoxan and CCNU, reported by Chahinian, to give a response rate of 46 percent and a median survival of 9 months.[56] However, when this combination was recently evaluated in a Group master protocol, the response rate fell to less than 20 percent and the use of this combination was accompanied by severe toxicity. No improvement in median survival was found in this latter study. These reports emphasize the importance of randomized, group-wide studies as opposed to single institution studies which frequently give inflated results.

SUMMARY

To date, most of the single agents and combinations utilized in the treatment of patients with nonsmall cell bronchogenic carcinoma have shown no major impact on median survival, and response rates in controlled studies have tended to be in the range of 20 percent or less. In many of these studies the higher response rates were usually accompanied by moderately severe toxicity. One of the lessons to be learned from the numerous studies carried out in patients with lung cancer by the Cooperative Groups has been that when agents, which have little or no significant activity when used alone, are utilized in combinations, the response rates rarely increase while toxicity often increases significantly. Therefore, there is presently a continued search for new agents and combinations of agents which will have significant antitumor effect with no major increase in toxicity. Two groups are carrying out Phase II studies utilizing a master protocol or pilot study approach which looks for major improvements in response rate and rapidly eliminates arms which do not appear to have significant activity. It is hoped that the master protocol approach will identify worthwhile leads which can then be studied in a Phase III approach which may require subdivision by cell type.

To quote from a recent review by Livingston, "Certain negative leads have now made themselves apparent as well. At least for the well differentiated squamous tumors and adenocarcinomas, very aggressive approaches with currently available drug combinations appear to be of no benefit to the patient population. The role of the standard alkylating agents in these tumors is very much open to question. Furthermore, in the opinion of this reviewer, the nitrosoureas have been exhaustively evaluated and found wanting. The design of future drug combinations in nonoat cell disease would probably benefit from their deletion."[57]

The fact that the Cooperative Groups have access to large numbers of patients with advanced lung carcinoma and the fact that the median survival in these patients is relatively short should result in the rapid accumulation of data regarding response and median survival, and hopefully the identification of combinations which give meaningful increases in survival, rather than just response rates that may look impressive in early pilot studies.

1. Green RA, Humphrey E, Close H, Patno ME: Alkylating agents in bronchogenic carcinoma. Am J of Med 46:516-525, 1969.
2. Yesner R, Gerstl B, Auerbach O: Application of the World Health Organization classfication of lung carcinoma to biopsy material. Ann of Thoracic Surg 1:1, 33-49, 1965.
3. Yesner R: Observer variability and reliability in lung cancer diagnosis. Cancer Chemother Rep 4:55-57, 1973.
4. Yesner R: Histologic typing of lung cancer with clinical implications. Front Radiation Ther Oncol 9:140-150, 1974.
5. Yesner R: Correlations of histopathology with manifestations and outcome of lung cancer. JAMA 211:2081-2086, 1970.
6. Steele JD, Kleitsch WP, Dunn JE Jr, et al: Survival in males with bronchogenic carcinoma resected as solitary pulmonary nodules. Ann Thoracic Surg 2:368-376, 1966.
7. Yesner R: Spectrum of lung cancer and ectopic hormones. Pathology Annual, Part 1, 13:217-240, 1978.
8. Hyde L, Yee J, Wilson R, Patno ME: Cell type and the natural history of lung cancer. JAMA 193:52-54, 1965.
9. Hyde L, Wolf J, McCracken S, Yesner R: Natural course of inoperable lung cancer. Chest 64:309-312, 1973.
10. Livingston RB, Moore TN, Heilbrun L, Bottomley R, Lehane D, Rivkin SE, Thigpen T: Small cell carcinoma of the lung: Combined chemotherapy and radiation. Ann of Intern Med 88:194-199, 1978.
11. Cohen MH, Ihde DC, Fossieck BE, Bunn PA, Matthews MJ, Shackney SE, Johnston AV, Minna JD: Cyclic alternating combination chemotherapy of small cell bronchogenic carcinoma. ASCO 19:359, 1978.
12. Shields T, Higgins GA, Keehn RJ: Factors influencing survival after resection for bronchial carcinoma. J of Thoracic and Cardiovascular Surg 64:391-399, 1972.
13. Higgins GA, Shields TW, Keehn RJ: The solitary pulmonary nodule. Arch of Surg 11:570-575, 1975.
14. Hughes FA, Higgins G: Veterans Administration Surgical Adjuvant Lung Cancer chemotherapeutic study: Present status. J of Thoracic and Cardiovascular Surg 44:295-308, 1962.
15. Shields TW, Humphrey EW, Eastridge CE, Keehn RJ: Adjuvant cancer chemotherapy after resection of carcinoma of the lung. Cancer 40:2057-2062, 1977.
16. Yalow RS, Eastridge CE, Higgins G, Wolf J: Plasma and tumor ACTH in carcinoma of the lung. Cancer 44:1789-1792, 1979.
17. Roswit B, Patno ME, Rapp R, et al: The survival of patients with inoperable lung cancer: A large-scale randomized study of radiation therapy versus placebo. Radiology 90:688-697, 1968.
18. Wolf J, Patno ME, Roswit B, D'Esopo N: Controlled study of survival of patients with clinically inoperable lung cancer treated with radiation therapy. Am J Med 40:360-367, 1966.
19. Perez CA, Stanley K, Mietlowski W: Radiation therapy in the treatment of non-small cell bronchogenic carcinoma. Preliminary report of two dose fractionation studies. In Lung Cancer: Progress in Therapeutic Approach, F Muggia and M. Rozencwig, eds., Raven Press, N.Y., pp. 295-314, 1979.
20. Petrovich Z, Mitelowski W, Ohanian M, Cox J: Clinical report on the treatment of locally advanced lung cancer. Cancer 40:72-77, 1977.
21. Cohen JL, Krant MJ, Shnider BI, Matias PI, Horton J, Baxter D: Radiation plus 5-Fluorouracil: Clinical demonstration of an additive effect in bronchogenic carcinoma. Cancer Chemother Rep 55:253-258, 1971.
22. Perez CA: Radiation therapy in the management of carcinoma of the lung. Cancer 39:901-916, 1977.
23. Moore TN, Livingston RB, Heilbrun L, Eltringham J, Skinner O, White J, Tesh D: The effectiveness of prophylactic brain irradiation in small cell carcinoma of the lung. A Southwest Oncology Group Study. Cancer 41:2149-2153, 1978.
24. Maurer LH, Tulloh M, Weiss RB, Blom J, Leone L, Glidewell O, Pajek TF: A randomized combined modality trial in small cell carcinoma of the lung: Comparison of combination chemotherapy-radiation therapy versus cyclophosphamide-radiation therapy effects of maintenance chemotherapy and prophylactic whole brain irradiation. Cancer, 45:30-39, 1980.
25. Einhorn LH, Fee WH, Farber MO, et al: Improved chemotherapy for small cell undifferentiated lung cancer. JAMA 235:1225-1229, 1976.
26. SWOG, Minutes, March 1979.
27. Moore TN, Livingston RB, Heilbrun L: An acceptable rate of complications in combined doxorubicin-irradiation for small cell carcinoma of the lung. A Southwest Oncology Group Study. Int J Radiation Oncol Biol Phys 4:675-680, 1978.
28. ECOG, Minutes, November 1978.
29. Wolf J, Spear P, Yesner R, Patno ME: Nitrogen mustard and the steroid hormones in the treatment of inoperable bronchogenic carcinoma. Am J of Med 29:1008-1016, 1960.
30. McCracken S, Aboody A: Continuous intravenous infusion of streptonigrin in patients with bronchogenic carcinoma. Cancer Chemother Rep 46:23-26, 1965.
31. Fink A, Finegold SM, Patno ME, Close HP, Whittington RM: Vinblastine sulfate in the treatment of bronchogenic carcinoma. Cancer Chemother Rep 54:451-452, 1970.
32. Mizgerd JB, Amick RM, Hilal HN, Patno ME: Clinical study of 5-(3,3-dimethyl-1-triazeno) imidazole-4-carboxamide in carcinoma of the lung. Cancer Chemother Rep 55:83-86, 1971.
33. Kaung DT, Sbar S, Patno ME: Treatment of nonresectable cancer of the lung with hydroxyurea given intermittently. Cancer Chemother Rep 55:87-89, 1971.

34. Whittington RM, Fairly JL, Majima H, Patno ME, Prentice R: BCNU in the treatment of bronchogenic carcinoma. Cancer Chemother Rep 56:739-743, 1972.

35. Kaung DT, Wolf J, Hyde L, Zelen M: Preliminary report on the treatment of nonresectable cancer of the lung. Cancer Chemother Rep 58:359-364, 1974.

36. Rohwedder JJ, Sagastume E: Heparin and polychemotherapy for treatment of lung cancer. Cancer Treat Rep 61:1399-1401, 1977.

37. Brindley CO, Griffin GP, Williams JS, Wolf J: An analysis of comparative trials of L-asparaginase, cyclophosphamide and placebo in patients with inoperable bronchogenic carcinoma using corrected survival estimates. Autorensonderdrucke aus Oncology Vol. 35, Heft 1/78.

38. Hyde L, Wolf J, Phillips R, Mietlowski W: Combined chemotherapy for squamous cell carcinoma of the lung. Chest 73:5, 603-607, 1978.

39. Kaung DT, Walsh WS, Sbar S, Patno ME: Hydroxyurea in therapy for nonresectable cancer of the lung. Cancer Chemother Rep 52:271-274, 1968.

40. Bickers JN: Phase II studies of hydroxyurea in adults: carcinoma of the lung. Cancer Chemother Rep 40:45-46, 1964.

41. Knight EW, Lagakos S, Stolbach L, Colsky J, Horton J, Israel L, Bennett J, Perlia C, Regelson W, Carbone PP: Adriamycin in the treatment of far-advanced lung cancer. Cancer Treat Rep 60:939-941, 1976.

42. Selawry O, Krant M, Scotto J, Kazam E, Schneiderman M, Olson K, Shnider B, Edmonson J, Holland J, Taylor S: Methotrexate compared with placebo in lung cancer. Cancer 40:4-8, 1977.

43. Wilson WL, Van Ryzin J, Weiss AJ, Frelick RW, Moss SE: A Phase III study in lung carcinoma comparing hexamethylmelamine to dibromodulcitol. Oncology 31:293-309, 1975.

44. Lerner H, Carbone P, Colsky J, Lurie P: BCNU effect in primary lung cancer --EST 0669. ASCO 19:344, 1978.

45. Perlia CP, Stolbach L: Adriamycin and cytoxan in the treatment of inoperable lung cancer. AACR 17:27, 1976.

46. Edmonson JH, Lagakos SW, Selawry OS, Perlia CP, Bennett JM, Muggia FM, Wampler G, Brodovsky HW, Horton J, Colsky J, Mansour EG, Creech R, Stolbach L, Greenspan EM, Levitt M, Israel L, Ezdinli EZ, Carbone PP: Cyclophosphamide and CCNU in the treatment of inoperable small cell carcinoma and adenocarcinoma of the lung. Cancer Treat Rep 60:925-932, 1976.

47. Edmonson JH, Lagakos S, Stolbach L, Perlia CP, Bennett JM, Mansour EG, Horton J, Regelson W, Cummings FJ, Israel L, Brodsky I, Shnider BI, Creech R, Carbone PP: Mechlorethamine plus CCNU in the treatment of inoperable squamous and large cell carcinoma of the lung. Cancer Treat Rep 60:625-627, 1976.

48. Hoogstraten B, Haas CD, Haut A, Talley RW, Rivkin S, Isaacs BL: CCNU and bleomycin in the treatment of cancer: A Southwest Oncology Group Study. Med Pediatr Oncol 1:95-106, 1975.

49. Armentrout S, Bateman J, Pajak T: Oral nitrosoureas in multiple drug programs for bronchogenic carcinomas. ASCO 16:242, 1975.

50. Livingston RB, Einhorn LH, Bodey JP, Burgess MA, Freireich EF, Gottlieb JA: COMB (cyclophosphamide, oncovin, methyl CCNU and bleomycin): a four-drug combination in solid tumors. Cancer 36:327-332, 1975.

51. Blum RH: An overview of studies with adriamycin in the United States. Cancer Chemother Rep 6:247-251, 1975.

52. Rozencweig M, Kenis Y: European studies with adriamycin in lung cancer. Cancer Chemother Rep 6:343-347, 1975.

53. O'Bryan R, Luce J, Talley R, Gottlieb J, Baker L, Bonadonna G: Phase II evaluation of adriamycin in human neoplasia. Cancer 32:1-8, 1973.

54. Livingston RB, Fee WH, Einhorn LH, Burgess MA, Freireich EJ, Gottlieb JA, Farber MO: BACON (bleomycin, adriamycin, CCNU, oncovin, nitrogen mustard) in squamous lung cancer. Cancer 37:1237-1242, 1976.

55. Livingston RB, Heilbrun L, Lehane D, Costanzi JJ, Bottomley R, Palmer RL, Stuckey WJ, Hoogstraten B: Comparative trial of combination chemotherapy in extensive squamous carcinoma of the lung: A Southwest Oncology Group Study. Cancer Treat Rep 61:1623-1629, 1977.

56. Chahinian AP, Arnold DJ, Cohen JM, Purpora DP, Jaffrey IS, Teirstein AS, Kirschner PA, Holland JF: Chemotherapy for bronchogenic carcinoma. JAMA 237:2392-2396, 1977.

57. Livingston RB: Combination chemotherapy of bronchogenic carcinoma. I. Nonoat cell. Cancer Treat Rev 4:153-165, 1977.

9

Gastrointestinal cancer

Charles G. Moertel, V.K. Vaitkevicius, George A. Higgins,
and Bernard Gardner

Gastrointestinal cancer afflicts more people and causes more cancer deaths than cancer taking origin in any other organ system. Routine surgical treatment has only had reasonable success in the infrequently encountered early stages of these diseases. National statistics show overall five-year survival rates of less than 15 percent for gastric cancer and less than 10 percent in carcinomas primary to the esophagus, liver, bile ducts, and pancreas. It is only in large bowel cancer that surgery has had a reasonable rate of success, but even here more than half of all diagnosed patients will die of their cancers. Since, from the standpoint of both incidence and mortality, gastrointestinal cancer represents the major malignant disease challenge in this country, it is appropriate that this group of cancers should receive commensurate interest and effort in the national Cooperative Group Program.

This report will encompass the documented accomplishments in gastrointestinal cancer of the currently active grant supported national Cooperative Groups. It was derived from 39 manuscripts and 19 abstracts submitted by the Group chairmen. Of these, 16 manuscripts and 14 abstracts will not be specifically referenced since they were either preliminary reports of data later published in final form, duplications of earlier publications, or reviews of previously published data. Therefore, this report is based on a total of 23 manuscripts and 5 abstracts reporting results of the 24 Group protocols in gastrointestinal carcinoma conducted over the past 21 years.[1-28] This report specifically will not refer to work of contract funded national Cooperative Groups, work of contract or grant funded individual institutions, or work of grant funded Cooperative Groups which are no longer active.

ADVANCED CANCER STUDIES

COLORECTAL CARCINOMA

Some of the earliest data recorded by Cooperative Groups regarding treatment of advanced colorectal cancer were those offered by the Veterans Administration Surgical Adjuvant Group for patients entered into their controlled trials, who were found to be eligible only for palliative resections. Indeed, these are among the very few studies in which chemotherapy is compared to no treatment in patients with advanced disease. Much of their initial data regarding Thiotepa and 5-FUDR were difficult to interpret because histologic proof of residual disease was frequently not obtained during the operative procedures. In their more recent short-term and prolonged 5-Fluorouracil (5-FU) trials, however, patients were specifically designated as histologically confirmed residual and in each of these trials the 5-FU treated patients had more favorable survival curves in comparison to randomized controls.[16] In both of these trials the number of patients with palliative procedures was relatively small and the differences between treated groups and control groups were not statistically significant. In short, the possibility that 5-FU treatment could add slightly to survival when compared to no treatment was suggested but not proven. One of the most striking features of these two consecutive trials, however, was the remarkable difference in survival of patients after palliative surgical procedures, even when patients were considered with comparable extent of disease. In their first trial the two-year survival for proven palliative resection was only 13.5 percent whereas, in their second trial the two-year survival in comparable patients was 30.0 percent. This is the most highly significant difference demonstrated in all of the Veterans Administration Surgical Adjuvant Group trials in colorectal cancer and clearly illustrates the total unreliability of historically controlled studies in the treatment of advanced gastrointestinal cancer.

With the exception of the VASAG, all other Cooperative Group trials for advanced colorectal cancer have addressed the patient with measurable disease and objective response has been the primary indicator of therapeutic effect.

One of the first randomized comparisons of single-drug treatment in colorectal cancer compared three antimetabolites, 5-FU, FUDR, and methotrexate, each given intravenously and by intensive course.[2] This study had the added sophistication of double blinding. It was marred, however, by a very high rate of ineligibility, 24 percent. Also, the dosage of FUDR was lower than that employed in other studies in which more favorable response rates were recorded. It must be noted that in this study a 25 percent reduction criterion was employed for declaring objective response, more liberal than the 50 percent reduction that is generally required by studies carried out today. Only 60 percent of the overall group of responders achieved a greater than 50 percent reduction. In this study 5-FU showed a significant superiority in response rate when compared to the other two agents (Table 1). The inadequacy of methotrexate for large bowel cancer has been rather clearly demonstrated by the whole of the literature. The low response rate for FUDR stands in contrast to other reports and may be related to an inadequate dosage. It is noteworthy that survivorship for these three treatment approaches was essentially identical.

TABLE 1
Randomized Comparison of Antimetabolites in Advanced Colorectal Carcinoma

Drug	Objective Response Rate*	Median Survival – weeks
5-FU	13/48 (27%)	23.4
FUDR	2/46 (10%)	21
Methotrexate	4/40 (4%)	22

*A 25% reduction criterion employed for objective response

Other single drugs evaluated by the Cooperative Groups in later studies are displayed in Table 2. For four of the drugs, procarbazine, thioguanine, β-2'-deoxythioguanosine, dianhydrogalactitol, these represented the initial Phase II studies in colorectal cancer. For five of the drugs, the results were confirmatory of work previously published by others. It is perhaps noteworthy that 76 percent of the 625 patients entered on these Phase II trials had had previous chemotherapy exposure. Among the 150 patients with no prior treatment an overall objective response rate of 13 percent was recorded. Among the 475 patients who had had prior chemotherapy the overall response rate was only 3.6 percent. These data bring into serious question the use of previously treated patients for evaluation of new agents in the more drug resistant malignant neoplasms. Of the nine drugs tested, only the nitrosoureas can be assumed to have some reasonable activity in colorectal cancer, and this primarily in previously untreated patients.

TABLE 2
Single-drug Phase II Studies in Colorectal Carcinoma

	Objective Response Rate		
Drug	No prior Rx	Previous Rx	All patients
Procarbazine	0/13	1/25 (4%)	1/38 (3%)
Streptozotocin	0/17	5/33 (15%)	5/20 (10%)
CCNU	5/18 (28%)	1/37 (3%)	6/55 (11%)
6-thioguanine	1/17 (6%)	3/37 (8%)	4/54 (7%)
methyl CCNU	13/85 (15%)	4/116 (4%)	17/201 (8%)
B-2'-deoxythioguanosine		1/99 (1%)	1/99 (1%)
VP-16		0/44	0/44
Diglycoaldehyde		2/45 (4%)	2/45 (4%)
Dianhydrogalactitol		0/39	0/39

TABLE 3
Randomized Controlled Studies of Drug Combinations in Colorectal Carcinoma

Drugs	Dosage Regimen	Objective Response	Median Survival (wks)
5-FU Oral	600 mg/M^2/wk	5/28 (18%)	32
vs.			
5-FU IV	600 mg/M^2/wk	6/39 (15%)	30
vs.			
5-FU Oral + Cyclophosphamide	600 mg/M^2/wk* 1,000 mg/M^2 q 8 wks	4/87 (5%)	29
vs.			
5-FU Oral + 6-thioguanine	600 mg/M^2/wk 40 mg/M^2/d x 14 q 8 wks	9/77 (12%)	31
vs.			
Methyl CCNU	175 mg/M^2 q 8 wks	13/85 (17%)	27
5-FU IV	400 mg/M^2/wk	4/42 (9.5%)	
vs.			No Difference
5-FU IV + Methyl CCNU	400 mg/M^2/wk 175 mg/M^2 q 6 wks	48/151 (32%)	
5-FU IV	15 mg/kg/wk	6/29 (21%)	36
vs.			
5-FU IV + Ara-C	15 mg/kg/wk 30-100 mg/kg/wk	5/43 (12%)	28

* Given on 2nd to 6th week of 8 week cycle.

The primary thrust of Cooperative Group studies in chemotherapy of colorectal cancer during recent years has been evaluation of drug combinations. Three of these studies were both randomized and controlled with 5-FU as a standard treatment. One looked at both oral and IV 5-FU given by weekly schedule without a loading course, weekly oral 5-FU in combination with cyclophosphamide, weekly oral 5-FU in combination with 6-thioguanine, and methyl CCNU used alone.[24] Neither of the drug combinations produced an objective response rate superior to 5-FU alone and, indeed, the combination of oral 5-FU and cyclophosphamide was significantly worse. All treatment arms were associated with comparable median survivals (Table 3).

The second study compared weekly 5-FU with weekly 5-FU + methyl CCNU.[8] Here the combination produced an objective response rate that was significantly superior to the single drug. The very low dose of weekly 5-FU used in the control arm may constitute a serious defect in methodology since it is questionable whether this represents the most ideal dosage or schedule for this agent. It is noteworthy that in spite of the superiority in objective response rate there was no superiority of survival associated with the combination drug treatment, 32 weeks versus 21 weeks for 5-FU (p = .20).

The third study compared weekly 5-FU alone with weekly 5-FU plus two dosage schedules of cytosine arabinoside.[4] Clearly the combination added nothing to either response rate or survival.

In all of these controlled studies of drug combinations in colorectal cancer a weekly schedule for 5-FU was employed. The choice of such a control might reasonably be questioned in light of the study by the no longer active Central Oncology Group showing the weekly method to be

TABLE 4
Drug Combination Studies in Colorectal Carcinoma

Drugs	Dosage Regimen	Objective Response
5-FU IV +	12 mg/kg/d × 4 then 6 mg/kg qod × 3	4/36 (11%)
Azapicyl	300 mg/m² days 1 and 21	
Methyl CCNU + B-2'-Deoxythio-guanosine	130 mg/m² q 8 wks 60 mg/m²/d × 5 q 4 wks	3/49 (6%)
5-FU + Methyl CCNU Daunomycin	350 mg/m²/wk 150 mg/m² q 8 wks 40 mg/m² q 4 wks	5/27 (19%)

substantially and significantly inferior to administration of 5-FU by intensive course.[29]

Three Phase II studies were carried out by the Cooperative Groups (Table 4). Neither of these had promising results although it must be remembered that only previously treated patients were entered.

Table 5 lists the Cooperative Group studies in advanced colorectal cancer in which two or more drug combinations were evaluated in

TABLE 5

Randomized Controlled Studies of Drug Combinations in Colorectal Carcinoma

Drugs	Dosage Regimen	Objective Response	Median Survival (wks)
5-FU 24 hr. IV + mitomycin-C	$1,000$ mg/M^2 x 4 q 4 wks 15-20 mg/M^2 q 8 wks	25/136 (18%)	43
vs.			
5-FU 24 hr. IV + Methyl CCNU	$1,000$ mg/M^2 x 4 q 4 wks 150-175 mg/M^2 q 8 wks	21/133 (16%)	43.5
5-FU IV + Methyl CCNU	325 mg/M^2 d x 5 q 5 wks 150 mg/M^2 q 10 wks	9/88 (10%)	26
vs.			
5-FU IV + Methyl CCNU + Vincristine	325 mg/M^2 d x 5 q 5 wks 150 mg/M^2 q 10 wks 1 mg/M^2 q 5 wks	10/81 (12%)	33
vs.			
5-FU IV + Methyl CCNU + DTIC	250 mg/M^2 d x 5 q 5 wks 100 mg/M^2 q 10 wks 100 mg/M^2 d x 2 q 5 wks	14/83 (14%)	41
vs.			
5-FU IV + Methyl CCNU + Vincristine + DTIC	250 mg/M^2 d x 5 q 5 wks 100 mg/M^2 10 wks 1 mg/M^2 q 5 wks 100 mg/M^2 d x 2 q 5 wks	11/71 (15%)	40
vs.			
5-FU IV + Hydroxyurea	600 mg/M^2 weekly 800 mg/M^2 q 8 hours 1 day/wk	15/73 (21%)	33
Methyl CCNU + Vincristine +	175 mg/M^2 q 8 wks 1 mg/M^2 q 2 wks	1/44 (2%)	17
vs.			
Methyl CCNU + DTIC	150 mg/M^2 q 8 wks 150 mg/M^2 d x 5 q 4 wks	8/53 (15%)	32
vs.			
Methyl CCNU + Vincristine + DTIC	150 mg/M^2 q 8 wks 1 mg/M^2 q 2 wks 150 mg/M^2 d x 5 q 4 wks	4/55 (7%)	24
vs.			
Methyl CCNU + β-2-deoxythio-guanosine	150 mg/M^2 q 8 wks 60 mg/M^2 d x 5 q 4 wks	1/53 (2%)	20

randomized trial but where no single drug was employed as a control. One study compared 5-FU plus mitomycin-C with 5-FU plus methyl CCNU.[21] In each combination 5-FU was given by 24-hour intravenous infusion. Essentially no differences were demonstrated in either response rate or survival, and one does not know how these results would have compared to a Group experience with 5-FU given by 24-hour infusion or with either of the other single drugs used alone.

One Group randomized some 400 previously untreated patients between five different 5-FU containing combinations and over 200 patients with prior chemotherapy exposure were randomized to four drug combinations not involving 5-FU.[19] Again there do not seem to be substantive differences among any of these treatment arms, and one does not know how these results might have compared to single-drug treatment in the same patient population.

Table 5 shows results of three additional combinations with data that the investigators reasonably concluded were unimpressive. The lack of value of combined methyl CCNU and β-2'-deoxythioguanosine would seem to be thoroughly established with a total of only four objective responses among 102 previously treated patients. [19 24]

GASTRIC CARCINOMA

As in colorectal carcinoma, the VASAG adjuvant studies in gastric carcinoma have provided some data comparing chemotherapy with no treatment for advanced disease in patients who had only palliative resections. [1,7] Survival curves for treatment with Thiotepa and with FUDR were both superior to no treatment controls. Regretably the number of patients studied was not adequate to confirm this suggestion of therapeutic effect at a statistically significant level.

Substantial interest in the chemotherapy of advanced gastric cancer has been shown by particularly two Groups. Because of the relatively rapid demise of these patients, survival data as well as objective response have been used to evaluate the effects of therapy. Group studies have been dominated by evaluation of drug combinations with very little data accrued regarding activity of single agents. Table 6 displays the results in advanced gastric carcinoma trials expressed in terms of objective response rate, and Table 7 shows the results expressed in terms of patient survival.

TABLE 6
Measurable Disease Studies in Gastric Carcinoma

Drugs	Dosage Regimen	Objective Response	
Methyl CCNU	200 mg/M^2 q 7 wks	3/37	(8%)
vs.			
Cyclophosphamide +	1,200 mg/M^2 once only	2/30	(7%)
Methyl CCNU	200 mg/M^2 q 7 wks		
vs.			
5-FU IV +	300 mg/M^2 d x 5 q 7 wks	12/30	(40%)
Methyl CCNU	175 mg/M^2 q 7 wks		
vs.			
Cyclophosphamide +	1,200 mg/M^2 once only	6/30	(20%)
5-FU IV +	300 mg/M^2 d x 5 q 7 wks		
Methyl CCNU	175 mg/M^2 q 7 wks		
5-FU IV	400 mg/M^2/wk	2/10	(20%)
vs.			
5-FU IV +	400 mg/M^2/wk	6/29	(21%)
Methyl CCNU	175 mg/M^2 q 6 wks		
5-FU 24 hr IV +	1,000 mg/M^2 d x 4 q 4 wks		19%
mitomycin-C	20 mg/M^2 q 8 wks	168	
vs.		total	
5-FU 24 hr IV +	1,000 mg/M^2 d x 4 q 4 wks	pts	14%
Methyl CCNU	175 mg/M^2 q 8 wks		
5-FU IV +	325 mg/M^2 x d x 5 q 5 wks	19/61	(31%)
mitomycin-C	3.75 mg/M^2 d x 5 q 5 wks		
vs.			
5-FU IV +	325 mg/M^2 d x 5 q 5 wks	13/55	(24%)
Methyl CCNU	150 mg/M^2 q 10 wks		
vs.			
adriamycin	60 mg/M^2 q 3 wks x 3 then q 4 wks	15/85	(18%)
5-FU IV	15 mg/kg/wk	2/9	(22%)
vs.			
5-FU IV +	15 mg/kg/wk	3/18	(19%)
Ara-C	30-100 mg/M^2/wk		
5-FU IV +	12 mg/kg d x 4 then 6 mg/kg q i d x 3 q 6 wks	1/7	(14%)
Azapicyl	300 mg/M^2 days 1 and 21		
Dianhydrogalactitol	25-30 mg/M^2 d x 5 q 5 wks	0/5	

The first study in Table 6 randomized patients with measurable disease only to either methyl CCNU used alone or to the combination of 5-FU and methyl CCNU.[9] Each of these groups was also randomized either to receive a single intravenous dose of cyclophosphamide as induction treatment or to receive no such induction therapy. In this study cyclophosphamide induction clearly added nothing to either response rate or survival; indeed, it seemed to detract. On the other hand, the combination of 5-FU and methyl CCNU produced a very favorable objective response rate of 40 percent associated with a significant survival increase when compared to results with methyl CCNU used alone. It is noteworthy, however, that in the fourth study a slightly modified version of the 5-FU methyl CCNU combination garnered a response rate of only 24 percent;[28] and that in employing nonmeasurable disease patients, the 5-FU methyl CCNU combination produced no advantage in patient survival when compared to treatment with 5-FU alone[23] (Table 7).

Weekly 5-FU alone was compared to weekly 5-FU plus methyl CCNU; and in contrast to the results in colorectal cancer, no difference was found in response rate between these two regimens,[8] nor did they demonstrate any survival difference.

The combination of 5-FU and mitomycin-C versus 5-FU and methyl CCNU with 5-FU given by 24-hour infusion in both combinations produced modest response rates and again no difference in survival was obtained.

One study compared combinations of 5-FU plus mitomycin-C, 5-FU plus methyl CCNU, and adriamycin used alone.[28] In the combinations 5-FU was given by rapid intravenous injection, and perhaps because of this, a somewhat higher response rate was garnered than in the preceding study. Again, however, there was no difference between these combinations either with respect to objective response rate or survival. Another study also confirmed the previously reported activity of adriamycin in gastric carcinoma.

In addition to comparing 5-FU alone versus 5-FU plus methyl CCNU, patients were also randomized to either concomitant testolactone or no testolactone.[23] This was based on a previously published report that the addition of "Lactones" to chemotherapy of gastrointestinal cancer produced a substantial improvement in survival.[30] Clearly this study did not validate such a claim (Table 7).

One must be cautious in interpreting the results of the small patient numbers in the last two studies of Table 6.[4,25] It would appear, however, that combinations of weekly 5-FU and cytosine arabinoside or

TABLE 7
Comparative Survival Studies in Gastric Carcinoma

Drugs	Patients	Median Survival (wks)
Cyclophosphamide induction	63	14
vs.		
No Cyclophosphamide induction	67	14
Methyl CCNU	63	13
vs.		
5-Fu + Methyl CCNU	55	20
Chemotherapy alone	84	32.5
vs.		
Chemotherapy + testolactone	95	30.5
5-FU	95	36.5
vs.		
5-FU + Methyl CCNU	84	25
5-FU	10	No difference
vs.		
5-FU + Methyl CCNU	29	
5-FU + Methyl CCNU	168 total patients	No difference
vs.		
5-FU + mitomycin-C		
adriamycin	37	16.3
vs.		
5-FU + Methyl CCNU	37	17.4
vs.		
5-FU + mitomycin-C	41	17.1
5-FU	9	31
vs.		
5-FU + Ara-C	15	21

of loading course 5-FU and azapicyl produce a bit less than spectacular results. The five-patient study of galactitol in gastric cancer does not offer sufficient experience to be classified as an adequate Phase II trial of this agent for this neoplasm.[27] In viewing all of the Cooperative Group advanced gastric carcinoma trials, it would appear that combinations of 5-FU plus methyl CCNU and perhaps 5-FU plus mitomycin-C, particularly if 5-FU is given by rapid intravenous injection and by intensive course, may produce some increase in response rate when compared to single agent chemotherapy. This conclusion, however, is not well established, and it would seem quite clear that none of the drugs or drug combinations tested have produced any important impact on patient survival.

PANCREATIC CARCINOMA

Advanced pancreatic carcinoma has been approached in five Group protocols evaluating two single drugs and seven drug combinations (Table 8). The single-drug studies showed a negligible response rate among 68 patients treated with methyl CCNU alone.[13] No responses were seen with dianhydrogalactitol for this neoplasm.[27]

In the combination drug studies, only 12 percent response rates were obtained with both 5-FU plus streptozotocin and cyclophosphamide plus streptozotocin.[15] Survival times in these measurable disease patients were very short. The combination of 5-FU plus streptozotocin produced no improvement in survival of patients with nonmeasurable disease when compared to treatment with 5-FU alone.[23]

A study involving only 22 patients showed modest response rates with both weekly 5-FU alone and weekly 5-FU plus methyl CCNU.[8] There was no difference in the response rates between these two arms and no difference in survival. In a later study, 24-hour infusion of 5-FU plus mitomycin-C produced a 30 percent objective response rate compared to only a 7 percent with 24-hour 5-FU plus methyl CCNU.[17] Again, however, there was no difference in patient survival.

In addition to the comparison of 5-FU alone versus 5-FU plus streptozotocin, one Group also addressed the question of whether the addition of spironolactone to chemotherapy of pancreatic carcinoma could have a favorable effect on survival,[23] this based on the historically controlled study of Waddell claiming striking survival improvement resulting from the addition of either spironolactone or testolactone or both to chemotherapy of pancreatic carcinoma.[30] As is so frequently the case when historically controlled studies are subjected to confirmation by randomized controlled trial, no confirmation was forthcoming.

TABLE 8
Pancreatic Carcinoma Studies

Drugs	Dosage Regimen	Objective Response	Median Survival (wks)
Methyl CCNU	200 mg/M^2 q 7 wks	4/68 (6%)	8
vs.			
5-FU IV +	400 mg/M^2 d x 5 q 6 wks	5/42 (12%)	13
streptozotocin	500 mg/M^2 d x 5 q 6 wks		
vs.			
Cyclophosphamide +	1,000 mg/M^2 q 3 wks	6/51 (12%)	9
streptozotocin	500 mg/M^2 d x 5 q 6 wks		
5-FU IV	400 mg/M^2/wk	1/6 (17%)	No difference
vs.			
5-FU IV +	400 mg/M^2/wk	3/16 (19%)	
Methyl CCNU	175 mg/M^2 q 6 wks		
5-FU 24 hr IV +	1,000 mg/M^2 d x 4 q 4 wks	(30%)	No difference
mitomycin-C	20 mg/M^2 q 8 wks		
vs.		144	
5-FU 24 hr IV +	1,000 mg/M^2 d q 4 wks	total (7%)	
Methyl CCNU	175 mg/M^2 q 8 wks	pts	
Dianhydrogalactitol	25-30 mg/M^2 d x 5	0/5	
5-FU IV	450 mg/M^2 d x 5 q 5 wks	No measurable disease	21
vs.			
5-FU IV +	450 mg/M^2 d x 5 q 5 wks		
Spironolactone	50 mg t i d		
vs.			
5-FU IV +	400 mg/M^2 d x 5 q 5 wks		18
streptozotocin	500 mg/M^2 d x 5 q 5 wks		
vs.		174	
5-FU IV +	400 mg/M^2 d x 5 q 5 wks	total	
streptozotocin +	500 mg/M^2 d x 5 q 5 wks	patients	
Spironolactone	50 mg t i d		

From an overall standpoint it is reasonable to conclude that the national Cooperative Group studies in advanced pancreatic carcinoma have thus far proved fruitless as has been the case for everyone else's studies of advanced pancreatic carcinoma.

HEPATOCELLULAR CARCINOMA

A unique feature of the national Cooperative Group studies has been the considerable work devoted to treatment of hepatocellular carcinoma, in spite of the relative rarity of this neoplasm in our country.

TABLE 9
Hepatocellular Carcinoma Studies

Drugs	Dosage Regimen	Objective Response American	African	All patients
adriamycin	25-75 mg/M^2 q 3 wks	4/22 (18%)	3/19 (16%)	7/41
adriamycin + 5-FU IV	30-60 mg/M^2 q 3 wks 500-600 mg/M^2 q 3 wks	5/38 (13%)		5/38
5-FU IV vs.	15 mg/kg/wk		0/22	0/22
5-FU IV + Ara-C	15 mg/kg/wk 30-100 mg/M^2/wk		1/16 (6%)	1/16
adriamycin vs.	40-60 mg/M^2 q 3 wks	6/37 (16%)	3/20 (15%)	9/57
5-FU Oral vs.	60 mg/M^2 d x 5 q 5 wks	0/34	0/14	0/48
5-FU Oral + streptozotocin vs.	600 mg/M^2 d x 5 q 5 wks 500 mg/M^2 d x 2 q 10 wks	4/22 (18%)	0/4	4/33
5-FU Oral + Methyl CCNU	500 mg/M^2 d x 5 q 5 wks 150 mg/M^2 q 10 wks	2/34 (6%)	0/14	2/48

This has been due in part to the participation of African investigators; but it does demonstrate, along with the studies in carcinoid tumor (vida infra), the ability of large Cooperative Groups to garner significant information regarding relatively uncommon tumors, information that could not be garnered by any one institution alone in a timely fashion.

The results summarized in Table 9 confirmed the significant activity of adriamycin in both American and African hepatoma.[11,22] It would seem quite clear that 5-FU given by weekly schedule and by oral route of administration are worthless for the treatment of this neoplasm. [4,22] The combination of weekly 5-FU with cytosine arabinoside also produced less than ideal therapeutic results.[4]

There is little advantage to be gained by combining 5-FU and adriamycin for hepatoma.[14] However, the dosage of 5-FU employed in this study is homeopathic in nature, and it would not seem that such a dosage regimen provides an appropriate evaluation for these drugs in combination.

The comparative survival statistics in Table 10 are of considerable interest, showing a significant survival advantage for both adriamycin alone and 5-FU plus streptozotocin in comparison to 5-FU alone in the

TABLE 10
Hepatocellular Carcinoma Survival Studies

	Median Survival - weeks	
Drug (s)	American	African
5-FU IV	—	8
vs		
5-FU IV + Ara C	—	8
Adriamycin	17	12
vs		
5-FU Oral	8	3
vs		
5-FU Oral + Streptozotocin	22	13
vs		
5-FU Oral + Methyl CCNU	19	6

treatment of African hepatoma.[22] The combination of 5-FU and methyl CCNU, as well as adriamycin alone and 5-FU plus streptozotocin, also produces a significant survival advantage in comparison to 5-FU alone for American hepatoma.   Hepatocellular carcinoma would seem to be one of the few gastrointestinal neoplasms in which a true addition to survival of advanced disease patients has been produced by appropriate chemotherapy.

METASTATIC CARCINOID TUMOR

One Group reported a remarkable large collection of 118 patients with metastatic carcinoid tumor who were randomized to treatment with streptozotocin combined with cyclophosphamide or streptozotocin combined with 5-FU.[20] Commonly experienced side effects included leukopenia, thrombocytopenia, nephrotoxicity, and very troublesome nausea and vomiting.   As displayed in Table 11 response rates with these combinations in small bowel carcinoids were 37 percent and 44 percent. Overall response rates among all carcinoid tumor patients were 26 percent and 33 percent. There was no significant difference in patient survival between the two treatment arms. Crossover treatment with 5-FU alone showed a modest response rate of 18 percent. There were no responses amongst eight patients treated with cyclophosphamide alone.   In this study urinary 5-HIAA excretion proved to be a useful biologic marker that correlated well with observed measurements of tumor bulk. Metastatic carcinoid tumor would seem to be a malignant

TABLE 11
Metastatic Carcinoid Tumor

PHASE II STUDY - UNTREATED PATIENTS

Primary	Objective Response Rate	
	Streptozotocin + Cyclophosphamide	Streptozotocin + 5-FU
Small bowel	7/19 (37%)	8/18 (44%)
Lung	0/10	2/7 (29%)
All others	5/18 (28%)	4/17 (24%)
All cases	12/47 (26%)	14/42 (33%)

PHASE II STUDY - PREVIOUSLY TREATED PATIENTS

	Cyclophosphamide	5-FU
All cases	0/8	2/11 (18%)

disease susceptible to chemotherapeutic approaches and continued investigation of the therapy of these neoplasms should be strongly encouraged.

SURGICAL ADJUVANT TRIALS IN GASTROINTESTINAL CARCINOMA

All completed and reported surgical adjuvant trials in gastrointestinal carcinoma conducted by currently active grant funded Cooperative Groups have been those of the VASAG, although other Cooperative Groups currently have such studies in progress. The studies of the VASAG will be reported in more detail in a separate report dealing with surgical activities of the Cooperative Groups. Only a brief summary will be offered here.

SURGICAL ADJUVANT TRIALS IN GASTRIC CARCINOMA

In gastric carcinoma the VASAG first evaluated Thiotepa given intra-peritoneally at surgery and intravenously on the first and second postoperative days.[1] In this study, involving 305 patients with curative resections, the early operative mortality for the treated group was significantly worse than for the controls - more than doubled. There was no significant difference in five-year survival between treatment and control groups. The second gastric surgical adjuvant study involved the use of FUDR in small dosage on postoperative days 1, 2, and 3 and in a more standard loading course beginning on the 35th day postoperatively.[7] In this study there was no difference in operative mortality between treated and control patients. Twenty-six percent of the treated patients showed leukopenia. Among 276 curative resections randomized to this study there was no significant difference in survival between treated and control patients. Utilizing data accrued from both of these studies the VASAG was able to obtain some quite authoritative data regarding prognostic factors. Those factors which had an adverse effect on survival at a p < .05 level were positive lymph nodes, adjacent organ involvement, posterior wall location of the primary lesion, serosal penetration, linitis plastica, resection of esophagus, and blood vessel invasion.

SURGICAL ADJUVANT TRIALS IN COLORECTAL CANCER

The initial surgical adjuvant trial of the VASAG in colorectal cancer involved the use of Thiotepa as described above for gastric carcinoma. The potential hazards of ineffective surgical adjuvant chemotherapy are clearly illustrated by this trial in which five-year survival was significantly better in control patients than in treated patients.[3] Subsequently, the VASAG has conducted three surgical adjuvant trials in colon cancer employing the fluorinated pyrimidines administered intravenously. One of these evaluated 5-FU given in a five-day course beginning on the fourteenth postoperative day and a second course initiated at six weeks.[16] One hundred sixty-five patients were entered into the treatment arm and 173 patients into the untreated control arm. A total of 7 percent of patients on the treated arm experienced leukopenia. There was no increase in postoperative complications and there was no significant difference in five-year survivorship between treatment and control arms.

The second trial involved two courses of FUDR, the first given on postoperative days 1, 2, and 3 and the second beginning on day 35 with five daily full doses followed by four doses given on alternate days.[5] The overall drug toxicity was not stated in the report but six of the treated patients were known to have died from drug toxicity. Survival curves of 276 treated patients and 273 controls were essentially identical. The third VASAG fluorinated pyrimidine surgical adjuvant trial involved five-day courses of 5-FU initiated 14 days postoperatively and repeated every six to eight weeks for 18 months.[16] In this trial the incidence of leukopenia was not stated but there was no increase in postoperative mortality. Two hundred fifty-seven patients were entered into treatment arm and 261 patients were entered into the control arm. There was no significant difference in five-year survival.

Whereas one may obtain statistical significance by adding up selected groups within each of these three fluorinated pyrimidine surgical adjuvant trials, it would seem appropriate to state that not one of the studies demonstrated a significant survival advantage associated with either 5-FU or FUDR therapy.

A fifth VASAG study of considerable interest is the evaluation of preoperative radiation therapy for rectal carcinoma.[26] This was a randomized study involving either no preoperative treatment or pre-operative radiation administered at a total dosage between 2,000 and 2,500 rads with surgery performed as soon as possible after completion of radiation therapy. A total of 700 patients were randomized to study. The resectability rate was equal in both groups. Four hundred fifty-three patients had curative resections. As in other uncontrolled preoperative radiation therapy studies, this controlled evaluation showed a definite reduction in positive regional lymph nodes in patients who had received radiation therapy when compared to the control group. Among patients who had curative resections the five-year survival for preoperative radiation was 48.5 percent and for untreated controls 39 percent. In further analysis of their data, it was found that the survival advantage was accrued only by patients who had AP resections. There was no difference in survival amongst patients who had other surgical procedures.

In the only other randomized study of this approach the New York Memorial Group found no evidence of therapeutic benefit for preoperative radiation.[31] The design of the VASAG study, however, would seem to be much cleaner than that of the New York Memorial Study which "randomized" on the basis of birth dates and thereby allowed knowledge of treatment arm assignment before the patient was entered on study. At this time it would be considered likely that preoperative radiation for rectal carcinoma does indeed produce significant benefit for patients. These results have stimulated a number of other studies involving both preoperative and postoperative radiation, and it is hoped that confirmation of these favorable results will soon be forthcoming. The VASAG has initiated a second study involving a larger preoperative radiation therapy dose of 3,150 rads administered over 24 days. At this time they have seen no increase in postoperative complications and a comparable reduction in regional node involvement to that observed in their first study. Followup is not, as yet, sufficiently complete to indicate any therapeutic results.

Utilizing their large patient population entered into colorectal cancer surgical adjuvant trials, the VASAG has conducted an extensive analysis of prognostic factors.   Those factors which they found to produce a significantly unfavorable effect on survival are the following: Previous decompression operation, primary rectal lesion, technical complications at surgery, serosal penetration, blood vessel invasion, lymphatic invasion, postitive lymph nodes, and cancer involving other organs.

CONCLUSIONS

In viewing the overall results of gastrointestinal cancer studies conducted by the currently active Cooperative Groups, it appears that little, if anything, of substantial value has been accomplished for patients with major types of advanced and metastatic diseases. Specifically, no evidence has been presented of any survival gain with chemotherapy of advanced and metastatic colorectal adenocarcinoma, pancreatic adenocarcinoma, and gastric adenocarcinoma. A more optimistic note may be sounding with regard to hepatocellular carcinoma. Here, adriamycin appears to produce an overall survival gain in African patients with hepatoma and adriamcyin as well as 5-FU nitrosourea combinations seem to produce a similar survival gain for American patients with hepatoma. Very high rates of response in patients with carcinoid tumor may also indicate a potentially fruitful area for future investigation.   In surgical adjuvant treatment of gastric cancer, approaches with both Thiotepa and one of the fluorinated pyrimidines, FUDR, have been unequivocal failures. For colorectal cancer any evidence of true therapeutic benefit from previous approaches must be considered highly equivocal.   In rectal carcinoma there is strongly suggestive evidence that preoperative radiation therapy is clinically tolerable and increases cure rates in patients undergoing anterior resections. Gastrointestinal cancer remains a major challenge for the Cooperative Groups, and it would seem evident that more innovative approaches than those applied in the past will be required before any major therapeutic accomplishment can be anticipated.

1.   VA Cooperative Surgical Adjuvant Study Group: Use of Thiotepa as an adjuvant to the surgical management of carcinoma of the stomach. Cancer 18:291-297, 1965.

2.   Eastern Cooperative Group in Solid Tumor Chemotherapy: Comparison of antimetabolites in the treatment of breast and colon cancer. JAMA 200:770-778, 1967.

3.   Dwight RW, Higgins GA, Keehn RJ: Factors influencing survival after resection in cancer of the colon and rectum. Am J Surg 117:512-522, 1969.

4.   Gailani S, Holland JF, Falkson G, Leone L, Burningham R, Larsen V: Comparison of treatment of metastatic gastrointestinal cancer with 5-Fluorouracil (5-FU) to a combination of 5-FU with cytosine arabinoside. Cancer 29:1308-1313, 1972.

5.   Dwight RW, Humphrey EW, Higgins GA, Keehn RJ: FUDR as an adjuvant to surgery in cancer of the large bowel. J Surg Oncol 5: 243-248, 1973.

6.   Horton J, Mittelman A, Taylor SG, Jurkowitz L, Bennett JM, Ezdinli E, Colsky J, Hanley JA: Phase II trials with procarbazine, streptozotocin, 6-thioguanine, and CCNU in patients with metastatic cancer of the large bowel. Cancer Chemother Rep 59:333-340, 1975.

7.   Higgins GA, Serlin O, Amadeo JH, McElhinney J, Keehn J: Gastric cancer. Factors in survival. Chir Gastroenterol 10:393-398, 1976.

8.   Baker LH, Talley RW, Matter R, Lehane DE, Ruffner BW, Jones SE, Morrison FS, Stephens RL, Gehan EA, Vaitkevicius VK: Phase III comparison of the treatment of advanced gastrointestinal cancer with bolus weekly 5-FU versus methyl CCNU plus bolus weekly 5-FU. Cancer 38:1-7, 1976.

9.   Moertel CG, Mittelman JA, Bakemeier, RF, Engstrom P, Hanley J: Sequential and combination chemotherapy of advanced gastric cancer. Cancer 38:678-682, 1976.

10. Douglass HO, MacIntyre JM, Evans JT, Kaufman J, Carbone PP: Methyl CCNU plus β-2'-deoxythioguanosine versus VP-16 or diglycoaldehyde in advanced previously treated colorectal adenocarcinoma: A Phase II study of the ECOG. ASCO 18:313, 1977.

11. Vogel CL, Bayley AC, Brooker RJ, Anthony PP, Ziegler JL: A Phase II study of adriamycin in patients with hepatocellular carcinoma from Zambia and the United States. Cancer 39:1923-1929, 1977.

12. Serlin O, Keehn RJ, Higgins GA, Harrower HW, Mendeloff GL: Factors related to survival following resection for gastric carcinoma. Cancer 40:1318-1329, 1977.

13. Moertel CG, Douglass HO, Hanley J, Carbone PP: Phase II study of methyl CCNU in the treatment of advanced pancreatic carcinoma. Cancer Treat Rep 60:1659-1661, 1976.

14. Baker LH, Saiki JH, Jones SE, Hewlett JS, Brownlee RW, Stephens RL, Vaitkevicius VK: Adriamycin and 5-Fluorouracil in the treatment of advanced hepatoma: A Southwest Oncology Group study. Cancer Treat Rep 61:1595-1597, 1977.

15. Moertel CG, Douglass HO, Hanley J, Carbone PP: Treatment of advanced adenocarcinoma of the pancreas with combinations of streptozotocin plus 5-Fluorouracil and streptozotocin plus cyclophosphamide. Cancer 40:605-608, 1977.

16. Higgins GA, Lee LE, Dwight RW, Keehn RS: The case for adjuvant 5-Fluorouracil in colorectal cancer. Cancer Clin Trials Spring:35-41, 1978.

17. Buroker T, Kim PN, Heilbrun L, Vaitkevicius V: 5-FU infusion with mitomycin-C versus 5-FU infusion with methyl CCNU in the treatment of advanced upper gastrointestinal cancer. A Phase III Study. ASCO 19:310, 1978.

18. Perry MC, White L, Kardinal C: 5-Fluorouracil, methyl CCNU, and daunomycin in advanced colorectal adenocarcinoma. ASCO 19:328, 1978.

19. Engstrom P, MacIntyre J, Douglass H, Carbone PP: Combination chemotherapy of advanced bowel cancer. ASCO 19:384, 1978.

20. Moertel CG, Hanley JA: Combination chemotherapy trials for metastatic carcinoid tumor. ASCO 19:322, 1978.

21. Buroker T, Kim PN, Groppe C, et al: 5-FU infusion with mitomycin-C versus 5-FU infusion with methyl CCNU in the treatment of advanced colon cancer. Cancer 42:1228-1233, 1978.

22. Falkson G, Lavin P, Moertel CG, Pretorius FJ, Carbone PP: Chemotherapy studies in primary liver cancer. A prospective randomized clinical trial. Cancer 42:2149-2156, 1978.

23. Moertel CG, Lavin PT, Engstrom P, Gelber RO, Carbone PP: 5-FU, nitrosourea, and "Lactone": Chemotherapy of gastric and pancreatic cancer - A controlled evaluation of combinations. Surgery, 85:509-514, 1979.

24. Douglass HO, Lavin PT, Woll J, Conroy JF, Carbone PP: Chemotherapy of advanced measurable colon and rectal carcinoma with oral 5-Fluorouracil, alone or in combination with cyclophosphamide or thioguanine, with intravenous 5-Fluorouracil or β-2'-deoxythioguanosine or with oral 3(4-methyl-cyclohexyl)-1(2-chorethyl)-1-nitrosourea: A Phase II-III Study of ECOG (EST-4273). Cancer, 42:2538-2545, 1978.

25. Haut A, Talley RW: 5-Fluorouracil and azapicyl in the treatment of adenocarcinoma of the stomach, colon, and rectum. Unpublished.

26. Higgins GA, Humphrey EW, Amadeo JH, Juler GL: Preoperative radiotherapy for colorectal cancer. Unpublished.

27. Hynes HE, Vaitkevicius VK, O'Bryan RM, Vaughn CB: Phase II trial of dianhydrogalactitol in patients with advanced gastrointestinal cancer. Unpublished.

28. Moertel CG, Lavin PT: Phase II-III chemotherapy studies in advanced gastric cancer. Unpublished.

29. Ansfield FJ, Kiotz J, Nealon T, Ramirez G, Minton J, Hill G, Wilson W, Davis H, Correll G: A Phase III study comparing the clinical utility of four regimens of 5-Fluorouracil. Cancer 39:34-41, 1977.

30. Waddell WR: Chemotherapy for carcinoma of the pancreas. Surgery 74:420-429, 1973.

31. Stearns MW, Deddish MR, Quan SH, Learning RH: Preoperative Roentgen therapy for cancer of the rectum and rectosigmoid. Surg Gynecol & Obstet 138:584-589, 1974.

10

Genitourinary cancer

William L. Caldwell, Lawrence Einhorn, and Ronald L. Stephens

To date studies of genitourinary cancer by the Cooperative Groups have been relatively limited. It is not entirely clear why the Cooperative Group activity in this field has not been more extensive, but there are several possible reasons:

1) Chemotherapy regimens have been relatively ineffective for most genitourinary tumors until recently.

2) Only recently have the Groups become multidisciplinary and even now there is not adequate multidisciplinary input into protocol design.

3) Most genitourinary tumors are seen by urologists and radiotherapists; it is oftentimes difficult to get agreement about the suitability of protocols within one discipline and between participants of two disciplines the problem is magnified two-fold. The increased interest in participation of medical oncologists in the GU patients may actually introduce some crystallization of opinions with a better acceptance of protocol studies than in the past.

4) Genitourinary Task Forces (e.g. bladder, prostate, renal) are engaged in studies which may make urologists less interested in studies which deviate from those of the Task Forces.

For regionally localized tumors improved radiotherapy techniques, which include fast neutron therapy, proton, helium, heavy particle and pi meson therapy, hypoxic cell sensitizers (e.g. misonidazole) and irradiation, hyperthermia and irradiation, hyperfractionated irradiation techniques, and irradiation integrated with resection, all show promise in pilot studies and are being evaluated in several Cooperative Groups. The goals of these studies are to establish treatment approaches which result in a higher local control rate, possibly even with the added benefit of reduced treatment-related morbidity. Some of these protocols currently utilize adjuvant chemotherapy. If an enhanced local control rate is demonstrated, then the role of adjuvant chemotherapy certainly will have to be evaluated since disseminated disease will then become a significant management problem.

The recent demonstration of the activity of cis-platinum in metastatic bladder cancer and the evidence showing potential value for cytolytic chemotherapy in prostate cancer has spurred renewed interest in these previously "chemoresistant" tumors. Although several original successful chemotherapy trials in testicular cancer were single institution studies, it is the task of the Cooperative Groups to confirm these positive studies and to demonstrate regimens that are maximally effective without producing unnecessary toxicity. Also, the question of the need for maintenance chemotherapy can be studied. It is unlikely any single institution can answer the important questions that remain in testicular cancer as well as a well-designed Cooperative Group or intergroup study can.

It is not anticipated that more radical operative approaches will be devised. More likely there will be a reduction in the extent of resections as the effectiveness of other modalities increases. Integrated therapy consisting of resection, irradiation, and chemotherapy will be more frequently utilized in many patients. The need for multidisciplined evaluation of such patients presumably will be demonstrated in some of the ongoing and many of the proposed studies.

In the following section the major current problems which persist for the various tumor types will be discussed. The approaches of the Cooperative Groups in addressing these questions will be considered by indicating ongoing as well as planned studies.

BLADDER CANCER

Superficial tumors, particularly when multiple or recurrent, present difficult problems for urologists who would like to be conservative in the management. The measures to delay or prevent recurrences more effective than thio-TEPA or other drugs currently in use, must be sought and evaluated. For example, 13-cis-retinoic acid shows considerable promise and should be evaluated in Cooperative Group studies; it is being used in a Bladder Study Group protocol. If such drugs are shown to be effective, subsets of patients which benefit need to be identified.

The more aggressive tumors (either high grade tumors or those with deep muscle involvement -- clinical Stages B_2 and C) are currently treated in this country with integrated therapy (usually with the irradiation being utilized preoperatively) in patients suitable for cystectomy; those who are over 65 to 70 years of age or with medical contraindications for cystectomy are usually irradiated. The controversies regarding integrated therapy are as follows: 1) the dose of irradiation, 2) the timing of the irradiation, and 3) the volume irradiated.

As part of an integrated therapy program preoperative irradiation has been utilized most frequently and continues to be the most common approach based on the benefits derived according to numerous literature reports.[1] Nevertheless, postoperative irradiation is not an unreasonable approach as well; the extent of disease can be better assessed, there is no delay before cystectomy which permits subsequently a more conventional irradiation dose and fractionation without distressing the urologists, and there are no treatment-related urinary symptoms or signs during the irradiation. An RTOG pilot study which utilizes both pre- and postoperative irradiation has almost concluded accruing patients; the pelvis is irradiated to 500 rad in a single dose the day before cystectomy and then two to three weeks after cystectomy a dose of 4,500 rad/5 weeks to the pelvis concludes the treatment.

Irradiation field sizes as part of integrated therapy vary in reported series from 10x10 cm to as large as 15x15 cm or even larger. Since irradiation probably is effective by virtue of eradicating small foci of tumor in the pelvis not removed at the time of cystectomy, it would seem necessary to irradiate this volume at risk. Fields of at least 14x12 cm are required to achieve this.

Of special interest to radiotherapists is the question whether or not continuous therapy or split course therapy is to be preferred. This was investigated in detail for five different disease sites in more than 600 patients.[2] Preliminary results for bladder cancer show no large differences in the severity of the reactions to the treatments and no significant difference in median survival, which is approximately nine months.

An important finding of the reports relating to integrated therapy is that patients so treated are more at risk of having their first recurrence by a manifestation of systemic disease rather than a local or regional recurrence (which is the case with either modality alone). An effective systemic adjuvant regimen is needed to impact further on the survival rate of these patients. The Groups are planning protocols to evaluate adjuvant chemotherapy with cis-platinum, adriamycin, and cytoxan in patients treated with preoperative irradiation and cystectomy.

The most effective cancer chemotherapeutic agents for transitional cell cancer of the bladder are adriamycin and cis-platinum. A dose response study of adriamycin was completed in 65 patients, and with doses ranging from 25 mg/M^2 to 50 mg/M^2 only 3 of 41 patients showed a response.[3] At 60 mg/M^2 there were 2 of 7 (29 percent) responses, and at 75 mg/M^2 the Group saw 6 of 17 (35 percent) responses for an overall response rate of 33.3 percent at these two dose levels.

Cis-diamminedichloroplatinum (cis-platinum) has considerable side effects and its nephrotoxicity causes special consideration in the management of genitourinary malignancies. Prehydration and treatment with mannitol are strongly advised. Rossof et al gave the cumulative data on reported responses in 52 patients.[4] There were 2 complete and 18 partial remissions for an overall response rate of 38.5 percent. A dose of 75 mg/M^2 was given every 3 weeks.

One Cooperative Group recently completed a randomized trial of adriamycin alone at 50 mg/M^2 every 3 weeks and adriamycin at the same dose on day 1 plus cis-platinum at 50 mg/M^2 on day 2. Renal toxicity was not a major problem in this study.[5] The response rate with adriamycin alone was 16.7 percent (8 of 48) and with the combination 33.3 percent (13 of 39). This difference in response rates was not translated in a difference in survival, which was 27 weeks.

The efficacy of 3 drugs, cyclophosphamide, 500 mg/M^2, adriamycin 50 mg/M^2 and cis-platinum 40 mg/M^2, was reported in 10 patients with metastatic disease.[6] There were 4 responses lasting 4 to 9 months. The range of the WBC nadirs was 300-7,100/mm^3 and of the platelet nadirs it was 39,000-392,000/mm.^{3} This combination, but with slightly different dosages, has also been reported by Troner.[7] In 42 eligible patients there were 8 responses for 19 percent. Median duration of response was 24 weeks.

PROSTATE CANCER

In the past decade new data regarding the natural history of cancer of the prostate, derived primarily from the VA trials, has impacted on its management. The hazards of elective DES therapy (5 mg po/day), the relatively good prognosis of patients who are treated only on definite indication (the placebo groups), and the derivation of the Gleason classification are some of the recent contributions to knowledge about prostate cancer. It is possible that subsets of patients can be identified who can be managed more conservatively than at the present time.

Also during the last decade interest has developed in implantation of the prostate with seeds of 125-I or 198-Au. This approach has been either in conjunction with radical lymphadenectomy as a definitive procedure or as a method of boosting the irradiation dose to the prostate with external irradiation being used to treat the regional lymphatics and lymph nodes. There has been no comparison of these techniques to date. One Group is at present enrolling patients in Phase III studies which evaluate conservative versus wide-field irradiation techniques for patients with clinical Stage B or C disease.

Traditionally, therapy for metastatic prostate cancer has consisted of DES and/or bilateral orchiectomy. Despite unquestionable and often dramatic subjective improvement with hormonal therapy, there has not been concomitant prolongation of survival.

Cyclophosphamide was considered the only worthwhile chemotherapeutic agent until adriamycin was investigated.[8,9] With adriamycin no responses were observed in 24 patients who received 50 mg/M^2 or less, but there were 14 partial responses amongst 54 patients (26 percent) treated with 60 or 75 mg/M^2 (Table 1). Cis-platinum at a dose of 75 mg/M^2 every three weeks resulted in 4 partial remissions in 21 patients with metastatic disease.[4] Other single agents such as streptozotocin, DTIC, procarbazine and hydroxyurea appear to have little efficacy. 5-Fluorouracil has a low level of activity.

Three trials with combination chemotherapy have been completed. Cyclophosphamide plus 5-FU resulted in 2 of 12 remissions,[10] while

TABLE 1
Efficacy of Single Agents in Patients With Advanced Prostatic Cancer

DRUG	PATIENTS	CR+PR	IMPROVED +STABLE	REFERENCES
Cyclophosphamide	53	4	18	8,9
Streptozotocin	41	-	10	8
DTIC	25	2	8	8
Procarbazine	20	-	5	8
5-FU	59	5	-	8
cis-Platinum	21	4	NG	4
Adriamycin				
25-50 mg/M^2	24	-	NG	3,10
60-75 mg/M^2	54	14	NG	3,10,11
Hydroxyurea	68	1	10	12

cytoxan + adriamycin had 4 responses and 23 improvements in 66 patients.[12] One Group studied the combination of adriamycin, BCNU and cyclophosphamide.[13] In 24 patients there were 7 responses and 3 improvements. These responses have, in general, lasted up to one year.

TESTICULAR CANCER

Effective management of Stages I and II pure seminomas is well established and although controversy persists as to the use of postorchiectomy radiation or of retroperitoneal lymphadenectomy, it is generally recognized that either therapy will result in a 5-year survival of over 90 percent of the patients. Initial presentation as Stage III disease is rare. This, as well as relapse after initial therapy, will benefit from an intergroup study.

Several controversies exist regarding the treatment of germ cell tumors. These include: 1) the accuracy of clinical staging, 2) most appropriate management of the regional lymph nodes (particularly in those with clinical Stage I or IIA disease), 3) the role of adjuvant chemotherapy in patients with Stage II disease, and 4) the best adjuvant and definitive chemotherapy regimen (including the role of maintenance therapy). The first and third questions are likely to be answered by the recently activated intergroup testicular protocol.

A study conducted at the Walter Reed General Hospital included patients with embryonal carcinoma, teratoma or teratocarcinoma alone or in combination with seminoma or choriocarcinoma.[14] Treatment consisted of orchiectomy followed by radiation to the drainage lymphatics of the testis or of radiation followed by orchiectomy plus lymphadenectomy and finally additional irradiation. The 3-year disease-free survival was 86 percent and 97 percent respectively for Stage I disease, 82 percent and 81 percent for Stage II disease. These results and those of other studies which show less favorable results in Stage II disease, indicate the need for additional chemotherapy in Stage II disease especially since favorable results have been obtained in Stage III disease.

Jacobs and Muggia have recently published a most comprehensive report of the role of chemotherapy in testicular cancer and the reader is referred to their article.[15] The most active single agents are cisplatinum, vinblastine, actinomycin-D and bleomycin. Nearly all combination chemotherapy trials conducted in the sixties contained actinomycin-D and resulted in 7 to 43 percent complete remissions. Bleomycin and vinblastine were added between 1970 and 1975. This led to an improvement in the overall response rates with 2 of every 3 patients achieving a remission. The complete remission rates also improved.   When cis-platinum and adriamycin were added the new combinations are produced objective response rates approaching 100 percent and CR rates in the range of 60 to 80 percent: The scope of this chapter does not permit a detailed report of the many studies which led to this significant advance.   Major contributors and a few representative references are Einhorn[16], investigators at Memorial Sloan-Kettering Cancer Center[17], as well as the Cooperative Groups[18-19]

RENAL CELL CARCINOMA

Surgical excision is still the only treatment for cure of renal cell carcinoma.   Postoperative irradiation has not been effective and although preoperative radiotherapy may decrease local recurrence it has not improved the five-year survival.   Identification of an effective chemotherapy regimen is a primary need for managing this cancer. However, no agent is at present capable of significantly altering the course of metastatic disease.

DeKernion and Berry[20] did not find a single objective response amongst 110 patients treated with progestational agents.   Although an occasional response is seen, it remains the anecdotal case.   Vinblastine has resulted in a few remissions, but adriamycin has been a disappointment,[3] 2 of 38 responses, and cis-platinum has equally poor activity[4]

One Cooperative Group has completed two large trials.   The first consisted of 165 patients who were evaluable for determining an objective tumor response.[20] Vinblastine alone gave 4 of 44 responses, methyl CCNU had 2 of 45 responses, vinblastine plus depo-provera saw only 3 of 38 decreases in tumor size and methyl CCNU + depo-provera resulted in 4 of 38 remissions. These responses were all of short duration.   The second study demonstrated very low orders of response for megestrol acetate, VP16-213, cyclophosphamide and galactitol[21]

This failure to find any active agent remains the major stumbling block in making a further impact on the treatment of renal cell carcinoma.

REFERENCES

1. Caldwell WL: Symposium on uroepithelial tumors - radiotherapy: Definitive, integrated and palliative therapy. Urol Clin N Amer 3:129-148, 1975.
2. RTOG, minutes. January 1979.
3. O'Bryan RM, Baker LH, Gottlieb JE, Rivkin SE, Balcerzak SP, Grumet GN, Salmon SE, Moon TE and Hoogstraten B: Dose response evaluation of adriamycin in human neoplasia. Cancer 39:1940-1948, 1977.
4. Rossof AH, Talley RW, Stephens R, Thigpen T, Samson MK, Groppe C, Eyre HJ and Fisher R: Phase II evaluation of cis-dichlorodiammineplatinum (II) in advanced malignancies of the genitourinary and gynecologic organs: A Southwest Oncology Group study. Cancer Treat Rep 63:1557-1564, 1979.
5. SWOG, Progress Report 1977 - 1979.
6. Troner M, Hemstreet G: Cyclophosphamide, adriamycin and cis-platinum (CAP) chemotherapy of metastatic transitional cell carcinoma (TCC) of the bladder. AACR 19:161, 1978.
7. Troner MB: Cyclophosphamide, adriamycin and platinum (CAP) in the treatment of urothelial malignancy. AACR 20:117, 1979.
8. Johnson DE, Scott WW, Gibbons RP, Prout GR, Schmidt JD, Chu TM, Gaeta J, Saroff J, Murphy GP: National randomized study of chemotherapeutic agents in advanced prostatic carcinoma: A progress report. Cancer Treat Rep 61:317-323, 1977.
9. Scott WW, Gibbons RP, Johnson DE, Prout GR, Schmidt JD, Saroff J, Murphy GP: The continued evaluation of the effects of chemotherapy in patients with advanced carcinoma of the prostate. J Urol 116:211-213, 1976.
10. Eagan RT, Hahn RG, Myers RP: Adriamycin versus 5-Fluorouracil and cyclophosphamide in the treatment of metastatic prostatic cancer. Cancer Treat Rep 60:115-117, 1976.
11. DeWys WD, Bauer M, Colsky J, Cooper RA, Creech R, Carbone PP: Comparative trial of adriamycin and 5-Fluorouracil in advanced prostatic cancer - progress report. Cancer Treat Rep 61:325-328, 1977.
12. SWOG, Minutes. October 1979.
13. van Amburg AL, Presant CA, Klahr C: Chemotherapy of advanced prostatic cancer with adriamycin, BCNU and cyclophosphamide. ASCO 20:321, 1979.
14. Maier JG, Mittemeyer B: Carcinoma of the testis. Cancer 39:981-986, 1977.
15. Jacobs EM, Muggia FM: Testicular cancer: Risk factors and the role of adjuvant chemotherapy. Cancer 45:1782-1790, 1980.
16. Einhorn LH, Donohue J: Cis-diamminedichloroplatinum, vinblastine and bleomycin combination chemotherapy in disseminated testicular cancer. Ann Int Med 87:293-298, 1977.
17. Cvitkovic E, Cheng E, Whitmore WF, Golbey RB: Germ cell tumor chemotherapy update. ASCO 18:324, 1977.
18. Samson MK, Stephens RL, Rivkin S, Opipari M, Maloney T, Groppe CW and Fisher R: Vinblastine, bleomycin and cis-dichlorodiammineplatinum (II) in disseminated testicular cancer: Preliminary report of a Southwest Oncology Group study. Cancer Treat Rep 63:1663-1667, 1979.
19. Blom J, Brodovsky HS: Comparison of the treatment of metastatic testicular tumors with actinomycin D or actinomycin D, bleomycin and vincristine. ASCO 17:290, 1976.
20. Hahn RG, Temkin NR, Savlov ED, Perlia C, Wampler GL, Horton J, Marsh J, Carbone PP: Phase II study of vinblastine, methyl CCNU and medroxyprogesterone in advanced renal cell cancer. Cancer Treat Rep 62:1093-1095, 1978.
21. Hahn RG, Bauer M, Wolter J, Creech R, Bennett JM, Wampler G: Phase II study of single-agent therapy with megestrol acetate, VP16-213, cyclophosphamide and dianhydrogalactitol in advanced renal cell cancer. Cancer Treat Rep 63:513-515, 1979.

11

Gynecologic cancer

George C. Lewis, Jr., Robert Slayton, Joseph Newall, and Robert Hilgers

INTRODUCTION

During the 20-year period, 1958 to 1978, clinical investigation in gynecologic cancer has expanded significantly. From 1958 to 1963, eighteen patients were entered into a handful of protocols, most of these dealing with solid tumors on a Phase II basis. From 1963 to 1968 a total of 827 entered protocols; 1,334 were studied in the next 5-year period; and from 1973 to 1978 no less than 6,335 patients were entered. This increase in interest in gynecologic malignancy is related to expanded multispecialty participation in Cooperative Group investigations and also reflects the recognition that gynecologic cancer constitutes a significant segment of all malignancies encountered in clinical practice. It should be noted that the American Cancer Society estimates the number of new malignancies for pelvic genital organs in females will exceed 69,000 per annum in 1978. Genital organ malignancies represent the third largest site for malignancy exceeded only by breast and all digestive organs combined. Large bowel, lung and ovarian cancer account for the three highest mortalities. The total mortalities for genital cancer is 22,500 per annum. Today, one out of every five women who get cancer will have a genital malignancy, excluding nonmelanoma skin cancer and carcinoma in situ of the uterine cervix. One out of every eight women with cancer will die of uterine or ovarian cancer. The American Cancer Society estimates that of the 49 million women currently 35 years of age or older, 700,000 will eventually develop cancer of the endometrium.

One might conclude with this background that a significant segment of Cooperative Group research has been devoted to gynecologic cancer over the past twenty years. This has not been the case, but the reasons are not readily apparent. Pelvic cancer has a long history of effective management by radiation and/or surgery. The 1940 to 1960 period saw the introduction of many technical improvements - transfusions, cytology, megavoltage equipment, etc. The application of these improvements to standard therapy reduced the pressure for research into new or different methods of treatment. In contrast, for the leukemias and in most solid tumors, there were no effective means for control. The Groups organized in the 1950's and 1960's saw these areas as their primary objectives.

A review of progress reports and minutes of Cooperative Group meetings revealed that initially gynecologic malignancy was handled in broad Phase II studies together with other malignancies, generally advanced or recurrent and not always identified as to origin. Because of this, it is difficult to accurately specify how many gynecologic malignancies were involved. There were a few, mostly cervical and ovarian in origin. The first gynecologic cooperative study was conducted from 1963 to 1968 by the Endometrial Adjuvant Study Group. In a trial involving over 700 patients, the Group found that adjuvant therapy with medroxyprogesterone acetate was no more effective than placebo following surgery and radiotherapy in Stage I disease. More importantly, the trial showed that practicing surgeons could collaborate with other physicians outside their own institution.

Between the 1960's and early 1970's, a few Phase III and Phase II trials involving gynecologic malignancy were developed by other Groups. Groups that initially concentrated on leukemia trials set up Solid Tumor

TABLE 1
Cooperative Group Protocols and Patient Entries
By Site of Malignancy; 1958-1978

SITE	# PROTOCOLS	# PATIENTS ENTERED BY NON-GYN GROUPS	# PATIENTS ENTERED BY GYN GROUPS	TOTAL # PATIENTS
Cervix	49	683	1944	2627
Ovary	74	1513	1788	3301
Tube	1	3	0	3
Uterus	35	221	2288**	2509
Vagina	2	2	0	2
Vulva	5	1	65	66
Gynecologic Site Not Specified	11	1	11	12
TOTAL	177	2424	6096	8520

Committees and conducted studies that included gynecologic tumors. These were expanded into disease-oriented committees, such as genito-urinary, gastrointestinal, breast, etc. Eventually some disease-oriented committees separated the Urologic Study Committees from the Gyne-cologic Study Committees. In 1970, a group specifically limited to gynecologic malignancy was formed, called the Gynecologic Oncology Group. The net result for all the Groups in the twenty-year period was the appearance of a variety of studies in all the areas of gynecologic oncology (Table 1).

To date, 135 protocols have been activated that included gynecologic patients, either partially or entirely (Table 2). Eight thousand five hundred and twenty patients have been entered and approximately 5,879 patients are evaluable. Most of the therapeutic procedures involved in protocols are for ovarian cancer. At least 103 protocols involve such malignancies, followed by 101 protocols divided almost evenly between endometrium and cervix. Eleven studies involve small numbers of vaginal, vulval, and tubal malignancies. Most studies involved drugs. Sixteen studies involved radiation, 8 surgery, and 6 pathology-cytology.

In the earlier studies, gynecologic cases were "also ran" cases. They were managed in essentially single modality, nongynecologic groups. With the addition of Genitourinary Committees and the establishment of Gynecologic Committees, general groups have become more multi-

TABLE 2
Number of Gynecologic Protocols and Patients Entered
by Cooperative Groups; 1958-1978

GROUP	# PROTOCOLS	# PATIENTS ENTERED	# PATIENTS EVALUATED
CALGB	7	92	92
ECSG	1	5	5
COG	3	58	41
ECOG	19*	1078	857
NCOG	2	6	---
RTOG	4*	220	170
SECSG	10	109	109
SWOG	24	817	663
WOG	5	39	38
EAG	1	700	525
GOG	59*	5396	3379
TOTAL	135	8520	5879

* Total Includes One Study Shared; Patients Counted Under Group Entered

disciplinary. To date, 11 Cooperative Groups, (Table 2), 8 of whom are still active, have activated protocols that include gynecologic patients. Three Groups have shared a gynecologic study of Stage II ovarian cancer. Liaison in gynecologic studies has been conducted or is being explored by six Groups.

The eight Groups have alone or together expanded from an occasional study, incidentally including gynecologic oncology 20 years ago, to over 40 studies currently devoted to the specialty. Multidisciplinary participation has received an increased emphasis. It is now possible to say that all stages and all cell types of gynecologic malignancy are receiving attention. While advanced ovarian cancer held most of the initial attention, the scope of work is now being broadened to include early ovarian cancer, endometrial lesions, cervical cancer and other lesions in significant numbers. This report describes the past and present efforts of Cooperative Groups in gynecologic oncology presented by the site of origin of the disease.

ADENOCARCINOMA OF THE OVARY

TRIALS INVOLVING SURGERY, CHEMOTHERAPY, RADIOTHERAPY AND IMMUNOTHERAPY

Ovarian cancer is a common malignancy, and is usually lethal. Successful treatment depends on accurate staging and the development of more effective cytotoxic agents whether they be chemical agents, forms of ionizing radiation or immune adjuvants. Localized disease is uncommon and is rarely encountered in large referral centers. Thus, the role of adjuvant therapy in the high-risk patient with early disease must be evaluated in a controlled cooperative clinical trial. The effectiveness of debulking surgery has been demonstrated in advanced disease but a large number of new agents remain to be tested, alone and in combination following reductive surgery. Only the Cooperative Group Program provides an adequate number of patients to conduct controlled trials, and investigators sufficiently aware of the importance of careful protocol design to test new methods of treatment.

SINGLE MODALITY

Early Disease - FIGO Stages I-II

In a trial designed to evaluate the role of adjuvant therapy in Stage IA and IB ovarian cancer, Hreshchyshyn et al[1] found fewer failures in the group receiving melphalan therapy (Table 3). No benefit was observed in the group receiving pelvic radiation. Cyst rupture and high tumor grade were unfavorable risk factors. Attachment to adjacent structures, and tumor size greater than 10 cm were also unfavorable factors, but a statistically significant difference could not be established.

TABLE 3
Adjuvant Therapy in Early Disease

	Number of Failures/At Risk	Percent
Observation	5/29	17.2%
Radiation Therapy (5,000 rads midpelvis)	7/23	30.4%
Melphalan 0.2 mg/kg x 5 days q 4 weeks x 18	2/34	5.8%

In an attempt to define more precisely the risk of failure in Stage I ovarian cancer, and to assess the value of adjuvant melphalan therapy in patients with low grade tumors, a protocol was designed requiring panhysterectomy, bilateral salpingo-oophorectomy and a staging procedure which includes partial omentectomy, multiple peritoneal biopsies, biopsy of suspicious paraaortic lymph nodes and cytologic examination of peritoneal fluid. This trial will include untreated controls.

Another trial compares melphalan and intraperitoneal radioactive phosphorus in patients with high grade Stage I tumors and in Stage II disease, and compares melphalan alone with melphalan plus pelvic radiation in Stage II disease with residual tumor after surgery.

Advanced Disease - FIGO Stages III-IV and Recurrent

In the trial comparing melphalan and chlorambucil in advanced ovarian cancer, Rossof et al[2] observed response in 12.5 percent of 24 patients with melphalan and in 22 percent of 23 patients receiving chlorambucil. Survival was prolonged (68 weeks median) in the melphalan group. Patients failing one drug failed to respond to the other on crossover.

In a larger trial using higher doses of melphalan, Brodovsky et al[3] observed response in 26 percent of 114 patients with advanced ovarian cancer. In this trial the combination of cytoxan, methotrexate, and 5-Fluorouracil produced responses in 41 percent of 110 patients, but no differences were observed in the number of complete responses with 19 in the single agent and 21 in the combination arm. The duration of complete response was longer in the single agent arm; more hemato- logic and gastrointestinal toxicity was observed in the combination arm. Stratification variables included prior radiation therapy and the pre- sence of measurable disease.

Early attempts to show a clinical advantage with combination chemo- therapy were also unsuccessful. Blom et al[4] compared several drug combinations with standard melphalan therapy. The overall response rate to melphalan was 27 percent, and was not enhanced by the addition of 5-Fluorouracil, or 5-Fluorouracil and actinomycin-D. Furthermore, the response to melphalan alone equalled the response to the combi- nation actinomycin-D, 5-Fluorouracil and cytoxan (AcFUCy). In addi- tion there was excessive toxicity in two of the combination arms.

In a further effort to document the superiority of combination therapy, Bruckner et al compared standard melphalan therapy with the Thiotepa- methotrexate regimen (TM) originally described by Greenspan[5] and with the combination cyclophosphamide, adriamycin, fluorouracil (CAF) and alternating sequences of TM and CAF.[6] The CAF regimen produced twice the number of responses compared to L-PAM and was also better than the other two treatment arms (Table 4).

TABLE 4
Chemotherapy in Advanced Ovarian Cancer

Treatment	# Patients	CR	PR	Percent CR + PR
L-PAM	70	4	4	11.4
TSPA + MTX	72	4	7	15.3
CAF	71	7	14	29.6
TSPA + MTX rotating with CAF	62	2	11	21.0

Based on a pilot study designed by Vogl[7] showing response in 19 of 21 (90.4 percent) previously untreated patients with advanced ovarian cancer, the combination of cyclophosphamide, hexamethylmelamine, adriamycin and cis-platinum (CHAD), is currently being evaluated comparing this combination with standard melphalan therapy in a randomized groupwide trial.

Phase II Trials

A number of single agents have been tested in refractory ovarian cancer including adriamycin,[8] cis-platinum,[9,10] CCNU and methyl CCNU,[11] dianhydrogalactitol,[12] hexamethylmelamine,[13] high-dose methotrexate with Leucovorin,[14] piperazinedione,[15] VP-16,[16] and Yoshi-864.[17] Except for cis-platinum, which gives responses in about 30 percent of the patients, the results have been disappointing.

Combinations which have been tested in refractory ovarian cancer include adriamycin/cis-platinum,[18] adriamycin/cis-platinum/hexamethylmelamine,[19] adriamycin/BCNU/cyclophosphamide,[20] and cis-platinum/hexamethylmelamine/5-FU with or without adriamycin.[21] This study resulted in 23 of 74 (31 percent) complete plus partial responses for the 3-drug combination and 14 of 29 (48 percent) for the 4 drugs. The median duration was 4.3 months for the former combination and 5.8 months for the latter.

COMBINED MODALITY TRIALS

In a randomized trial comparing radiation therapy, chemotherapy and combined therapy, Miller et al[22] reported no advantage in untreated Stage III disease with combination therapy (Table 5).

TABLE 5
Radiotherapy and Chemotherapy in Stage III Ovarian Cancer

Treatment	Response Rate	Median Survival
Abdominal radiation (3,500 rads midplane)	9/17 (52%)	94.9 weeks
Chlorambucil 0.2 mg/kg daily for 8 weeks	9/18 (50%)	33.5 weeks
Combination of the above	11/16 (69%)	42.2 weeks

Although survival appeared to be prolonged in the group receiving radiotherapy alone, differences in response rates were small. The chemotherapy group received treatment for only eight weeks, making it difficult to draw definitive conclusions.

In a trial comparing melphalan alone, pelvic and abdominal radiation and combined melphalan-radiation therapy in patients with Stage III disease, stratified into optimal (residual masses less than 3 cm diameter) and suboptimal (greater than 3 cm) categories, no survival benefit was found from combined therapy, although time to progression was prolonged in both disease categories.[23]

Only two chemoimmunotherapy studies have been completed. Treatment in one consisted of either adriamycin + cyclophosphamide (AC) or AC + BCG.[24]   The response rates are 36 percent and 53 percent respectively (p = .05) in 154 patients studied. Response duration is slightly longer with BCG added (median 9.5 months). However, the important aspect of the outcome of this study was the prolongation of the median survival resulting from AC + BCG (23 months) as compared to 13 months for AC alone (p = .004). If confirmed in subsequent studies this result indicates an important contribution of BCG. In the other study, which was nonrandomized, melphalan plus C parvum,[25] there were 26 of 45 (53 percent) responses with a median duration of 12 months. The median survival is 24 months. These results were an improvement over melphalan alone.

Germ Cell Tumors of the Ovary

Slayton, et al[26] treated 27 patients with malignant germ cell tumors of the ovary with vincristine, dactinomycin, and cyclophosphamide and 12 patients with other combination therapy; 14 tumors were pure endodermal sinus tumors, two were embryonal carcinomas, 11 were mixed germ cell tumors, and 12 were immature teratomas. Of 23 patients with surgically resected disease (Stage I-IIIA), seven failed with a median followup of 24.5 months for the 16 patients remaining free of disease. There were eight responses in 16 patients with advanced disease (Stages IIB, III and recurrent) and median followup for patients remaining free of disease was 26.5 months. Four of eight patients with tumors containing endodermal sinus elements responded to chemotherapy and remained disease-free. Grade III hematologic toxicity was seen in eight patients, and dose-limiting G.I. toxicity in five patients.

ENDOMETRIAL ADENOCARCINOMA

TRIALS INVOLVING SURGERY, CHEMOTHERAPY, RADIOTHERAPY AND IMMUNOTHERAPY

Carcinoma of the endometrium has received increasing attention because of an apparent rising incidence even though this may only be the result of an aging population.

The development of competitive clinical trials has been complicated by a number of factors. Among these are:

1)   The disease is predominantly one of older women.

2)   The prognosis is generally favorable and the disease slow growing.

3)   Various methods of treatment appear to be equally effective in the limited tumor and the specific roles of surgery and radiotherapy are not clearly demarcated.

As a result of this confusion, it was clear that an accurate under-standing of the natural history of the disease was necessary. A study of Stage I disease with regard to grade of tumor, depth of myometrial invasion, uterine size, pelvic and paraaortic lymph node metastasis was inaugurated and a preliminary report published in 1976.[27] Lymph node metastasis appears to correlate well with the first three factors, an important finding in terms of realistic local management.

Hormone Therapy

At the time of the inception of the Cooperative Groups, progestational agents were the mainstay of the management of the advanced case even though some doubt existed as to their real efficacy. A study, investigating the response of patients with advanced endometrial can-cer to progestin therapy, reported objective response in 30 percent. A second study assessed the value of the agents as adjuvant therapy but reported no benefit following 14 weeks of progesterone when used with surgery plus irradiation in Stage II disease.[28]

More recently, a study was introduced[29] to determine if the presence of specific cytoplasmic progesterone receptors could predict a response to progestin therapy. High progesterone receptor activity was found to be related to the tumor grade in well differentiated tumors and did appear to predict response.

Combination Chemotherapy

A number of agents used either singly or in combination have been tested. A study using adriamycin showed that 17 of 49 patients responded to the drug (including 7 complete responses) when a dose of 60 mg/M^2 was used. Fourteen had had prior progestin therapy and 3 chemotherapy.[30] Median duration of partial response was 4 months, and 5 months for those with complete response. The treatment involved moderate hematological toxicity with one death from cardiac failure.

A separate trial[31] reported responses in 4 of 21 patients (19 percent) using adriamycin 50 mg/M^2 every 3 weeks, but no responses were seen in 19 patients receiving cyclophosphamide 600 mg/M^2 IV every 3 weeks. White counts below 2,000 were seen in 5 of 20 patients treated with adriamycin and in 3 of 15 treated with cyclophosphamide. There was no overt cardiac toxicity; one patient receiving cyclophosphamide developed severe cystitis. All 4 patients who responded to adriamycin had favorable performance status and disease located outside the pelvis, suggesting the importance of these factors as strata for future studies.

Two studies have been designed to evaluate combinations of 5-Fluorouracil, adriamycin and a mustard with megestrol acetate (Megace), a progestin. A third clinical trial has been designed to evaluate BCG vaccination in combination with adriamycin and cyclophosphamide. A fourth trial, soon to be activated, will reevaluate the role of progestin therapy in untreated patients, and will compare combined adriamycin-cyclophosphamide therapy with adriamycin alone in progestin failures.

SQUAMOUS CELL CARCINOMA OF THE CERVIX

TRIALS INVOLVING SURGERY, CHEMOTHERAPY, RADIOTHERAPY, AND IMMUNOTHERAPY

Single Agent Therapy

The number of randomized controlled clinical trials in cervical cancer is small. Those utilizing single agent chemotherapy include a report by Stolinsky and Bateman[32] who report response in 8/35 with hexamethylmelamine 12 mg/kg daily for 21 days with a four-week rest period. All had received prior irradiation; three had received prior chemotherapy. Nausea and vomiting were frequently dose-limiting; four reported a mild peripheral neuropathy. Two of nine patients had a WBC below 2,000, and 0 of 9 had platelets below 60,000.

In a Phase II trial involving patients with epidermoid and transitional cell carcinoma, Panettiere et al[33] reported response in 9 of 34 patients (26 percent) with squamous cell carcinoma treated with porfiromycin 7.5-10.5 mg/M^2 twice weekly. Median response duration was 93 days. Severe thrombocytopenia was common and dose-limiting with this schedule, and severe soft tissue necrosis from extravasation of the drug was seen in six patients. This agent is not recommended for further use.

Thigpen et al[34] reported response in 8 of 18 (44 percent) with two complete responses with cis-platinum 50 mg/M^2 every three weeks. At the time of the report, it was too early to assess duration of response or survival. Two of nineteen patients had severe nausea and vomiting; five developed azotemia, requiring interruption of treatment in two. Myelo-suppression was insignificant.

Delgado et al[15] reported 2 of 33 responses (6 percent) with one complete response to piperazinedione at 9 mg/M^2 every 3 weeks. Severe leukopenia was observed in 8 of 19 patients, two of which were fatal. Severe thrombocytopenia was observed in 8 of 15, was life-threatening in one, and was fatal in two. An additional eight patients developed anemia while receiving treatment.

Omura et al[35] reported responses in 2 of 58 patients (3.4 percent) treated with CCNU 100 mg/M^2 every six weeks and in 3 of 62 patients (4.8 percent) with methyl CCNU 130 mg/M^2 every six weeks. Seven of 34 patients receiving CCNU had a WBC below 2,000 or platelets below 50,000; 8 of 26 receiving methyl CCNU had similar toxicity. Nausea was common but not dose-limiting.

Morrow et al[36] found responses in 2 of 16 patients with advanced squamous cell carcinoma of the cervix with continuous pelvic arterial infusion of bleomycin at 20 mg/M^2 per week for a total of 10 weeks. The average dose of bleomycin was 221 units (range 80 to 320 units). Severe stomatitis and skin blisters in two patients made it necessary to stop therapy. Pulmonary fibrosis or pneumonitis was seen in four. The investigators could find no clinical advantage of this treatment method.

Combination Chemotherapy

Trials evaluating drug combinations in advanced squamous cell carci-noma of the cervix include the one by Wallace et al[37] (Table 6).

Cycles were repeated every 3 to 4 weeks in each regimen. Time to progression was chosen as the primary end point owing to the difficulty in evaluating response in areas previously operated and heavily irra-diated.

TABLE 6
Adriamycin and Combination Chemotherapy
in Advanced Cervical Carcinoma

	Median Time to Progression	Median Survival
Adriamycin 60 mg/M^2	3.7 months	6.0 months
Adriamycin 60 mg/M^2 plus Vincristine 1.5 mg/M^2	4.2 months	5.0 months
Adriamycin 50 mg/M^2 plus Cytoxan 500 mg/M^2 I.V.	5.7 months	7.8 months

Greenberg et al[38] report partial response in 5 of 9 patients (56 percent) receiving adriamycin every three weeks in escalating doses, starting at 30 mg/M^2, and in 0 of 11 patients receiving adriamycin combined with bleomycin 10 units/M^2 weekly IV. All five responses to the single agent were seen in metastatic lesions in areas not previously irradiated; all were observed early, and were of short duration. Median survival was only 4.0 months in the responding group, and 4.3 months in the group showing no response.

In a Phase II trial, Baker et al[39] reported responses in 52 of 115 patients (45 percent) with advanced squamous cell carcinoma of the cervix with a combination of mitomycin-C, vincristine and bleomycin. Bleomycin was given by weekly injection (24 patients), twice weekly injection (50 patients), and by continuous 96-hour infusion (41 patients) six hours after administration of vincristine. Response was present in 6 of 24 (25 percent) with the weekly schedule of bleomycin, in 30 of 50 (60 percent) with twice weekly bleomycin with eight complete responses, and in 16 of 41 (39 percent) with six complete responses with bleomycin infusion. Median duration of response was longer with infusion, 16 weeks versus 9 weeks with twice weekly bleomycin and was 11 weeks with the weekly dose. The incidence of severe peripheral neuropathy and muscle weakness in the twice weekly group caused investigators to abandon this schedule.

Radiotherapy for Carcinoma of the Cervix

In the area of radiation therapy of cancer of the cervix, split-course irradiation has been stated to be as effective as the conventional continuous course of treatment but better tolerated by the patient. In order to evaluate this hypothesis, a trial for Stage III carcinoma of the cervix was activated in 1971 and later modified to include Stage IVB disease.[40] Preliminary results indicate that the tumor control rate in the two groups is similar; severe treatment reactions, namely fibrosis, radiation cystitis and proctitis, edema and soft tissue necrosis, are similar in both groups. Median survival is 26 months.

Another area of radiation therapy investigation involves the evaluation of altered radiosensitivity by changes in cellular oxygen concentration. A trial is underway using high-pressure oxygen in Stages IIB, III, and IVA carcinoma of the cervix.[41] Treatment failure was 16 percent for hyperbaric oxygen and 48 percent for air. The 3-year survival rates are similar, 56 percent and 49 percent. One of the earliest radiosensitizers to be tested under controlled clinical conditions was hydroxyurea. A study of this drug combined with radiotherapy compared to radio-therapy with placebo has been completed in Stages IIB, III, and IVA.[42] The response rate was 56.5 percent for the placebo group and 74 percent for hydroxyurea. Median survivals in Stage IIIB patients were 13 and 23 months respectively. Toxicity was significantly greater in hydroxyurea patients.

In the surgery and surgical pathology areas, one study included patients thought to have microinvasive carcinoma of the cervix. These patients were subject to thorough evaluation of cone and hysterectomy speci-mens. In this retrospective study, nodal involvement was determined and survival was compared with the pathology findings.[42] Two hundred thirty-five evaluable patients were studied and the major conclusion was the difficulty in making a diagnosis of microinvasive carcinoma by many of the pathologists in the country. Half of the patients were rejected by the review pathologists. It was noted that successful management of the patients was largely related to both depths of penetration and the width of the area involved by microinvasive penetration. Another protocol dealt with 292 evaluable patients in whom tumor spread, particularly involvement of the pelvic or para-aortic nodes, was contrasted with the clinical stage of the disease. Further studies are being done to evaluate survival and complications from the surgical evaluation of the patient who subsequently receives radiation therapy. The results of this study have not been published but it is quite apparent that the clinical staging is far from satisfactory in establishing programs of treatment. Traditional radiation ports are destined to treatment failure when the disease extends to the para-aortic lymph nodes.

UTERINE SARCOMA

Omura and Blessing[43] reported a response in 14 of 51 (27.5 percent) patients with Stages III-IV uterine sarcoma (leiomyosarcoma, heterologous mixed mesodermal sarcomas, stromal sarcoma) using adriamycin 60 mg/M^2 every 3 weeks, and in 11 of 40 patients (27.5 percent) with adriamycin 60 mg/M^2 plus dimethyl triazeno imidazole carboxamide (DTIC) 250 mg/M^2 times five every 3 weeks. There was no significant difference in estimated median duration of response (4.2 months versus 5.3 months). In patients without measurable disease there was no significant difference in time to progression or in survival between the two groups, and since the addition of DTIC increased the incidence of serious G.I. toxicity from 18 percent to 51 percent and serious hematologic toxicity from 31 percent to 53 percent, the use of adriamycin alone appears advisable for uterine sarcoma.

MISCELLANEOUS

Only 83 patients have been registered in studies which did not involve uterus, cervix, and ovary. Most of the 65 patients with vulvar cancer were entered into staging and therapy programs, irradiation versus surgery. In general, tube, vagina and nonspecified cases have been entered into Phase II studies, there not being enough patients to conduct any site-oriented trial.

SUMMARY

It is apparent that pelvic malignancy is a significant segment of the cancers involving women. Despite this significance, relatively little emphasis has been placed upon gynecologic oncology in the past, but this deficiency is currently being corrected. It is apparent that through one Group concentrating on gynecologic oncology and several other general Groups including gynecologic oncology in their trials, a broad multidiscipline attack is being made. Progress is occurring. With increased concentration in this area, Groups can advance from earlier studies aimed only at disposing of empirical therapeutics, to trials that bring to the public the most effective techniques and agents that will reduce the burden of pelvic cancer in women.

Larger numbers of women need to be involved in clinical trials so that study completion time can be reduced. This will permit the evaluation of more new therapies effectively and promptly for the transfer of information, to benefit the general public, to physicians who deal with patients throughout the United States. The various Groups have as immediate objectives the pilot studying of new approaches, the Phase II testing of many new agents and the Phase III testing of newly found therapeutic measures.   Through large scale efforts of clinical investigation, the Groups should be able in the future to improve control in late cancers to such a degree that more emphasis can be placed upon the discovery and management of early cancers.   Hopefully, at the same time, new procedures will be developed for the early detection of malignant and premalignant conditions so that massive, toxic and injurious therapy, too frequently required now, will be a thing of the past.

REFERENCES

1. Hreshchyshyn MM, Norris HJ: Postoperative treatment of women with resectable ovarian cancer with radiotherapy, melphalan or no further therapy. AACR 18:195, 1977.
2. Rossof AH, Drukker BH, Talley RW, Torres J, Bonnett J, Brownlee RW: Randomized evaluation of chlorambucil and melphalan in advanced ovarian cancer. AACR 17:300, 1976.
3. Brodovsky H, Temkin N, Sears M: Melphalan versus cyclophosphamide methotrexate and 5-Fluorouracil in women with ovarian cancer. ASCO 18:308, 1977.
4. Blom J, Park R, Blessing J: Treatment of women with disseminated and recurrent ovarian cancer with single and multichemotherapeutic agents. ASCO 19:338, 1978.
5. Greenspan EM: Thiotepa and methotrexate chemotherapy of advanced ovarian carcinoma. Mt Sinai Hospital Journal 35:52-67, 1968.
6. Bruckner HW, Pagano M, Falkson G, Creech R, Arseneau JC, Horton J, Brodovsky H, Davis TE, Slayton RW, Greenspan E: Controlled prospective trial of combination chemotherapy with cyclophosphamide, adriamycin and 5-Fluorouracil for the treatment of advanced ovarian cancer: A preliminary report. Cancer Treat Rep 63:297-299, 1979.
7. Vogl S, Berenzweig M, Kaplan BH, Moukhtar M, Bulkin W: The CHAD and HAD regimens in advanced ovarian cancer: Combination chemotherapy including cyclophosphamide, hexamethylmelamine, adriamycin and cis-diamminedichloroplatinum (II). Cancer Treat Rep 63:311-318, 1979.
8. O'Bryan RM, Luce JK, Talley RW, Gottlieb JA, Baker LH, Bonadonna G: Phase II evaluation of adriamycin in human neoplasia. Cancer 32:1-8, 1973.
9. Rossof AH, Talley RW, Stephens RL: Phase II evaluation of single high dose cis-diamminedichloroplatinum (II) in gynecologic and genitourinary neoplasia. AACR 18:97, 1977.
10. Thigpen T, Shingleton H, Homesley H, Lagasse L, Blessing J: Cis-diamminedichloroplatinum (NSC 119875) in treatment of gynecologic malignancies. Phase II Trials by the Gynecologic Oncology Group. Cancer Treat Rep 63:1549, 1979.
11. Omura G, DiSaia P, Blessing J, Boronow R, Hreshchyshyn M, Park R: Chemotherapy for mustard-resistant ovarian adenocarcinoma: A randomized trial of CCNU and methyl CCNU. Cancer Treat Rep 61:1533-1535, 1977.
12. Blom J: GOG Protocol 26E.
13. Omura G: Personal Communication.
14. Parker LM, Griffiths CT, Yankee RA, Knapp RC, Canellos GP: High-dose methotrexate with leucovorin rescue in ovarian cancer: A Phase II study. Cancer Treat Rep 63:275-279, 1979.
15. Delgado G, Thigpen T, Dolan T, Morrison F: Phase II trial of piperazinedione in treatment of advanced ovarian carcinoma. ASCO 19:332, 1978.
16. Slayton R, Creasman W, Bundy B: Phase II trial of VP-16 in treatment of advanced squamous cell carcinoma of the cervix. ASCO 20:365, 1979.
17. Altman SJ, Metter GE, Nealon TF, Weiss AJ, Ramirez G, Madden RE, Fletcher WS, Strawitz JG, Multhauf PM: Yoshi-864, a Phase II study in solid tumors. Cancer Treat Rep 62:389-395, 1978.
18. Briscoe K, Pasmantier M, Brown J, Kennedy BJ: Cis-diamminedichloroplatinum (II) and adriamycin in the treatment of advanced ovarian carcinoma. ASCO 19:378, 1978.
19. Vogl SH, Greenwald G, Moukhtar M, Wollner D, Kaplan BH: Ovarian cancer: Effective treatment of alkylating agent failures. JAMA 241:1908-1911, 1979.
20. Presant CA: SEG Protocol 76 OVCA 0202.
21. Alberts DS, Hilgers RD, Moon TE, Martimbeau PW, Rivkin S: Combination chemotherapy for alkylator-resistant ovarian carcinoma: Preliminary report of a Southwest Oncology Group Trial. Cancer Treat Rep 63:301-306, 1979.
22. Miller SP, Brenner S, Horton J, Stolbach L, Schnider BI, Pocock S: Comparative evaluation of combined radiation-chlorambucil treatment of ovarian carcinomatosis. Cancer 36:1625-1630, 1975.
23. Brady L, Blessing J, Homesley H, Lewis GC: Radiotherapy (RT), chemotherapy (CT) and combined therapy in Stage III epithelial ovarian cancer. AACR 20:218, 1979.
24. Alberts D, Moon T, Stephens R, Wilson H, Oishi N, Hilgers R: A randomized study of chemoimmuno-therapy for advanced ovarian carcinoma: Preliminary report of a Southwest Oncology Group Study. Cancer Treat Rep 63:325-331, 1979.
25. Creasman W, Gall SA, Blessing JA, Schmidt HJ, Abu-Ghazaleh S, Whisnant JK, DiSaia PJ: Evaluation of combination chemotherapy and immunotherapy in Stage III epithelial cancer of ovary. Cancer Treat Rep In Press.
26. Slayton RE, Hreshchyshyn MM, Silverberg SG, Shingleton HM, Park RC, DiSaia PJ, Blessing JA: Treatment of malignant ovarian germ cell tumors. Cancer 42:390-398, 1978.
27. Creasman WT, Boronow RC, Morrow CP, DiSaia PJ, Blessing JA: Adenocarcinoma of the endometrium: Its metastatic lymph node potential. Gynecol Oncol 4:239-243, 1976.
28. Lewis GC Jr, Black NH, Mortel R, Bross ID: Adjuvant progesterone therapy in the primary definitive treatment of endometrial cancer. Gynecol Oncol 2:368-376, 1974.
29. Ehrlich CE, Young PC, Cleary RE: Progesterone receptors - A new approach to recurrent endometrial cancer. AACR 18:7, 1977.
30. Thigpen T, Torres J, Buchsbaum H: Phase II trial of adriamycin in the treatment of advanced endometrial adenocarcinoma. ASCO 18:352, 1977.
31. Horton J, Begg CB, Arseneault J, Bruckner H, Creech R, Hahn RG: Comparison of adriamycin with cyclophosphamide in patients with advanced endometrial cancer. Cancer Treat Rep 62:159-161, 1978.
32. Stolinsky DC, Bateman JR: Further experience with hexamethylmelamine in the treatment of carcinoma of the cervix. Cancer Chemother Rep 57:497-499, 1973.

33. Panettiere FJ, Talley RW, Torres J, Lane M: Porfiromycin in the management of epidermoid and transitional cell cancer: A Phase II study. Cancer Treat Rep 60:907-911, 1976.

34. Thigpen T, Shingleton H: Phase II trial of cis-platinum in the treatment of advanced squamous cell carcinoma of the cervix. ASCO 19:332, 1978.

35. Omura GA, Shingleton HM, Creasman WT, Blessing JA, Boronow RC: Chemotherapy of gynecologic cancer with nitrosoureas: A randomized trial of CCNU and methyl CCNU in cancers of the cervix, corpus, vagina, and vulva. Cancer Treat Rep 62:833-835, 1978.

36. Morrow CP, DiSaia PJ, Mangan CE, Lagasse LD: Continuous pelvic arterial infusion with bleomycin for squamous carcinoma of the cervix recurrent after irradiation. Cancer Treat Rep 61:1403-1405, 1977.

37. Wallace HJ, Hreshchyshyn MM, Blessing JA: Comparison of therapeutic effects of adriamycin versus adriamycin and vincristine versus adriamycin plus cyclophosphamide in the treatment of advanced carcinoma of the cervix. AACR, 18:131, 1977.

38. Greenberg BR, Kardinal CG, Pajak TF, Bateman JR: Adriamycin versus adriamycin and bleomycin in advanced epidermoid carcinoma of the cervix. Cancer Treat Rep 61:1383-1384, 1977.

39. Baker LH, Opipari MI, Wilson H, Bottomley R, Coltman CA: Mitomycin-C, vincristine and bleomycin therapy for advanced cervical cancer. Am J Obstet Gynecol 52:146-150, 1978.

40. RTOG, Minutes, June 1979.

41. RTOG, Progress Report 1976-1978.

42. GOG, Minutes, January 1978

43. Omura GA, Blessing JA: Chemotherapy of Stage III, IV and recurrent uterine sarcomas: A randomized trial of adriamycin (AD) versus adriamycin plus dimethyl triazeno imidazole carboxamide (DTIC). AACR 19:26, 1978.

12

Malignant melanoma

John J. Costanzi, Thomas J. Cunningham, and Charles M. Balch

INTRODUCTION

Melanoma accounts for only one percent of all cancers and it is therefore difficult for a single institution to perform clinical studies with adequate patient numbers to permit randomization. It is only through Cooperative Group efforts that valid studies, by all disciplines, can be prospectively performed.

The overall history of Cooperative Group contributions to the management of malignant melanoma reflects the history of Cooperative Groups in general. Almost all Groups initially began with one discipline and the majority of the original studies involved drug testing in the treatment of various stages of malignant melanoma. Over the last five years or so, the Groups began including other modalities and disciplines. Radiotherapy was one of the first disciplines to be included, followed by surgery, immunotherapy, pathology and various basic sciences involved in drug development and pharmacokinetics.

In the early days of Cooperative Group studies a number of single chemotherapeutic agents were tested primarily in the disseminated form of melanoma. These studies continued until imidazole carboxamide (DTIC) became available and appeared to be the single agent of choice. Subsequent studies attempted to utilize DTIC in various schedules and in combinations. At the same time new single agents that became available were widely tested by the Groups seeking drugs equal to or more effective than DTIC. Also during this time, a few studies showed potential promise in the use of immunotherapeutic agents in both disseminated and early high-risk melanoma. The

Cooperative Groups undertook various studies including immunotherapy alone and in combination with various chemotherapeutic agents for the treatment of these two categories. The major impetus for studying the immunotherapeutic agents was the fact that the majority of the positive studies published suffered from small numbers of patients and lack of adequate prospective controls. They used historical controls. Much more data was gleaned from these Group studies than just response rate and survival.

The statistical offices of the Cooperative Groups became very integral parts of the treatment team. With their highly sophisticated methods of evaluation, numerous prognostic factors were identified which aided the investigators in proper stratification of patients. These prognostic factors, which will be discussed, have arisen not only from the pure chemotherapy studies but also more recently from the studies involving immunotherapy. Radiotherapy began playing an integral role in some Cooperative Group melanoma studies, primarily in attempts to better manage the patient with metastatic melanoma to the brain. More recently, surgeons have played an important role. For years there has been a school of thought which has utilized regional limb perfusion for the treatment of Stage II disease. Although this technique and method has its disciples, it has unfortunately never been put to a prospective, randomized test. Such studies are now underway.

Therefore, in general, the major advantages of Cooperative Group evaluation in the treatment of melanoma is the fact that a large number of patients can be studied in a short period of time in prospective randomized trials. These prospective randomized trials make the results, whether they be negative or positive, more significant.

EARLY SINGLE DRUG STUDIES

From July, 1967 to June, 1970, a large number of single agents were tested. At first the results were rather bleak since no objective or subjective responses were noted. The drugs tested included ThioTEPA, 5-Fluorouracil, 5-Fluorouracil plus warfarin, phenylalanine mustard, cyclophosphamide, vinblastine, cytosine arabinoside, 3022AB, methotrexate, hexamethylmelamine and azotomycin.[1] In this study one partial response was noted among seven evaluable patients receiving hydroxyurea, and there were three partial responses out of seven evaluable patients receiving BCNU.

Subsequently, hydroxyurea was extensively studied. Patients received either intravenous or oral hydroxyurea in pulse doses every 8 hours for 5 days repeated every 2 weeks. The doses ranged from 1.5 to 3 mg/M^2/day. Of 19 patients receiving 51 courses one partial remission and two improvements were observed.[2]

IMIDAZOLE CARBOXAMIDE (DTIC) FOR
DISSEMINATED MELANOMA

In 1970, a Phase I study of intravenous DTIC was performed.[3] The drug was administered in 100-250 ml of 5% dextrose and water over a 15-30 minute period for 5 days every three weeks. The initial dose level was 70 mg/M^2/day and was progressively increased. Myelosuppression and antitumor effects were first noted at 150 mg/M^2/day but most patients subsequently received a dose of 250 mg/M^2/day for 5 days. Therefore, in future studies, when DTIC was used alone it has been given at 250 mg/M^2/day for 5 days and when used in combination with other agents it was given at a dose level of 150 mg/M^2/day. The major toxic effects of DTIC were nausea and vomiting which began 1-3 hours after drug administration, was most severe after the first dose, and diminished after subsequent doses on the five-day course. Leukopenia and thrombocytopenia occurred in equal frequency and were the second most common side effects. Leukopenia was maximum at 25 days with a complete recovery by day 40. The thrombocytopenic time sequence was similar. Other toxic effects included pain along the injected vein, usually occurring after direct IV injection, a flu-like syndrome, and a suggestion of hepatic toxicity as noted by reversible enzyme elevations. A total of 110 patients with disseminated malignant melanoma were treated in this study and a response rate of 19 percent was noted. Other Phase I studies of DTIC showed similar results.[4]

Two different dose levels of DTIC were then studied in malignant melanoma. A prospective randomized study of 155 patients receiving either 2.0 or 4.5 mg/kg for 10 successive daily intravenous doses was conducted.[5] An objective response rate of 28 percent was noted in 115 evaluable patients, 21 percent in all cases with 24 percent for the 2.0 mg and 17 percent for the 4.5 mg. The 2.0 mg schedule produced a significantly greater duration of response than did the 4.5 mg schedule, exceeding 6 months, in half of the responding patients. Toxicity was definitely greater in the 4.5 mg regimen but in general it was mild. There were no drug related deaths.

Triazeno imidazole carboxamide mustard, a related compound was compared to DTIC in a prospective randomized study of 178 patients.[6] The dose of DTIC was 150 mg/M^2/day x 5 repeated every 30 days. The response rate for DTIC was 18 percent, whereas for TIC mustard it was a low 6 percent (p = .03). The duration of response was brief at 15 weeks for patients responding to DTIC and 4 weeks for the TIC mustard patients. Although the response rate was low for this very difficult tumor, the Cooperative Groups had establised a standard treatment agent with DTIC. In addition they had shown that extent of disease, patient performance status, and disease response to treatment influenced the length of survival.

NEWER SINGLE AGENTS

New promising single chemotherapeutic agents can be easily and quickly studied in Cooperative Groups since patient numbers are large and accrual is fast. This offers a definite advantage in that the effectiveness or the noneffectiveness of a compound can be determined rather quickly.

Dianhydrogalactitol (DAG) was studied in patients with advanced malignant melanoma.[7] Of the patients receiving this drug, at 25 mg/M^2/day, 19 had progressive disease, three demonstrated stable disease after two or more cycles of drug, and two were inevaluable for response. Toxicity included leukopenia and thrombocytopenia. DAG appears insignificantly active in the therapy of malignant melanoma.

Cyclocytidine at 240 mg/M^2/day for 10 days was studied in 29 patients with metastatic malignant melanoma[8] and one achieved a partial remission. Toxicity included delayed thrombocytopenia, orthostatic hypotension and jaw pain. VP-16-213 was administered at 45 mg/M^2 daily x 5 every three weeks in 29 patients with malignant melanoma.[9] All of these patients had extensive prior therapy. No responses were noted and the major toxic effect was myelosuppression. Cis-platinum was evaluated in a randomized trial with or without mannitol diuresis.[10] There were 1 of 25 (4 percent) responses in patients receiving cis-platinum and mannitol. Of importance, renal toxicity was worse in the patient who received no mannitol.

Piperazinedione has been studied in 28 patients and there were no responders noted.[11] Forty-two percent of these patients noted leukopenia, 60 percent thrombocytopenia, 35 percent anemia and 18 percent nausea and vomiting. Another study showed two partial responders out of 41 evaluable patients.[12] Overall piperazinedione is not a useful drug in the management of drug-resistant melanoma. Other drugs which are currently being examined by Cooperative Groups to determine if they have efficacy in disseminated melanoma include diglycoaldehyde, tamoxifen and gallium.

COMBINATION CHEMOTHERAPY

Since the response rate of disseminated melanoma to DTIC was positive, combination chemotherapy programs were soon begun. In a prospective study of 275 patients comparing DTIC alone versus DTIC plus BCNU versus DTIC + methyl CCNU the response rates were very similar, i.e., 16 percent on DTIC alone, 17 percent of 93 patients with DTIC + BCNU and 16 percent of 114 patients receiving DTIC + methyl CCNU.[13] There appeared to be a longer duration of response for the DTIC + methyl CCNU arm when compared to the other two but this was not statistically significant. The significant prognostic factors as they relate to response were site of involvement, sex, and ambulatory status. Age, prior treatment or time from first symptoms were not important.

DTIC at 150 mg/M^2/day for 5 days was then added to vincristine 1.4 mg/M^2 on day 1 and 5 and BCNU at 150 mg/M^2 on day 1. Treatment was administered every 28 days.[14] A response rate of 21 percent was observed with 16 percent noting stable disease (Table 1). The median survival was 42 months from diagnosis and 5.3 months from the onset of treatment. These results did not significantly differ from DTIC alone. Of interest and of possible future significance, this study demonstrated that patients with lymphopenia prior to the onset of therapy had a similar response rate to other patients but had a shorter median survival (4.4 months versus 7.8 months). This is significant at the .03 level. This group subsequently added chlorpromazine to the three-drug regimen of BCNU, vincristine and DTIC.[15] This addition to the BVD regimen produced a response rate of 22 percent with 28 percent of the patients having stable disease. Of importance in this study was the observation that patients who exhibited any degree of improvement during their first course of treatment had the highest overall response rate (72 percent) to the BVD regimen. In those patients who did not have any improvement in the first course, a change in therapy should probably be instituted. The median survival from the onset of therapy was 6 months for all patients and 18 months for patients who responded. The response rate and duration were not different from BVD alone. It

TABLE 1
Combination Chemotherapy in Advanced Melanoma

	BVD	BVD-C	BHD $\pm$ V
Patients entered	144	121	506
Complete Remission	9 (6%)	12 (10%)	35 (7%)
Partial Remission	22 (15%)	15 (12%)	103 (20%)
Median Duration (Months)			
CR	--	10	12
PR	--	6	4
Median Survival	5.3	6.0	5.5

B = BCNU; D = DTIC; V = Vincristine; C = chlorpromazine;
H = hydroxyurea

was noted that patients with absolute lymphocyte counts above 2700/cc had significantly higher response rates and longer survivals than patients with lower initial lymphocyte counts. These were significant at the .05 level.

DTIC was then studied in combination with BCNU and hydroxyurea versus the same three drugs with vincristine[16] The response rate of the three-drug regimen was 27 percent. The addition of vincristine did not improve the response rate (30 percent). These response rates include all patients (including those lost-to-followup and early deaths). If the early deaths were not considered, the overall response rate was 38 percent. Further important prognostic factors were elucidated in this study. The best responses were noted in patients with skin, lung and/or lymph node involvement, but the presence of liver and brain involvement heralded poor responses. The response rate in this study was independent of age, sex or previous therapy. The median survival for all evaluable patients was 5.5 months from start of therapy and was independent of the regimen utilized. In this study 7 percent of the patients achieved a complete response with 20 percent achieving partial response. The duration of response in these two groups showed a statistically significant longer duration in complete responders than in partial responders (Figure 1). Subsequent studies utilizing BCNU,

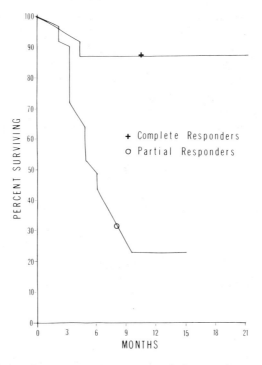

Fig. 1. Duration of response computed from date of response to last followup in complete and partial responders

hydroxyurea and imidazole carboxamide have consistently shown that about one-third of the patients respond and the responders have a longer survival than nonresponders.

This BHD experience prompted it to be compared with other regimens by another group.[17] In this study patients were randomized to DTIC alone, DTIC, CCNU and vincristine, DTIC, BCNU and vincristine and DTIC, BCNU and hydroxyurea. Two hundred seventy patients were studied and the overall response rate was 17.3 percent for the evaluable patients and 15.5 percent for all patients entered. There was no statistically significant difference in the response rate among the four treatment arms. The response rate to BHD in this study was less than previously described for the higher dose regimens (17 percent versus 30 percent). This suggested that in order to elicit a better response rate, a high enough drug dose should be given to at least produce mild to moderate leukopenia. This Cooperative Group then conducted a study to determine whether escalating drug doses to toxicity or to complete regression would improve the rate and duration of response to DTIC alone or a combination of DTIC, CCNU and vincristine.[18] In this study, there were 337 evaluable patients. The overall response rate was 20.2 percent and there was no statistical difference between DTIC alone or the three-drug combination. There was a slight increase in the regression rate for DTIC alone but the remission duration and survival was not improved. The authors concluded that the usage of DTIC alone or in combination with a nitrosourea and vincristine had reached its maximum benefit over a wide range of DTIC dosage.

In order to determine whether a more convenient treatment schedule is effective, a study was performed comparing single high-dose DTIC plus cyclophosphamide versus the standard 5-day DTIC plus cyclophosphamide in disseminated metastatic melanoma.[19] Forty-two patients received cytoxan at 600 mg/M^2 plus DTIC at 600 mg/M^2 on day 1, and 88 patients received cytoxan at 600 mg/M^2 plus DTIC at 200 mg/M^2 daily x 5. Response rates were 19 percent and 18 percent. In this study, patients with metastases confined to skin or lymph nodes had a 40 percent response, while in patients with visceral metastases response rates were 19 percent. In those with good performance status (above 70) response rates were 28 percent. Seventy-two percent of the patients demonstrated toxicity which included granulocytopenia, thrombocytopenia, nausea and vomiting. It was felt that a single administration of high-dose DTIC was equally effective to the five-day treatment, a schedule which was studied by other Groups.

IMMUNOTHERAPY

During the time that these large-scale studies were being performed, various studies were being conducted at individual institutions exami-

ning the efficacy of chemotherapy plus immunotherapy in the treatment of disseminated melanoma.[20] In 1974, a report was published in
which DTIC was combined with fresh Pasteur BCG given by scarification in patients with disseminated melanoma.[21] This combination
produced a response rate of 27 percent (5 percent complete responses,
22 percent partial responses).   The major results reportedly showed
increased remission rates in those patients receiving the BCG near the
region of metastatic involvement, prolonged remissions with chemoimmunotherapy compared to chemotherapy used alone (historical control), and significantly prolonged overall survival of patients receiving
chemoimmunotherapy compared to the survival of patients receiving
chemotherapy alone (historical controls).   This group of investigators
then added methyl CCNU to the DTIC, BCG regimen and noted a
similar 27 percent response rate. The major difference in this study
compared to the past DTIC + BCG combination was that half of the
remissions were complete for an overall complete remission rate of
13.5 percent. Once again they demonstrated that patients treated with
BCG plus chemotherapy had significantly longer remission durations
than groups of patients previously treated with DTIC alone (historical
controls).

Intradermal metastases of malignant melanoma when treated with
intralesional injections of BCG[22] showed significant toxic effects including fever, nausea, rash, local skin necrosis and lymphopenia. No
clinically significant systemic BCG infection was identified. Nine such
patients were treated, with 7 of the 9 having local regression of the
BCG treated lesions and 2 of the 7 experiencing complete regression of
lesions which had not been treated. Four of the responding patients and
both of the nonresponding patients had had negative PPD skin tests
prior to treatment. Conversion to positive PPD after BCG treatment
was noted only in the 4 patients who responded to treatment.   This
study prompted a comparative study of two different methods of
administration of BCG in malignant melanoma.[23] Fifty-nine patients
with local intradermal metastases with no distant metastases were
randomly treated with either .1 ml of TICE BCG intralesionally or .3 -.5
ml of BCG given by intradermal multipuncture technique (TINE) in
rotating deltoid or thigh sites. No lethal or life-threatening toxicity
was noted. Ten of 32 patients showed pretreatment anergy to a battery
of skin tests recall antigens and 7 of 7 who tested PPD negative
converted to positive with BCG. Objective regressions were seen in 43
percent (12 of 28) of intralesionally treated patients, 5 of whom had
regression of uninjected lesions. Only 2 out of 25 (8 percent) patients
receiving intradermal punctures had a partial response. Median survival
times of 21.1 and 13.3 months in intralesions and intradermal patients
respectively were not significantly different. The higher repsonse rate
of those treated with intralesional injections was not reflected in an

increased overall survival for this group but complete responders achieved a significantly superior survival.

Since these early immunotherapeutic programs appeared beneficial, the use of BCG was then studied in disseminated malignant melanoma in a prospective randomized fashion. The study randomized patients with disseminated melanoma to the BHD regimen versus the BHD + BCG administered on days 7, 14 and 21, versus the regimen reported by Gutterman et al, utilizing DTIC at 250 mg/M^2 daily for 5 days plus BCG on days 7, 14, and 21.[24] This study was recently updated. Three hundred fifty-one eligible patients were entered on the study and the randomization occurred in a 1:2:2 fashion. Of importance is the better objective regimen in the BHD group (35 percent) as compared to the DTIC plus BCG group (19 percent) (p=0.04) (Table 2). The addition of BCG to the BHD regimen resulted in a 27 percent response rate. This was also significant at the 5 percent level when compared to the DTIC + BCG group. There was no difference among the groups with respect to length of remission or survival from the start of treatment.

Significant subgroups were noted in this study which will alter stratification for future studies. The response rate in males was 33 percent for BHD which was significantly higher than the 15 percent for DTIC + BCG (p=0.02). For females the differences between rates were much less. They were 26 percent, 28 percent and 22 percent respectively for BHD, BHD + BCG and DTIC + BCG. Another important observation was the response with decades of age. There was an advantage of BHD over DTIC plus BCG in the third, fourth and fifth decades. This was absent in younger and older patients and even appeared to reverse for those patients over 70 years of age for whom the response was 9 percent with BHD and 36 percent for DTIC + BCG. This was not statistically significant (p=0.31). The advantage of BHD plus BCG relative to DTIC + BCG was somewhat diminished for patients 40 years and younger and those over 70. In short, for the BHD group the response rates first increased then decreased with the peak occurring in the fourth and fifth decades. A similar pattern holds true for the BHD + BCG arm except

TABLE 2
Chemoimmunotherapy in Advanced Melanoma

	BHD	BHD+BCG	DTIC+BCG
Total Patients	82	150	119
CR	9 (11%)	20 (13%)	9 (8%)
CR + PR	29 (35%)	44 (29%)← p=.05 →23 (19%)	

p=.04

that the rates increased more slowly, peaking in the sixth decade. The rate for the DTIC, BCG group increased more slowly and did not peak until the last decade reported. The p value associated with comparisons of these patterns are 0.11 for BHD versus BHD + BCG, 0.02 for BHD versus DTIC + BCG and 0.21 for BHD + BCG versus DTIC + BCG. This is an important observation and it appears that future studies should take age into consideration for stratification. Toxicity in this study was similar to the original BHD study except for dermatitis, chills and fever which were confined to the two arms receiving BCG. In the BHD + BCG arm, there were 5 cases of dermatitis, two of them severe, and 11 cases of chills and fever with 3 being severe. Dermatitis was reported 4 times in the DTIC + BCG arm, while chills and fever were noted 11 times. Therefore, this BCG toxicity at least demonstrates a pathophysiologic effect of the innoculation.

Although there were no differences in survival, median 25 weeks in the three groups, there were significant differences in small subgroups. Patients over the age of 60 in the DTIC + BCG group had longer remission than their counterparts in the BHD and the BHD + BCG groups (p=0.02). In patients with lung involvement, the BHD treated group had poorer survival experience than the BCG treated patients (p=0.08) and the same finding held (p=0.05) for patients with nodal

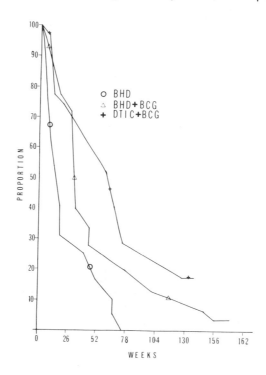

Fig. 2. Survival from treatment start, by treatment, patients older than 60 years

involvement. Among patients over 60 years of age, both the BHD + BCG and the DTIC + BCG patients survived significantly longer (p=0.01) than the BHD patients (Fig. 2).

Therefore, this study has demonstrated that the addition of BCG to chemotherapy in the treatment of disseminated melanoma does not increase response rates of survival but offers an advantage in small subgroups, specifically in those patients who have pulmonary involvement and in those patients over the age of 60 years.

Corynebacterium parvum was also studied in disseminated malignant melanoma.[25] An update of this study has 65 patients receiving cyclophosphamide at 600 mg/M^2 on day 1 plus DTIC at 200 mg/M^2 on days 1 through 5 and 55 patients were treated with the same chemotherapy plus corynebacterium parvum at 5 mg/M^2 IV on days 8 and 15. Courses were repeated every three weeks. Responses were noted in 28 percent of patients on chemotherapy alone and 33 percent on chemotherapy + C parvum. Duration of remission and survival in both groups were equal. There was no therapeutic advantage in frequency of response, duration of survival or length of remission for the immunotherapy limb when patients were analyzed according to the presence or absence of visceral metastases, pretreatment performance status or pretreatment evaluation of delayed hypersensitivity. Although myelosuppression was equal in both regimens, blood pressure changes, fever, chills and azotemia were more frequent and more severe in patients on the immunotherapy limb. This study also showed a benefit in response rates of chemoimmunotherapy in the few patients over 60 years of age (chemotherapy alone - 11 percent, chemoimmunotherapy - 33 percent).

Chemotherapy with or without MER was studied in patients with disseminated melanoma.[26] Patients receiving the three-drug combination consisting of procarbazine, vinblastine and dactinomycin had a 22 percent response rate (9 of 41), and patients receiving a similar combination of chemotherapy plus MER had a 15 percent response rate (6 of 40). Not only did the addition of MER decrease the response rate but it did not increase the duration of remission in the responders.

Some of the immunotherapeutic studies in melanoma by Cooperative Groups looked at immunologic prognostic factors in these patients. The value of pretherapy total peripheral lymphocytes and white blood cells was noted in patients receiving BCG.[27] Total peripheral lymphocytes and white blood cells were measured in patients receiving combination chemotherapy versus combination chemotherapy plus BCG. Patients with less than 1,000/cmm lymphocytes had a response rate of 24 percent, 1,000 to 2,000/cm had 19 percent while those with lymphocyte counts greater than 2,000/cmm had a response rate of 32 percent (p=0.03). There was no difference in survival for the three lymphocyte levels.

The prognostic value of skin tests was also evaluated.[28] There were no significant differences noted between the overall response to therapy and the number of positive skin tests. Patients with anergy had a median survival of 26 weeks, those with 1 or 2 positive tests 32 weeks, and those with 3 or more positive tests 48 weeks (p=0.05). No difference in survival was found between patients with a negative or positive reaction to PPD, dermatophyton, varidase or candida. There were statistical differences in the survival of patients with a positive reaction to mumps (p=0.02) or to PHA (p=0.02). Of those patients that were treated with BCG and had a pretreatment PPD negative, 74 percent changed to positive on a repeat test during treatment. These patients had a median survival of greater than 63 weeks while those that remained negative during the treatment had a median survival of 31 weeks (p=0.01). If there is any prognostic value of these delayed hypersensitivity studies, it appears to be confined to mumps and PHA skin tests.

COMBINED MODALITY STUDIES

The Cooperative Groups initially began as primary vehicles to perform chemotherapeutic studies. During the last 5 years with the increasing role of immunotherapy, this discipline has been added and more recently all major medical disciplines including surgery and its various subspecialties, radiotherapy and pathology have begun to play roles in Cooperative Group studies. One of the first studies tested the efficacy of radiotherapy in melanoma.[29] An attempt was made to evaluate the response to whole brain radiation with chemotherapy and/or cortico-steroids. Forty-one patients with cerebral metastases from melanoma were analyzed. These patients received a median tumor dose of 3,000 rads delivered to the entire brain over a two-week period. Twenty-four patients received concomitant chemotherapy and corticosteroids and 14 others received either chemotherapy or corticosteroids. The median and mean survival from completion of irradiation for all patients was 86 and 103 days respectively. Thirty-nine percent of the patients showed definite neurological improvement and had a median survival of 131 days. The median survival of the 25 nonresponding patients was only 17 days (p=0.002). The most frequently seen responses included return of limb function, disappearance of confusion, and cessation of other CNS manifestations. Since most chemotherapeutic regimens do not affect brain metastases, whole brain radiation has been instituted as stratification for all patients with disseminated disease who have brain metastases. Investigatively, the Cooperative Groups are studying various radiotherapy dosages and schedules to see if indeed an improvement in response rate and also in survival can be obtained.

Another extremely important clinical manifestation of disseminated melanoma is the presence of symptomatic bulky disease in lymph node areas and in organs such as the liver. In those patients in which surgery is not feasible, attempts at cytoreduction with varying doses and schedules of radiotherapy are studied.

An early Group study demonstrated that intraarterial administration of DTIC was feasible and could produce good local control of disease.[30] In this study 17 patients with advanced regional melanoma were treated with intraarterial DTIC in doses ranging from 75 mg/M^2 for 10 days to 400 mg/M^2 daily for 5 days. Six partial responses and one complete remission was noted for an overall response rate of 41 percent. The local control of melanoma by this modality was impressive and toxicity was much less than that which is usually seen with systemic chemotherapy utilizing DTIC. Some current Phase III studies in disseminated melanoma now stratify the patients with massive liver metastases to receive DTIC per hepatic artery infusion at 250 mg/M^2/day for 5 days.

The surgical discipline of Cooperative Groups is playing a greater role in studies in melanoma. Besides the previously mentioned perfusion studies, there has been widespread use in numerous centers of regional limb perfusion for invasive melanomas. Unfortunately the proponents of such a technique have never compared the efficacy of regional perfusion to wide excision alone. Such a study is now being undertaken.[31] It is a randomized study in which patients receive wide excision alone versus wide excision followed by regional perfusion with L-PAM at 1.2 mg/kg (48 mg/M^2). The perfusion time is 45 minutes and regional perfusion of the extremity should take place no more than 12 weeks after the wide excision of the primary lesion. A large group of surgeons are involved in this study. One of the questions that was raised was the similarity of techniques being used at various institutions. The surgeons who do this procedure at the member institutions met for a workshop of perfusion techniques in one laboratory. Following this, a standard technique was adopted to be utilized by all the surgeons.

Several Groups have studied the potential influence of chemotherapy and/or immunotherapy following resection of local disease. One group randomized 165 patients to chemotherapy alone versus no therapy for Stage I, II or III melanoma with all evidence of disease being removed and no evidence of metastases noted by extensive studies.[32] The chemotherapy patients received DTIC at 4.5 mg/kg IV daily for 10 days in the second, fifth, eighth, and eleventh postoperative months. At 150 weeks, 38 out of 84 no treatment patients and 46 out of 81 receiving DTIC were dead. There were no significant differences among males, but females showed a significantly longer disease-free interval in the no treatment arm. This study further showed that initial stage was significant as far as disease-free interval was concerned. Patients with Stage I had a markedly longer disease-free interval than those with Stage II and III (p value = 0.0003). There was no difference in the disease-free interval between Stage II and III patients. In the Stage II and III patients who had significant thrombocytopenia, disease-free interval was prolonged over those not noticing any toxicity and the control group, with a p value of .02 comparing toxic versus nontoxic and .007 comparing toxic with control.

BCG as adjuvant treatment in patients with Stage I and II was also studied.[33] The full participation of surgeons and pathologists was enlisted and although initially accrual was of great concern, through cooperative interaction a total of 707 patients were entered. In this study patients were grouped A through D. Group A patients were Stage I level 3 and 4, Group B were Stage I level 5, and Group C were extremity and head and neck Stage II with local or nodal recurrences. These groups were further stratified by skin reactivity, sex, node dissection (Group A & B) and surgery less than four weeks or greater than 4 weeks. Group D were Stage II patients with recurrence within 5 cm of the primary or in adjacent nodes. These patients were stratified to skin reactivity, sex and treatment beginning less than 4 weeks from surgery or greater than 4 weeks. Groups A, B, and C were randomized to no BCG or to BCG utilizing lyophilized Tice BCG administered intradermally, weekly for 4 weeks within the regional lymph node area and thereafter by rotating quadrants for a total of 18 months. Group D patients received DTIC + BCG or BCG alone. DTIC was administered at 200 mg/M^2 IV daily x 5 every 4 weeks. The median time to recurrence is similar in all groups and the proportion of patients free of tumor is statistically the same for the randomized treatments. This large study does not support the beneficial effects of BCG reported in nonrandomized trials by a single institution.

Another important adjuvant study is now being conducted.[34] All patients in this study have had surgery with all evidence of diseae removed. Studies must indicate no residual disease. Class I patients are identified as those with localized melanoma without any evidence of satellite lesions or regional or distant metastases. Class II patients are those with regional or distant metastases with all evidence of tumor being removed. The Class I patients are receiving BHD or no therapy. The chemotherapy limb has 46 patients, the control limb has 49. At three years there have been 7 failures in the chemotherapy limb (15 percent) and 12 failures in the control limb (24 percent). At this point there does not appear to be any significant difference in sex, age, primary site of tumor, depth of invasion at diagnosis and whether the primary was nodular or superficial spreading. The study must, of course, continue.

The Class II patients number 103 on the chemotherapy alone arm and 91 on chemotherapy plus BCG. The chemotherapy is the BHD regimen. On the chemotherapy alone limb 47 percent of patients have relapsed; on the chemotherapy + BCG limb 50 percent. The median disease-free survival for BHD is 97 weeks versus 63 weeks for BHD + BCG (p=0.09). The overall median survival for BHD has not yet been reached with a followup of 3 years, while that for BHD + BCG is 90 weeks. This difference has reached statistical significance (p=0.01)

Although the majority of the adjuvant studies performed by the Cooperative Groups are early, an advantage of these Group studies is that a large number of patients can be accrued to answer these very critical questions. At this time, there does not appear to be any advantage to chemotherapy versus no treatment in completely removed Stage I patients, while the addition of BCG to chemotherapy in Stage II patients with all disease removed appears to be disadvantageous. However, it is important to remember that these patients had minimal disease in which BCG is supposed to work at its best. Of course, a longer observation period is definitely necessary for these conclusions to be solidified.

PROGNOSTIC FACTORS

The major advantage in Cooperative Group studies is that a disease such as melanoma can be studied from a large patient population accrued over a relatively short period of time. Although priority is given to response rate, duration of remission, overall survival and drug toxicity, considerable data is being accrued concerning prognostic factors that will help better patient stratification in future Cooperative Group studies and independent studies. Knowledge of these prognostic factors will minimize differences in response rates which might be due to intrinsic factors of the patients rather than the alternative treatments under study.

Melanoma is a capricious malignant neoplasm with many variables which seem to influence survival. Factors that have been described as having prognostic value include such clinical parameters as stage of disease, sex, anatomical location, type of surgical treatment, immuno-competence as well as pathological parameters such as level of invasion (Clarks' microstaging), tumor thickness (Breslow's microstaging), growth pattern, ulceration, angioinvasion or lymphocytic infiltration. When numerous factors appear to influence survival rates, a multifactorial analysis may help delineate the dominant variables with independent predictive value. A multifactorial analysis is thus a powerful statistical method that minimizes selection bias, permits a more sophisticated examination of clinicopathological correlates and discriminates those factors that independently influence survival rates.

STAGE I MELANOMA

The four prognostic parameters that independently influence survival rate in Stage I melanoma are: 1) tumor thickness, 2) type of initial surgical treatment (i.e. whether or not an elective lymphadenectomy has been performed), 3) melanoma ulceration and 4) anatomical location.[35] The Clark's level of invasion significantly correlates with survival. However, comparative analyses have shown that its predictive value appeared generally to correlate with lesion thickness. Furthermore, it appeared that the actual histological structures invaded by the melanoma (i.e. level of invasion) were less predictive than the measured thickness in some instances. Thickness thus appears to be the dominant prognostic factor and should be accounted for in stratifying Stage I melanoma patients. There is still considerable controversy about whether elective lymphadenectomy should be performed for clinical Stage I patients. At least one Group institution has suggested that there is a subgroup of melanoma patients who benefit from this procedure; these patients have melanoma thickness between .77 and 4.0 mm.[36] Until this controversy has been resolved, it is important for Cooperative Group studies to account for this variable in analyzing their adjunctive therapy data.

Ulceration of the epithelium overlying the primary cutaneous melanoma is also an important prognostic indicator. Furthermore, melanomas located on the upper and lower extremities have a statistically better survival rate than melanomas in axial locations (i.e. trunk and head and neck). Trunk lesions have the worst prognosis of any of the major anatomical groups analyzed. The majority of patients with extremity melanomas were female, whereas the majority of patients with trunk and head and neck lesions were males. It seems probable that most studies that are stratified according to the sex of the patient, have in fact, accounted for differences in anatomical location of the melanomas. Ideally this latter parameter should be accounted for separately.

STAGE II MELANOMA

In patients who have documented regional node metastases, the following prognostic parameters appear to be important stratification purposes: 1) the number of metastatic lymph nodes, 2) ulceration, 3) anatomical location and 4) whether the nodal metastases were synchronous or matachronous with the primary melanoma. Several studies have indicated that the number of lymph node metastases correlate with survival and should be accounted for in clinical trials. The most significant breakdown of nodal metastases was 1 versus 2-4 versus > 4 metastatic lymph nodes. Almost all studies to date have agreed that greater or less than 4 lymph nodes is an important breakpoint for stratification purposes.

STAGE III MELANOMA

The two most important variables in patients with distant metastatic disease are: 1) the sites of involvement, and 2) the ambulatory status. Some studies have suggested that sex, age, and initial drug response are important variables but this has not been corroborated by all of the Cooperative Group studies. When accounting for metastatic sites of involvement, the most important categories to delineate were skin, subcutaneous tissue and nodal metastases versus visceral metastases. The visceral lesions can be further subdivided into brain and liver metastases versus other visceral sites. The patient's ambulatory status (as measured by the Karnofsky criteria) were also important parameters that influenced drug response. Sex and patient age have not been important predictors of survival in some clinical trials although data from individual Group studies have indicated that the response rate in males was higher for chemotherapy and for chemoimmunotherapy while such differences were not noted among females.[24] This study also demonstrated that the advantage of chemoimmunotherapy was greatest for patients between 40 to 70 years and was diminished for those outside these age limits. Most studies to date have indicated that the disease-free interval prior to metastatic disease does not influence the outcome of drug treatment.

FUTURE DIRECTIONS

1. The significant role of Cooperative Group studies in melanoma in the past decade is unquestioned. For the future, Phase III studies should look toward more extensive stratification of host characteristics so that important subgroups can be better identified and treatment modalities can be tailored to those subgroups. This type of extensive stratification can only be performed in a situation where a large number of patients are studied and randomized such as is achieved by the Cooperative Groups as they exist today.

2. The role of immunotherapy in the treatment of early or disseminated melanoma is very limited. As this report has shown, it appears that it may increase survival and response times in small subgroups of patients. This important observation must be pursued in a larger number of patients to determine the exact efficacy of immunotherapy in man.

3.   Newer drugs will continue to be studied in a Phase II fashion. It is obvious from some past studies that many of these drugs are tested in patients who are nonresponsive or who have relapsed on higher priority treatment programs. Future studies will begin to incorporate these newer drugs as primary therapy compared to existing standard therapy since this will be a better test of the drug.

4.   New combinations of drugs or drugs with other modalities are constantly being sought as pilot studies and ultimately brought to Cooperative Groups to determine efficacy. Certain key institutions in various Cooperative Groups have the capabilities of doing indepth cell kinetic studies. When these data become available, hopefully the design of Phase III studies and combination studies will be done with more rationale and they can be tested in a larger group of patients. In the meantime, limited institutional studies are being encouraged in all Cooperative Groups in order to come up with leads that may be effective. These leads then should be brought to the entire Group so that the questions can be answered with larger numbers of patients.

REFERENCES

245

1. Larsen RR, Hill GJ: Improved systemic chemotherapy for malignant melanoma. Am J Surg 122:36-41, 1971.
2. Gottlieb JA, Frei E, Luce JK: Dose schedule studies with hydroxyurea in malignant melanoma. Cancer Chemother Rep 55:277-280, 1971.
3. Luce JK, Thurman, WG, Isaacs BL, Talley RW: Clinical trials with the antitumor agent 5-(3,3-dimethyl-1-triazeno) imidazole-4-carboxamide. Cancer Chemother Rep 54:119-124, 1970.
4. Johnson RO, Metter G, Wilson W, Hill G, Krementz E: Phase I evaluation of DTIC and other studies in malignant melanoma in the Central Oncology Group. Cancer Treatment Rep 60:183-187, 1976.
5. Nathanson L, Wolter J, Horton J, Colsky J, Shnider BI, Schilling A: Characteristics of prognosis and response to imidazole carboxamide in malignant melanoma. Clin Pharmacol Ther 12:955-962, 1971.
6. Costanza M, Nathanson L, Costello W, Wolter J, Brunk F, Colsky J, Hall T, Oberfield R, Regelson W: Results of a randomized study comparing DTIC with TIC mustard in malignant melanoma. Cancer 37:1654-1659, 1976.
7. Thigpen T, Morrison F, Baker L: Phase II evaluation of dianhydrogalactitol in treatment of advanced malignant melanoma. AACR 18:240, 1977.
8. McKelvey EM, Hewlett JS, Thigpen T, Whitecar J: Cyclocytidine chemotherapy for malignant melanoma. Cancer Treat Rep 62:469-471, 1978.
9. Cecil JW, Quagliana JM, Coltman CA, Al-Sarraf M, Thigpen T, Groppe CW: Evaluation of VP-16-213 in malignant melanoma. Cancer Treat Rep 62:801-803, 1978.
10. Al-Sarraf M: Clinical trial of cis-Platinum: Hydration with or without Mannitol in patients with previously treated advanced malignant melanoma. A Southwest Oncology Group study. AACR 20:185, 1979.
11. Al-Sarraf M, Thigpen T, Groppe CW, Haut A, Padilla F: Piperazinedione in patients with metastatic malignant melanoma. Cancer Treat Rep 62:1101-1103, 1978.
12. Presant C, Bartolucci A, Ungaro P, Oldham R: A Phase II trial of Piperazinedione in malignant melanoma. Cancer Treat Rep 63:1367-1369, 1979.
13. Carbone PP, Costello W: Eastern Cooperative Oncology Group studies with DTIC. Cancer Treat Rep 60:193-198, 1976.
14. McKelvey EM, Luce JK, Talley RW, Hersh EM, Hewlett JS, Moon TE: Combination chemotherapy with BCNU, vincristine and DTIC in disseminated malignant melanoma. Cancer 39:1-4, 1977.
15. McKelvey EM, Luce JK, Vaitkevicius VK, Talley RW, Bodey GP, Lane M, Moon TE: BCNU, vincristine, DTIC and chlorpromazine for disseminated malignant melanoma. Cancer 39:5-10, 1977.
16. Costanzi JJ, Vaitkevicius VK, Quagliana JM, Hoogstraten B, Coltman CA, Delaney FC: Combination chemotherapy for disseminated malignant melanoma. Cancer 35:342-346, 1975.
17. Carter RD, Krementz ET, Hill GJ, Metter GE, Fletcher WS, Golomb FM, Grage TB, Minton JP, Sparks FC: DTIC and combination therapy for malignant melanoma. Studies with DTIC, BCNU, CCNU, vincristine and hydroxyurea. Cancer Treat Rep 60:601-609, 1976.
18. Hill GJ, Metter GE, Krementz ET, Fletcher WS, Golomb EM, Ramirez G, Grage TB, Moss SE: DTIC and combination therapy for melanoma. II. Escalating schedules of DTIC with BCNU, CCNU and vincristine. Cancer Treat Rep, 63:11-12, 1979.
19. Presant CA, Bartolucci A: Comparison of cyclophosphamide plus 1-day DTIC or 5-day DTIC in metastatic melanoma. AACR 19:320, 1978.
20. Gutterman JU, Mavligit GM, Reed R, Burgess MA, Gottlieb J, Hersh EM: BCG in combination with DTIC for the treatment of malignant melanoma. Cancer Treat Rep 60:177-182, 1976.
21. Gutterman JU, Mavligit GM, Gottlieb JA, et al: Chemoimmunotherapy of disseminated malignant melanoma with DTIC and BCG. New Eng J Med 291:592-597, 1974.
22. Nathanson L: Regression of intradermal malignant melanoma after intralesional injection of microbacterium Bovis Strain BCG. Cancer Chemother Rep 56:659-665, 1972.
23. Nathanson L, Schoenfeld D, Regelson W, Colsky J, Mittleman A: Prospective comparison of intralesional and multipuncture BCG in recurrent intradermal melanoma. Cancer 43:1630-1635, 1979.
24. Costanzi JJ: Chemotherapy and BCG in the treatment of disseminated malignant melanoma. In Immunotherapy of Cancer: Present Status of Trials in Man, WD Terry, D, Windhorst, eds. New York: Raven Press, pp 87-93, 1978.
25. Presant CA, Bartolucci AA, Smalley RV, Vogler WR: Effects of Corynebacterium parvum on combination chemotherapy of disseminated malignant melanoma. In Immunotherapy of Cancer: Present Status of Trials in Man, WD Terry, D Windhorst, eds. New York: Raven Press, pp 113-121, 1978.
26. Kostinas JE, Leone LA, Rege VB: Procarbazine, vinblastine and dactinomycin in Stage III and IV melanoma with or without MER. ASCO 19:355, 1978.
27. Al-Sarraf M, Costanzi JJ: Prognostic value of pretherapy total peripheral lymphocytes and white blood cells in patients with advanced malignant melanoma treated with chemotherapy and BCG - a Southwest Oncology Group Study. ASCO 19:310, 1978.
28. Al-Sarraf M, Costanzi JJ: The value of cellular mediating immunity in patients with disseminated melanoma treated with chemoimmunotherapy - A Southwest Oncology Group Study. AACR 19:13, 1978.
29. Gottlieb JA, Frei E III, Luce JK: An evaluation of the management of patients with cerebral metastases from malignant melanoma. Cancer 29:701-705, 1972.
30. Einhorn LH, McBride CM, Luce JK, Caoili E, Gottlieb JA: Intra-arterial infusion therapy with DTIC for malignant melanoma. Cancer 32:749-755, 1973.

REFERENCES

31. Boddie AW, Dixon D: A randomized prospective study of regional limb perfusion and wide excision vs. wide excision alone for invasive melanomas of the lower extremity. SWOG Agenda, November, 1978.

32. Hill GJ: Minutes of Central Oncology Group: Study COG-7040.

33. Cunningham TJ, Schoenfeld D, Nathanson L, Wolters J, Patterson WB, Cohen MH: A control study of adjuvant therapy in patients with Stage I and II malignant melanoma. In Immunotherapy of Cancer: Present Status of Trials in Man WD Terry, MD Windhorst, eds. New York: Raven Press, pp. 19-25, 1978.

34. Tranum B, Quagliana J, Neidhart J, Dixon D: SWOG Study 7521, Agenda of SWOG Meeting, September, 1979.

35. Balch CM, Murad TM, Soong SJ, Ingalls, AL, Halper NB, Maddox WA: A multifactorial analysis of melanoma. I. Prognostic histopathological features comparing Clark's and Breslow's staging methods. Ann Surg 188:732-742, 1978.

36. Balch CM, Murad TM, Soong S, Ingalls AL, Richards PC, Maddox WA: Tumor thickness as a guide to surgical management of clinical Stage I melanoma patients. Cancer 43:883-888, 1979.

13

Sarcomas of soft tissue and bone

Cary A. Presant, Ernest C. Borden, Laurence Baker, Mark E. Nesbit, and
Wataru W. Sutow

INTRODUCTION

Sarcomas of soft tissues and bone are uncommon malignancies. Malignant tumors of bone account for 0.5 percent of malignancies, and have an age adjusted incidence of 1 per 100,000 (1.1 per 100,000 for males, and 0.8 per 100,000 for females). Approximately 2,000 new cases are diagnosed annually in the United States. Malignant tumors of soft tissues account for 0.9 percent of malignancies and have an age adjusted incidence of 2.5 per 100,000 (3 per 100,000 for males, and 2 per 100,000 for females). Approximately 4,500 new cases occur annually (Table 1).

These tumors are of greater importance than their low frequency suggests, since they frequently occur in young individuals. Forty percent of malignant tumors of bone and 17 percent of soft tissue sarcomas occur before the age of 25. Furthermore, mortality rates have, in the past, been high for all such tumors. Long-term survival occurs in only 25 percent of patients with bone sarcomas and in only 35 percent of patients with soft tissue sarcoma.

The Cooperative Groups are necessary for a significant impact on treatment programs for these diseases. The underlying reasons are several. First, since these tumors are intrinsically uncommon, testing of any therapeutic intervention in a randomized prospective study requires input of multiple institutions to access sufficient patients to meet statistical validity. Second, since the histological subtypes of soft tissue sarcomas are so numerous, multiple institutions are required to

TABLE 1
Impact of Groups on New Cases of Sarcoma

	Estimated No. New Cases Annually	Estimated No. Deaths Annually	Estimated No. Cases Studied by Groups	Percent of Patients Cared for by Cooperative Groups	
				Primary	Metastatic
Bone Sarcomas	2000	1500	330	9%	10%
Soft Tissue Sarcomas	4500	2900	735	5%	18%

define the natural history of any subtype. If a retrospective analysis were performed utilizing patients from only one institution, several decades would be required, during which time standard therapy changes would make it impossible to determine whether prognostic variables were related to the nature of the disease process or to the changing therapeutic interventions.

The Cooperative Group activities have provided current, critically reviewed, and quality controlled therapy for a significant fraction of patients with these diseases. As indicated in Table 1, the Groups treated approximately 17 percent of patients in the United States with malignant tumors of bone (9 percent of patients requiring primary management, and 10 percent of patients requiring palliative therapy) and provided care for 16 percent of patients with soft tissue sarcomas (approximately 5 percent of patients requiring primary management, and 18 percent of patients requiring palliative therapy). Therefore, one of every six patients at some time during the course of his disease receives treatment organized by sarcoma specialists within the Cooperative Groups. With the gradually increasing size of many of the Groups, this impact can be expected to increase in the future.

ADJUVANT THERAPY OF OSTEOSARCOMA

Primary adjuvant chemotherapy for patients with nonmetastatic osteosarcoma is now considered by most oncologists to be "standard therapy". Meaningful data are available to support its apparent effectiveness in lengthening the duration of disease-free survival and even more important, in increasing the survival rate.[1-4] Following is a review of the significant participation of Cooperative Groups and Group-affiliated institutions in the development of current treatment attitudes in osteosarcoma. Much work done in affiliated institutions actually constitutes one phase of Group activity and eventually becomes incorporated into Group programs. The major contributions from two institutions not affiliated with Groups must be recognized: First, the pioneering work with the high-dose methotrexate and with citrovorum factor (HD-MTX-CF) regimens at Sidney Farber Cancer Center;[3],[5] and, secondly, the extensive programs with multidrug regimens conducted at Memorial Sloan-Kettering Cancer Center.[6],[7] References will be made to data from these two institutions wherever it appears that the inclusion of those data is necessary to provide proper perspective.

Historically, osteosarcoma had long been considered to be chemo-resistant.[8],[9] Prior to 1970, Phase II studies in metastatic and advanced cases had demonstrated no consistently effective chemotherapeutic agents. However, sporadic regressions, occasionally of impressive degree, had been reported following the administration of such drugs as mitomycin-C[10] and phenylalanine mustard (PAM).[11] Follow-up studies with the same agents unfortunately indicated that good responses were very infrequent.[12,13] The historical survival rate, when various series spanning several decades were averaged, was at best less than 20 percent regardless of the therapy.[1,2,3,9] Table 2 summarizes statistics from several reports to provide control data on survival in osteosarcoma prior to the introduction of effective adjuvant chemotherapy.

ADJUVANT CHEMOTHERAPY

The Cooperative Group studies are shown in Table 3. Adjuvant chemotherapy in nonmetastatic osteosarcoma was first attempted in 1962 utilizing single agent administration of PAM.[14] Of 14 patients

TABLE 2
Survival in Osteosarcoma Prior to 1970

Source	Reference	Number of Cases	Survival
Compiled data	9	1286	20%(at 5 yrs)
Sidney Farber Cancer Center	3	48	15 to 20%
M.D. Anderson Hospital	1	89*†	20% (at 4 yrs)
Memorial Sloan-Kettering Cancer Center	2	210*†	21% (at 5 yrs)

* Age under 21 years

†Extremity primary lesions only

TABLE 3

Cooperative Group Activities in the Development of Adjuvant Chemotherapy Programs for Osteosarcoma

Cooperative Group	Activities
SWOG (Pediatric Division)	1. Phase I—II trials
	2. Concept of adjuvant chemotherapy
	3. Multidrug adjuvant chemotherapy (CONPADRI— COMPADRI studies)
	4. Pharmacologic studies- high-dose MTX
SWOG (Adult Division)	5. Adriamycin-DTIC studies
	6. Phase I-II trials with new drugs
CALGB	1. Adriamycin studies (Phase II)
	2. Adriamycin adjuvant chemotherapy
	3. Cis-platinum
COG	1. CONPADRI—I trial
	2. Phase I & II trials
CCSG	1. Phase I & II trials

treated, only two survived for five years. By 1965, the marked
effectiveness of VAC combination chemotherapy (vincristine, actinomycin-D and cyclophosphamide) had been demonstrated in childhood
rhabdomyosarcoma.[15] Dosage studies with cyclophosphamide had also
indicated that large-dose intermittent pulses seemingly improved the
therapeutic effectiveness of the drug.[16] Consequently, the original
VAC schedule was modified to include cyclophosphamide in pulses
(pulse-VAC) and the new regimen was utilized in adjuvant chemotherapy in nonmetastatic osteosarcoma from about 1968 until 1971.
From a total of 12 patients so treated, four remain free of disease.[14]

Early indication that adriamycin had considerable activity in metastatic
osteosarcoma was noted around 1970.[17,18] Adriamycin, vincristine,
cyclophosphamide, and PAM were then combined into a 4-drug regimen
(CONPADRI),[19-21] and this new adjuvant chemotherapeutic program
was first utilized in the treatment of nonmetastatic osteosarcoma in
March 1971. Of the first 18 patients treated, 10 (56 percent) have
remained disease-free 4 years or longer after amputation.[22]

Adriamycin was also utilized as a single agent in the adjuvant chemo-therapy of non-metastatic osteosarcoma.[4,23-27] The 5-year follow-up report of 88 patients showed a disease-free survival of 39 percent.[4] The main factors that appeared to influence significantly the disease-free rate were age under 16 years and adherence to protocol requirements for adriamycin dosage and surgical guidelines. The relapse-free rate in 47 patients with no protocol violation was 66 percent.[4]

When the regimen utilizing high-dose methotrexate with citrovorum factor (HD-MTX-CF) was shown to have significant antitumor activity in patients with metastatic osteosarcoma,[5] HD-MTX-CF pulses were added to multiagent programs that included adriamycin.[28-30] In one such program (COMPADRI-II), modification of the schedule (from CONPADRI-I) resulted in decreased dosage of adriamycin (Figure 1). It is assumed that the disappointing disease-free survival in COMPADRI-II and particularly the emergence of late metastases were the con-sequences of the dosage reduction.[29,31]

The effectiveness of HD-MTX-CF utilized as a single-agent adjuvant chemotherapy regimen has been evaluated particularly at the Sidney Farber Cancer Center. Of 12 patients treated, five (42 percent) remain free of disease.[6]

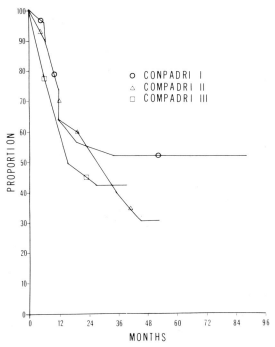

Fig. 1. Disease-free survival in osteosarcoma

TABLE 4
Overall Survival in Osteosarcoma Treated After 1970

| Institution | Survival Data | |
	No. Of Patients	Projected Survival (%)
M.D. Anderson Hospital	36	81
Sidney Farber Cancer Center	34	80
Memorial Sloan-Kettering Cancer Center	31	77

A valid measure of the effectiveness of treatment for any malignant tumor is the ultimate number of patients surviving the disease. Three sets of currently available data that can be used to estimate the projected overall survival rate in patients with osteosarcoma, non-metastatic at diagnosis are given in Table 4.

In comparison with the overall survival rate of less than 20 percent prior to 1970, the current 5-year survival rate approximating 80 percent would seem to constitute evidence that therapy after 1970 has become significantly effective. In the interpretation of these data, however, it must be kept in mind that overall survival includes the results of therapy instituted after the development of metastases. Thus, not all of the improved survival may be attributable to adjuvant chemotherapy during the nonmetastatic phase. On the other hand, the possibility exists that adjuvant chemotherapy programs may, in themselves, have improved the effectiveness of postmetastatic therapy. For example, earlier diagnosis of metastases could result from better follow-up studies. Chemotherapy could have changed the pattern of metastases from diffuse spread to more treatable fewer discrete nodules.[32]

CURRENT STUDIES

The paucity of significantly effective new chemotherapeutic agents for the treatment of osteosarcoma is a major bottleneck in the development of more effective adjuvant programs.[8,9] Table 5 indicates that practically every drug that has had at least moderate activity has been incorporated into one or more multidrug adjuvant regimens. The one exception is the combination of adriamycin and DTIC. Gottlieb and

TABLE 5
Development of Adjuvant Programs

Drug/Combinations	Phase II Effectiveness in Osteosarcoma	Incorporation in Adjuvant Programs
1. PAM	Moderate	Yes
2. Vincristine	Minimal	Yes
3. Cyclophosphamide	Some	Yes
4. VAC	Not Tested	Yes
5. Adriamycin	Good	Yes
6. DTIC	Minimal	No
7. Adria-DTIC	Good	Pilot studies
8. Cis-platinum	Moderate	Yes
9. Mitomycin-C	Minimal	No
10. 5-FU	Minimal	No
11. Hexamethylmelamine	Minimal	No

colleagues have demonstrated that in metastatic sarcomas the combination of adriamycin with DTIC was more effective than adriamycin used singly.[33-35] Although there is an ongoing study using adriamycin with DTIC in nonmetastatic osteosarcoma, other regimens use adriamycin without concomitant DTIC.

Although HD-MTX-CF regimens were used initially as single agent chemotherapy, the current programs utilized at the Sidney Farber Cancer Center now include both HD-MTX and adriamycin.[3,5,32] The investigators at Memorial Sloan-Kettering Cancer Center started with a multidrug approach and have now added bleomycin and actinomycin-D to a 5-drug regimen.[6] Whether increasing the number of agents in a given regimen or increasing its dose and/or frequency of administration will increase the effectiveness of treatment remains to be demonstrated.

The preoperative administration of chemotherapy has a logical outgrowth, the limb salvage approaches with en bloc resection and prosthetic bone replacement.[36,37] Also the possibility of prophylactic pulmonary irradiation is being reexamined. A prior negative study had utilized pulmonary irradiation without concomitant chemotherapy.[38]

One of the significant correlates of high-dose methotrexate therapy in osteosarcoma has been the development of pharmacologic laboratory support. While the primary purpose of such laboratories concerns the monitoring of the clinical course of patients undergoing protocol therapy, considerable basic pharmacokinetic research of methotrexate has also been generated. This represents a model multidisciplinary collaboration in which the good of the patient was the prime concern but in which the clinically-oriented laboratory activity in turn generated basic research problems.

There has been one discordant note in the general belief that the natural history of a malignant tumor such as osteosarcoma could not change suddenly. In a provocative report, Mayo Clinic investigators suggested that there was a significant improvement in the metastasis-free interval and survival time from 1963 to 1974 without the use of adjuvant chemotherapy.[39,40] This data questions the validity of the "historical controls" used in the previously cited studies and thus casts doubt on the effectiveness of adjuvant chemotherapy programs. In this respect, it is unfortunate that no direct comparative (randomized) studies were initiated in the early seventies so as to establish with greater certainty the therapeutic efficacy of adjuvant chemotherapy. On the other hand, the data from the M.D. Anderson Hospital,[1] Memorial Sloan Kettering Center,[2] and Sidney Farber Cancer Center[3] do not show an improvement in survival over the years without the use of adjuvant chemotherapy as was seen at Mayo Clinic.

ADJUVANT THERAPY OF EWING'S SARCOMA

The treatment of Ewing's sarcoma of bone has paralleled that of many of the other solid tumors in children in the last 20 years. During the 1950's and early 1960's, the prognosis was poor when the tumor was treated with local radiotherapy, or surgery or both. In a review of six series a total of only 36 out of 374 children (10 percent) survived five years. Early and often clinically undetectable metastases appeared to be the most important factor leading to the tumor's poor prognosis. The primary tumor could often be controlled by radiotherapy but local relapses occurred in 25 to 50 percent of reported cases. Doses of radiotherapy greater than 6,000 rads were usually associated with better local control. After the success of adding systemic chemotherapy to the treatment of Wilms' tumor and rhabdomyosarcoma was demonstrated, a similar approach in Ewing's sarcoma was taken. Initial studies were with single drugs and subsequently with a combination of drugs. The agents that were found to be effective were vincristine, cyclophosphamide, 5-Fluorouracil, BCNU, actinomycin-D, and adriamycin. With the addition of systemic chemotherapy to local treatment, the local relapse rate decreased to between 10 and 20 percent. Traditionally, the whole bone was irradiated but several studies suggested that a shrinking field technique rather than the uniform dose of radiation to the whole bone might give equally good results while allowing a decrease in local toxicity and late effects. Questions that were unanswered were: 1) what dose of radiotherapy would best control the primary lesion when combined with chemotherapy, 2) can individualization of radiation to different locations of primaries produce better results, and 3) what volume of radiation should be used for the treatment of primary lesion? It was at this point that a more coordinated effort began for the treatment of Ewing's sarcoma throughout the United States. It had the advantage of collecting large numbers of Ewing's sarcoma for the assessment of treatment results, as well as the study of epidemiological factors, pathologic patterns and prognostic variables.

INTERGROUP EWING'S SARCOMA PROTOCOL 1973-1978

A protocol was developed in January, 1973 which received the approval of three national study groups: Childrens Cancer Study Group, Southwest Oncology Group, and Cancer and Leukemia Group B. Participating institutions subscribed to one of two concurrently run studies. In some institutions, patients were randomized to receive either no chemo-

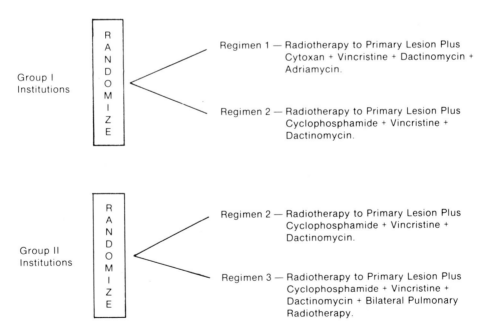

Fig. 2. Outline of study design for nonmetastatic Ewing's sarcoma of bone

therapy or combination chemotherapy consisting of vincristine, actinomycin-D, and cyclophosphamide (VAC). In other institutions patients
were randomized to receive VAC or VAC plus prophylactic bilateral
pulmonary irradiation. These treatments were adjuvant to local irradiation (vide infra).

By November, 1973, two-thirds of the patients who had received no
chemotherapy already had evidence of dissemination of their tumor. It
was decided to close randomization to the no chemotherapy arm. A
modification was developed so that there was randomization between a
four-drug chemotherapy program which included adriamycin in addition
to the VAC regimen and VAC alone (Figure 2). The randomization
continued for the group of institutions studying the difference between
VAC and VAC plus bilateral pulmonary irradiation.

By 1976, those patients who received VAC alone were found to have a
survival rate significantly lower than those who received either four
drugs or those with VAC plus bilateral pulmonary irradiation.[41] There
was no difference in the survival between the other two arms. Thereafter, patients were randomized to one of the two latter groups. The
rest period between the chemotherapy cycles was shortened from six
weeks to three weeks. The entire protocol was closed to further entry

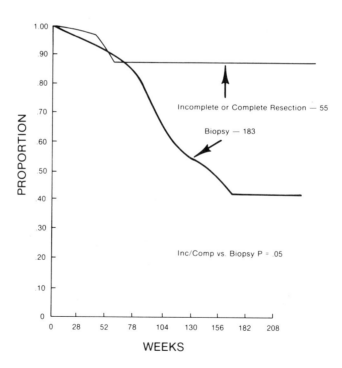

Fig. 3. Survival experience by initial surgical history by life table

of patients in November 1978 when final approval of a new study was completed (Study II) and the objectives of the initial study had been reached.

In the Intergroup Ewing's Sarcoma Protocol, the surgery is limited to a diagnostic biopsy only. However, during the period of time that this protocol was entering patients, there was a resurgence of interest in surgical procedures, and especially during the last several years, more aggressive surgery has been performed on the primary lesion. Twenty-two or 9 percent had complete resection of the primary lesion, and 32 or 13 percent had incomplete resection. Biopsy alone was performed in 183 patients. When analyzed by a multivariate method, these surgical differences, along with the primary site, sex, and treatment regimen, were significant factors in outcome. Patients with incomplete or complete resection had significantly better survival than patients with biopsy only (p = 0.05, Figure 3). They also have a longer disease-free survival (p = 0.12).

Overall, 314 evaluable patients were studied. One hundred of these were treated with VAC plus adriamycin, 60 with VAC alone, and 75 with VAC plus bilateral pulmonary irradiation.[42,43] The results demonstrated:

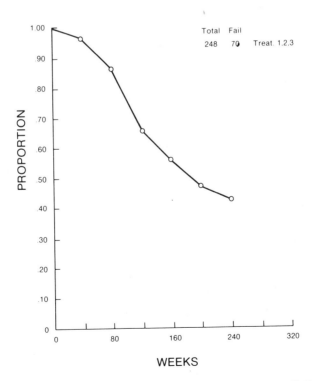

Fig. 4. Intergroup Ewing's sarcoma study; Survival for all 3 treatments combined

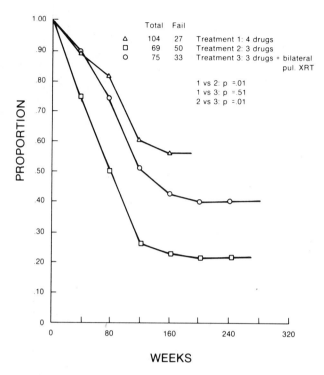

Fig. 5. Intergroup Ewing's sarcoma study; Time to relapse

1)   The overall survival was 58 percent at three years (Figure 4).

2)   The addition of adriamycin or bilateral pulmonary irradiation to VAC chemotherapy improved significantly the disease-free and overall survival (Figure 5). There was no statistically significant difference between the disease-free and overall survival for those patients who received VAC plus adriamycin and those who recieved VAC plus bilateral pulmonary irradiation. For these latter two groups of patients, the incidence and time to pulmonary metastases was the same. With longer followup (18 months longer), the median relapse-free survival has still not been reached with Treatment 1 and the difference with Treatment 3 has now reached the p = .11 level.

3)   Reducing the interval between the chemotherapy courses from six weeks to three weeks improved survival.

4)   Four patient characteristics (age, sex, primary site, surgical history) and the three treatment regimens were tested for

their relationship to time to relapse and to survival using Cox's regression model. The unfavorable characteristics were: primary site pelvis or proxima extremity, treatment with VAC alone and surgical history of biopsy only.[42]

LOCAL CONTROL IN THE INTERGROUP EWING'S SARCOMA STUDY

Patients all received a standard dose of radiation therapy, a tumor dose of 4,500 to 5,000 rads to the whole plus an optional boost dose of 1,000 rads to the radiographic extent of the lesion with 5 cm margin. Lower doses were given for younger children. This practice was based on the assumption that Ewing's sarcoma spreads along the medullary cavity to either end of the bone. In this study, clinically evident local relapse occurred in 12 percent of patients. Though there was not a significant advantage to higher doses, there was a trend relating higher dose to better local control with each increment in the dose of radiotherapy (Table 6). Patients with pelvic and humeral primaries had a relatively high rate of local relapse (16 and 21 percent respectively), while other lesions including the skull or spine had local relapse in only 4 to 10 percent. This included rib lesions which in the past were thought to have a very poor prognosis. Twelve cases did not have whole bone radiation but the primary lesion was treated with at least a 5 cm margin. The local control achieved in this group was similar to the group in which the whole bone was treated. In contrast, of the 28 patients in whom there was not at least a 5 cm margin around the area of destruction, the local relapse rate increased to 21 percent (Figure 6). The addition of adriamycin to VAC significantly reduced the local recurrence rate (Figure 7).

This study significantly changed the therapy of Ewing's sarcoma. As a result, the following recommendations were made:

1)   The most effective treatment consists of radiotherapy with 5,000 to 6,000 rads in combination with four-drug chemo-

TABLE 6
Intergroup Ewing's Sarcoma Study: Correlation of Local Control With Dose of Irradiation and Treatment Regimen

Tumor Dose (RADS)	Regimen I	Regimen II	Regimen III
3000 to less than 4000	4/4	1/1	1/1
4000 to less than 5000	19/21 (90%)	9/12 (75%)	9/10 (90%)
5000 to less than 6000	30/31 (97%)	25/30 (83%)	25/30 (83%)
6000 and greater	17/17 (100%)	20/21 (95%)	13/15 (87%)
Total	70/73 (96%)	55/64 (86%)	48/56 (86%)

therapy: actinomycin-D, vincristine, cyclophosphamide and adriamycin.

2)   The use of radiation therapy alone as local treatment for pelvic and humeral lesions should be questioned and possibly supplemented by the use of surgical resection since those lesions had a high local recurrence rate with radiotherapy alone.

3)   Whole bone irradiation including both epiphyseal centers may not be necessary for all primary lesions.

INTERGROUP EWING'S SARCOMA STUDY II

The major conclusions concerning the importance of the location of the primary, interval between treatment courses, initial surgical history, and effectiveness of four drugs (VAC + adriamycin) were taken into consideration as the basis for Study II. Pelvic primaries were separated

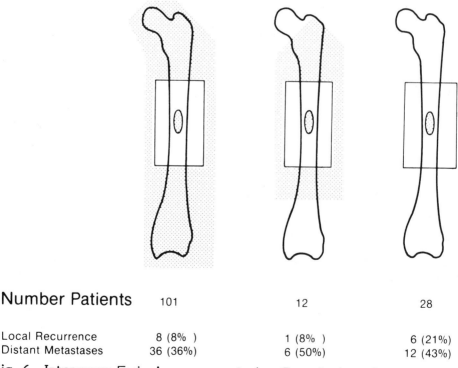

Number Patients	101	12	28
Local Recurrence	8 (8%)	1 (8%)	6 (21%)
Distant Metastases	36 (36%)	6 (50%)	12 (43%)

Fig. 6. Intergroup Ewing's sarcoma study: Correlation of treated volume with incidence of local recurrence and distant metastases

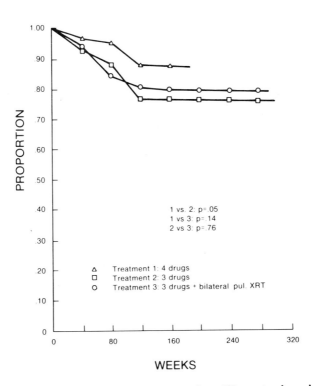

Fig. 7. Intergroup Ewing's sarcoma study: Time to local recurrence

from other primary locations because of their poorer prognosis. The study for nonpelvic primaries involved a comparison of two forms of chemotherapy: a four-drug chemotherapy program (VAC + adriamycin) given in a weekly fashion compared to the same four-drug chemotherapy (VAC + adriamycin) but given in a high-dose intermittent schedule.

For pelvic primaries, patients were given a six-week course of high dose intermittent chemotherapy followed by surgical resection, if possible. If the tumor was totally excised, no radiation therapy was given, and high dose intermittent chemotherapy was continued for an additional 70 weeks. If no surgery was attempted or if there was incomplete surgical resection, radiation therapy was administered to the area of the primary lesion, followed by high-dose intermittent chemotherapy for an additional 70 weeks.

Study II remains active at the present time. This study should answer questions on individualization of treatment by primary site, and on optimization of chemotherapy dose and schedule.

THERAPY OF ADVANCED BONE SARCOMAS

OSTEOSARCOMA AND CHRONDROSARCOMA

Survival with metastatic osteosarcoma is almost always less than 12 months in the absence of successful surgical or chemotherapeutic intervention.[44-46] Lung and/or pleura are the commonest sites of metastases being detected in over 70 percent of patients premortem and over 95 percent at autopsy. Less common sites (20 to 35 percent at autopsy) of metastatic disease include other thoracic structures (diaphragm, mediastinum, heart), bones, and lymph nodes. Infrequently, (10 percent at autopsy) other organs are involved.

Patients with recurrence presenting as discrete pulmonary metastases after an extended disease-free interval may be converted to long-term survivors by resection of the pulmonary nodules.[47,48] Such patients may also benefit from administration of chemotherapy following resection of the pulmonary nodules.[49]

Cooperative Group studies of metastatic osteosarcoma have focused on defining active chemotherapeutic agents. Among the earliest studies to demonstrate activity of adriamycin in this disease was a Phase II study of a Cooperative Group.[50] Adriamycin given every three weeks at 75 mg/M^2 for good-risk patients or 60 mg/M^2 for poor-risk patients resulted in 5 of 9 partial responses. A subsequent study at the same doses resulted in 0 of 4 responses for an overall response rate of 38 percent. The median duration of survival of responders was 8 months, and of nonresponders 3 months. Subsequent Cooperative Group studies of adriamycin in metastatic osteosarcoma have confirmed its activity as a single agent but with lower response rates. Using a weekly dosage schedule of 0.6 mg/kg in good-risk patients or 0.4 mg/kg in poor-risk patients after a short loading course led to an objective response rate of 14 percent in 22 patients.[51] Using a total dose of 60 mg/M^2 divided into 3 daily doses every three weeks resulted in an objective response rate of only 8 percent. The cumulative pooled response rate for adriamycin given every three weeks at 60 to 75 mg/M^2 in a Cooperative Group series has been six partial responses of 27 reported patients (22 percent).

High-dose methotrexate with leucovorin rescue, which is reported to have a 40 percent response rate in metastatic osteosarcoma,[52] has been successfully used by Cooperative Group members at individual institutions. It has not yet been extensively incorporated into Group studies, in part, because of concern about toxicity risks. However it has been incorporated into the adjuvant studies of osteosarcoma (COMPADRI) of one group.[53] No undue toxicity resulted.

Activity of a number of other chemotherapeutic agents has been explored in Phase II Cooperative Group trials in osteosarcoma. Alkylating agents have received the most attention. Phenylalanine mustard (L-PAM) resulted in three partial responses in 26 treated patients.[54] Cyclophosphamide resulted in one response in 11 patients,[55] uracil mustard was ineffective in 10 patients,[55] and mitomycin-C resulted in no responses in 13 patients.[56] DTIC (dimethyl triazeno imidazole carboxamide) in various Cooperative Groups and institutional trials has been slightly active with 2 of 14 patients treated having partial responses. Results of an ongoing trial with cis-platinum diammine dichloride (CPDD) suggests this drug may have therapeutic activity in osteogenic sarcoma.[57] One of eight patients previously treated with adriamycin and high-dose methotrexate had a complete response. An institutional trial with CPDD resulted in even better response rates (1 CR and 3 PR's of 8 treated patients).[58] However, in the evaluation of new agents for osteosarcoma it is important to note that occasionally remarkable responses have resulted from modalities, which with further evaluation have not had significant activity. Mitomycin-C, hexamethylmelamine, 5-Fluorouracil, and radiation therapy have all resulted in long-term complete responses (presumed cures). Other chemotherapeutic agents evaluated in prior Cooperative Group trials have not had significant activity. Thus adriamycin and high-dose methotrexate with leucovorin rescue are the most active compounds with L-PAM, DTIC, and CPDD resulting in lower objective response rates.

Combination chemotherapy, utilizing adriamycin together with other compounds, has been evaluated in several prior studies and remains under investigation. Adriamycin (60 mg/M^2) in combination with DTIC (250 mg/M^2 daily for five days) resulted in an objective response rate of 39 percent of 33 treated patients.[59] Three had complete responses and 10 had partial responses; the duration of survival in responding patients exceeded 11 months. In a subsequent study, vincristine was added to the combination. No increase in response resulted (3 PR's of 13 patients treated). Combining the results of these two studies utilizing adriamycin and DTIC, the overall response rate was 35 percent.[60] Median survival of the complete responders exceeded 15 months. Cyclophosphamide has been added to the adriamycin, DTIC and vincristine combination, but no further improvement in response rate has occurred. Seven of 29 patients responded with only one patient obtaining a complete response. The combination of cyclophosphamide, adriamycin, actinomycin-D and vincristine resulted in 2 CR's and 3 PR's of 20 treated patients. A combination employing adriamycin (60 mg/M^2), methotrexate (25 mg/M^2), and cyclophosphamide (600 mg/M^2) resulted in one complete and four partial responders of 12 treated patients.

The combination chemotherapy results give some support to the postulate that higher doses of adriamycin are more effective in inducing responses in osteosarcoma.[60] Other factors which may have influenced response rates include age, sex, prior therapy, disease-free interval, metastatic sites, and histologic subtypes. Patients with longer disease-free intervals had a higher objective response rate and had a significantly greater chance of obtaining a complete response in one study. Histopathologic review suggested that patients with the osteoblastic variant might have a higher response rate than chondroblastic osteosarcoma.[60]

In addition to basic pathologic differences, chondrosarcoma differs markedly from osteosarcoma in its clinical features. Age, site of origin, recurrence patterns, and rate of progression are all strikingly different. This tumor is one of adult life and older age, occurs predominantly in the trunk, frequently recurs locally, has a five-year survival even with inadequate primary surgical treatment of 38 percent and has a median survival time with metastatic disease of approximately 18 to 24 months.[61-63]

Adriamycin has been felt to have only limited activity in metastatic chondrosarcoma. However, Cooperative Group chemotherapy evaluations of adriamycin as a single agent have not borne this out. The overall reported response rate to adriamycin given at either 60-70 mg/M^2 every three weeks has been 40 percent (4 PR's of 10 treated patients). No other single agent has demonstrated significant activity in Cooperative Group trials. Addition of methotrexate, vincristine, actinomycin-D, cyclophosphamide, or DTIC to adriamcyin has seemingly decreased the single agent response rate of adriamycin.[59] Only 3 of 29 patients have had partial responses to adriamycin combination therapy.

Thus, Cooperative Group trials have clearly established the efficacy of adriamycin in metastatic osteosarcoma. No clear cut superiority of chemotherapeutic combinations to adriamycin alone given at optimal doses or to high-dose methotrexate with leucovorin rescue has been observed. Future studies of metastatic osteosarcoma may evaluate combinations such as cis-platinum and adriamycin or newer therapeutic modalities such as interferon.[64]

The future should see an increased number of intergroup studies. The rarity of osteosarcoma and chondrosarcoma limits the number of patients which can be entered in a reasonable period even by the largest Groups. Combined modality trials, such as the value of adjuvant chemotherapy following resection of discrete pulmonary metastases, will require intergroup collaboration. Determination of prognostic variables in metastatic disease will benefit from histopathologic reviews, which are already underway, and also from intergroup studies.

ADJUVANT THERAPY OF SOFT TISSUE SARCOMAS

The natural history of soft tissue sarcomas treated only with surgery is difficult to assess from retrospective review of the literature. Considering only resectable cases operated on for cure, the range of 5-year survivals for specific histological subtypes is considerable. For example, in synovial sarcoma the range of 5-year survival is 20 percent to 40 percent,[65-67] and in liposarcoma it is 32 percent to 47 percent.[68-69] Most recurrences are observed to be within 2 years of surgery. In some series it is difficult to identify radically versus locally resected cases and local versus local-plus-distant versus distant-only recurrences. Most confusing of all is the changing "state of the art" for nomenclature of histological subtypes. The recent emphasis on malignant fibrous histiocytoma as a distinct pathological entity creates a situation where the most commonly diagnosed soft part sarcoma has a poorly documented natural history since these patients had been previously classified within the older histological types.

Two important questions emerge:

1) What is the "natural history" of a given histological type of soft tissue sarcoma given adequate surgical management? Since the range is relatively large, no answer is possible without more sophisticated discriminant analysis to define clinical and surgical therapeutic prognostic factors.

2) What is the impact of pathological reclassification on the accepted natural history as reflected in previously published manuscripts? This cannot be assessed since few patients in any study could be reclassified by a pathologist or group of pathologists using current histological criteria and since current cases with adequate histological classification have obviously not been followed for a sufficient length of time to have adequate survival data.

The implication of these questions is that nonrandomized studies using "historical" controls will be nearly impossible to evaluate, unless "historical" controls have similar histological classification, clinical evaluation, and standard therapeutic intervention prior to the use of the modality being evaluated. Prospective randomized trials with authoritative pathological review will therefore be necessary to demonstrate the effect of any therapeutic intervention in this heterogenous group of disorders termed collectively "soft tissue sarcomas".

Recently, a staging system has been accepted for soft tissue sarcomas based on histopathological type and grade of malignancy, location and

TABLE 7
American Joint Committee Staging of Soft Tissue

Stage	Survival	
	2 Year	5 Year
I	85%	75%
II	73%	55%
III	45%	29%
IV	19%	7%

invasiveness of tumor, age of patient, and size of tumor.[70] This staging system has allowed discrimination of four groups of patients in the 702 cases reviewed (Table 7). The system remains limited by the lack of specific guidelines for grading the degree of malignancy within any given histological type and the lack of evaluation of therapy given patients included in the study on which the grading system was being formulated. Both limitations are being approached in current studies.

Given this background, what information exists from randomized or adequately controlled studies of adjuvant therapy in adult soft tissue sarcomas? Two adult studies are relevant.

VACAR study of soft tissue sarcomas.[71] Between 1973 and 1976, 75 patients with Grade II or Grade III soft tissue sarcoma were randomized to receive postoperative radiation therapy alone or postoperative radiation therapy plus chemotherapy (Table 8). Surgery was "conservative". Chemotherapy was given concurrently with radiation therapy unless the radiation therapy portal included more than 35 percent of bone marrow. It is important that all 8 head and neck and 4 abdominal tumors received chemotherapy. Chemotherapy doses were high: the median nadir granulocyte count was $400/mm^3$ with 3 infections requiring hospitalization, and 3 patients developed congestive heart failure. Of 47 patients with trunk or extremity tumors randomized on the study with a followup of 9 to 34 months, 67 percent of chemotherapy patients were free of disease versus 85 percent of control patients.

While this study appears to indicate no value of adjunctive chemotherapy, several criticisms are appropriate: a) Followup on this study is short- only 15 patients had been followed for 24 months; b) The number of patients was small, and therefore the number with any histological

TABLE 8
VACAR Protocol for Soft Tissue Sarcomas

Control	Surgery (no gross residual tumor)
	6,500 Rads in $6\frac{1}{2}$ weeks
Therapy	Surgery (no gross residual tumor)
	6,500 Rads in $6\frac{1}{2}$ weeks

Vincristine 1.5 mg/M^2 (maximum 2 mg) IV
day 1, then weekly x 9; then day 1 every 4 weeks
(8 weeks with actinomycin-D)

Cyclophosphamide 200 mg/M^2 PO days
3, 4, 5 every 4 weeks (8 weeks with
actinomycin-D)

Adriamycin 60 mg/M^2 IV day 2 every 4
weeks x 7; then actinomycin-D 0.3 mg/M^2
(maximum 0.5 mg) days 1-5 every 8 weeks

type was low; and c) if chemotherapy is more effective in only some histological types then the study is incomplete and potentially misleading. This means that the goals of this kind of study can be met only by a multiinstitutional approach.

It is important to note the comparison of the current results of the VACAR study with the "historical" control patients treated prior to the current study at the same institution. At 18 months after surgery, survival free of disease for the historical control group was 24 out of 53 (45 percent), compared to 10 out of 12 for control patients (83 percent), and 16 out of 21 for chemotherapy patients (76 percent). The VACAR study patients survived "significantly" better ($p < 0.005$), although "historical" patients also received surgery plus radiation therapy. This observation underscores the importance of not using historical controls to reach definitive conclusions.

Study of Uterine Sarcomas: Beginning in 1973, 101 patients with Stage I or Stage II uterine sarcomas were randomized to receive adriamycin 60 mg/M^2 IV every 3 weeks x 8 or no further therapy. Sixty patients were evaluable in 1977 (Minutes, Soft Tissue Sarcoma Discussion Meeting, October 1977). In the chemotherapy group, 4 of 24 patients (17 percent) have recurred, compared to 11 of 36 patients (31 percent) in the control group. Although this suggests some advantage for chemotherapy, several problems exist: a) Follow-up times were not stated, but were obviously still short; b) Histological diagnoses were varied with small numbers in each histological group and the patients had not at that time been classified according to histological grade of malignancy; and c) Since half the recurrences were in the pelvis and preoperative therapy was given to only half the patients, the study must still be analyzed for interaction among the following important variables as well as the contribution of each to the disease-free survival: preoperative radiotherapy, chemotherapy, stage, and histological grade of tumor.

It is important to note the advances made in pediatric rhabdomyosarcomas by the Intergroup Rhabdomyosarcoma Study.[72] Since the group is studying a single tumor type (albeit with histological variability) in a restricted age population, analysis of the results of adjuvant trials is more definitive than the studies currently in progress with adult soft tissue sarcomas. In prospective randomized trials, the Intergroup Rhabdomyosarcoma Study has demonstrated similar disease-free survival in patients with fully resectable tumors treated with postoperative radiotherapy, or postoperative vincristine, actinomycin-D plus cyclophosphamide. In patients with microscopic residual tumors following resection, postoperative radiation therapy plus chemotherapy produced equal survival regardless of whether cyclophosphamide was added to actinomycin-D plus vincristine or not.

Adjuvant trials in progress should help to establish the role of certain chemotherapy regimens in adult soft tissue sarcomas. Concurrent pathology review and standardization of nonchemotherapy treatment should also further define the current natural history of the diseases in question and the role of the American Joint Committee staging system in patient management.

THERAPY OF MALIGNANT MESOTHELIOMA

Mesotheliomas are neoplasms with unique pathologic and clinical features.[73,74] They arise in the serous lining of pleural or peritoneal cavities and have a histological appearance which may sometimes be variable and difficult to diagnose. Their spread is primarily by local invasion with only a limited propensity for more distant involvement. Symptoms usually come from compromise of local organ function, frequently from pleural effusion or ascites. Median survival from the onset of symptoms is approximately 12 months, with few patients surviving beyond two years. Local modalities such as surgery or radiation are sometimes of palliative benefit in treatment and in an occasional patient may have significant impact on disease progression.[75] However, the diffuse nature of the neoplastic process makes more systemic forms of therapy such as intracavitary isotope or chemotherapy potentially more advantageous.

Cooperative Groups have considered malignant mesothelioma as a mesenchymal neoplasm and have usually incorporated it as part of sarcoma trials. Thus, adriamycin has received the most extensive evaluation. As a single agent at 60-75 mg/M^2 every three weeks, adriamycin has had an overall response rate of 3 of 17 or 18 percent with one of the responders being a CR.[76,77] The only other compound which has completed Cooperative Group evaluation as a single agent has been cycloleucine, which resulted in partial responses in 2 of 7 patients. Combination chemotherapy with adriamycin and DTIC (both with and without vincristine) resulted in 4 of 15 responses (26 percent). Addition of cyclophosphamide to this combination may have further increased this response rate (2 of 6 PR's). Use of cyclophosphamide with vincristine and adriamycin without DTIC resulted in 4 of 7 (57 percent) responses.[77] Adriamycin, cyclophosphamide plus methotrexate produced two responses in eight patients (25 percent).[78] The overall response rate to adriamycin either alone or in combination in these trials has been 30 percent (17 of 56).

The clinical and pathological differences between malignant mesothelioma and soft tissue sarcomas warrant future development of separate Cooperative Group protocols. This is accentuated by its special association with asbestos exposure. Because of its infrequency (estimated at 500 new cases annually in the United States), only with intergroup collaboration will this be feasible. Recent leads from Cooperative Group studies with chemotherapy and institutional trials with intracavitary isotope and external radiation suggest that such an effort, particularly with pathological review and multimodality approaches, would prove rewarding.[75,77]

THERAPY OF ADVANCED SOFT TISSUE SARCOMAS

Several Cooperative Groups are currently studying therapy of advanced soft tissue sarcomas. Schemata for these major studies are presented in Table 9. The questions being asked by the current studies include:

1) What is the best dose and schedule of adriamycin?

2) Is a combination containing adriamycin superior to adriamycin alone?

3) What is the best adriamycin combination?

4)   Can remissions be prolonged by introduction of other drugs during maintenance therapy?

5)   What is the best dose and schedule of DTIC?

6)   Are there any useful agents?

These questions are based upon advances that have been made in the management of soft tissue sarcomas. These include: a) the demonstration that adriamycin is the single most important drug in the management of these diseases; b) a steep dose response relationship exists between adriamycin and response in soft tissue sarcomas, which is not

TABLE 9
Therapy of Advanced Soft Tissue Sarcoma
Multiinstitutional Trials in Progress

Cooperative Group/Schema: Randomization Arms

Cooperative Group	Schema: Randomization Arms
CALGB	A. Adriamycin 75 mg/M² x 1 every 28 days x 7, then cyclophosphamide, DTIC plus Vincristine B. Adriamycin 25 mg/M² x 3 every 28 days x 7, then cyclophosphamide, DTIC plus Vincristine
ECOG	A. Adriamycin 75 mg/M² q 3 weeks versus B. Adriamycin 20 mg/M² day 1-3 then weekly versus C. Adriamycin 60 mg/M² + DTIC 250 mg/M² day 1-5
SWOG	A. Adriamycin + DTIC x 6, then alternate with Cyclophosphamide, DTIC plus Actinomycin-D B. Adriamycin + DTIC + Cyclophosphamide C. Adriamycin + DTIC + Actinomycin-D
SECSG	Induction A. Adriamycin + Cyclophosphamide + Methotrexate B. Adriamycin + Cyclophosphamide + Methotrexate + Amphotericin B Maintenance A. Actinomycin-D B. Actinomycin-D + Amphotericin B

apparent in other diseases; c) a small fraction of patients will enjoy complete clinical remission of their disease; d) patients with complete clinical remission have significantly prolonged survival and, in some patients this survival has been sufficiently long to suggest cure; and e) treatment of pediatric soft part sarcomas with a multimodality approach has been successful.

Most of the advances have resulted from the work of Cooperative Groups since 1970. As a result of the success by pediatric oncologists in the management of certain soft tissue sarcomas, the common approach in the community at large for the management of soft tissue sarcomas prior to 1970 was the combination of vincristine, actinomycin-D and cyclophosphamide (VAC). However in a randomized study one group clearly demonstrated the superiority of adriamycin or adriamycin combination over VAC therapy (Table 10). The inability of actinomycin-D to add to the antitumor effect of an adriamycin combination was demonstrated most recently in a study completed comparing cyclophosphamide, vincristine, DTIC, and adriamycin (CYVADIC).[34] There was significant superiority to the CYVADIC arm both in terms of response and survival.

TABLE 10
Chemotherapy of Soft Tissue Sarcomas

Treatment	Complete Response	Partial Response	Evaluable Patients	% Response
Adriamycin	4	10	50	28%
Adriamycin, Vincristine, Cyclophosphamide	3	9	56	21%
Actinomycin D, Vincristine, Cyclophosphamide (VAC)	2	1	59	5%

The important role adriamycin plays in the management of soft tissue sarcomas has been demonstrated predominantly in a Cooperative Group setting. In 1971, a group performed a Phase II study of adriamycin in which 49 evaluable patients were treated, and complete responses were seen in two and partial remissions in 13, for an overall response rate of 31 percent.[18] Two years later, in trying to assess the dose response relationship of adriamycin, this group again confirmed a high response rate with adriamycin as a single agent. It also made the initial suggestion that response and survival in soft tissue sarcomas was function of dose and resulting toxicity of adriamycin. This observation was recently confirmed with the observation which clearly demonstrated the relationship between leukopenia and response as well as

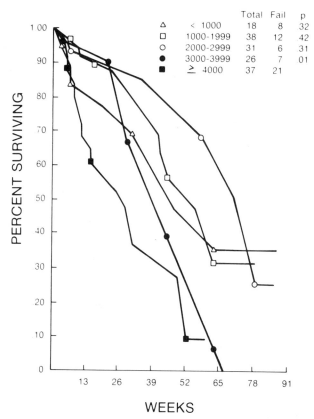

Fig. 8. Survival of sarcoma patients by WBC nadir

survival (Figure 8). Survival improves with lower nadirs until counts between 2,000 and 3,000 are reached. With lower nadirs, and the accompanying complications and dose reductions, the survival becomes worse again. In a recent report, the Mayo Clinic was unable to confirm the high response rate of adriamycin-DTIC combination chemotherapy of sarcomas. However, the results are not surprising in light of the dose and frequency of adriamycin administration chosen for their study.

Following the introduction of adriamycin into the management of soft tissue sarcomas, various combinations containing adriamycin have been employed. DTIC was selected for use in combination because of a preceeding Phase II study demonstrating an overall response rate of 17 percent in metastatic sarcomas with this agent.[79] Although the studies were of a sequential nature (not randomized), adriamycin plus DTIC demonstrated a response rate nearly 10 percent greater than the previous adriamycin study and a doubling of survival for the responding patients.[35] The survival advantage of DTIC combination is illustrated in Figure 9.

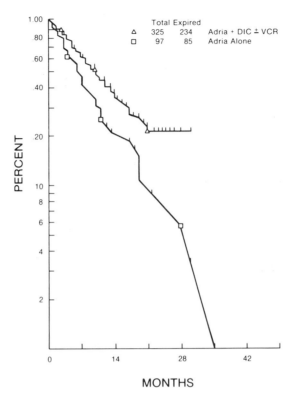

Fig. 9. Survival of metastatic sarcoma treated with adriamycin alone or in combination

Following adriamycin-DTIC, several other combinations have been developed, with three primary motivating factors: a) could a non-DTIC containing combination be as effective and avoid the severe gastro-intestinal toxicity associated with DTIC; b) could other drugs added to adriamycin-DTIC further enhance response rate and survival or; c) could the cycling of combinations improve the complete response rate observed? One group developed the combination of adriamycin, cyclo-phosphamide, and methotrexate, and analysis of their study suggests that this three-drug combination produces an overall response rate of 30 percent with a complete response rate of 6 percent. Further, the study indicated that remission duration was longest if adriamycin and cyclophosphamide plus methotrexate were used as maintenance ther-apy, compared to alternating with or switching to actinomycin-D, vincristine plus DTIC (Figure 10). After testing adriamycin-DTIC, the addition of vincristine to that combination was studied, followed by the addition of cyclophosphamide and vincristine to adriamycin-DTIC, and then a comparative trial of cyclophosphamide, vincristine, adriamycin and DTIC versus cyclophosphamide, vincristine, adriamycin, actinomycin-D. Figure 11 shows the overall results in terms of survival

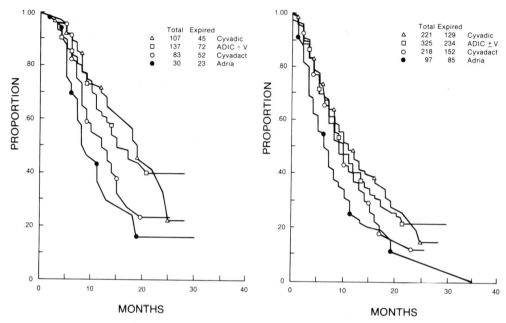

Fig. 10. Survival of responding patients with sarcomas in sequential SWOG studies

Fig. 11. Survival of all sarcoma patients in sequential SWOG studies

from these various combinations. Except for adriamycin alone, the differences are insignificant.

PATHOLOGY REVIEW OF SOFT TISSUE SARCOMA

The Sarcoma Committees of the various multiinstitutional groups have been instrumental in incorporating pathologists into Cooperative Group efforts. In the analysis of soft tissue sarcomas, histological confirmation of diagnosis was found to be essential to the understanding of the natural history of these diseases. Previously, the clinical approach to sarcoma assumed that the various histologic subtypes behaved essentially the same and, therefore, warranted similar therapeutic approaches. Since it was difficult for any single institution to collect enough patients within a particular histological type, it remained for the Cooperative Groups to demonstrate the prognostic value of proper classification.

In six studies completed by one of the groups, the histological subtypes of 742 patients with soft tissue sarcomas were reviewed. This revealed that the most common type of disseminated soft tissue sarcoma was leiomyosarcoma, representing 25.4 percent of all patients treated (Table 11). This was in contrast to three large published series on the frequency of soft tissue sarcomas which suggested that liposarcoma was most common (23 percent) followed by fibrosarcoma (21 percent) and that leiomyosarcoma represented only 5 percent of patients (Table 12). This observation may be of potential importance in designing treatment strategies for leiomyosarcoma but requires histological confirmation by other Groups.

Further review of the 742 Cooperative Group patients suggested that although the overall response rate varied little among the sarcoma histological subtypes (46 to 60 percent), complete responses varied from 6 percent to 20 percent (Table 11). This finding requires that the patients in this large series have pathology review to define precisely the association between complete response and histological type. Such an association would be very relevant to adjuvant study planning and evaluation.

With the emergence of this data, as well as the establishment of cooperation among the Cooperative Groups, it was realized by all that there must be communication among pathologists from each of the Groups concerned with the sarcomas. In March of 1977, a meeting was held in Detroit, Michigan, at which close cooperation was pledged by each pathology representative from the respective Groups. The need

TABLE 11
Disseminated Soft Tissue Sarcoma Therapy; 1970-1975

	No. of Patients	CR%	CR + PR%
Angiosarcoma	42 (5.6)	7.1	54.8
Fibrosarcoma	117 (15.7)	12.8	47.0
Leiomyosarcoma	189 (25.4)	12.1	45.5
Liposarcoma	95 (12.8)	12.6	50.5
Fibrous Histiocytoma	16 (2.1)	6.2	50.0
Neurofibrosarcoma	61 (8.2)	14.6	47.5
Rhabdomyosarcoma	80 (10.7)	17.5	55.0
Synovial sarcoma	35 (4.7)	20.0	60.0
Undifferentiated Sarcoma	86 (11.5)	14.0	51.1
Other	22 (2.9)	4.5	31.8
Total	742	13.0	49.2

( ) = % of total

TABLE 12
Frequency of histological types

	Memorial	Columbia	M.D. Anderson	Cum. Total	% of Total Pts.
Angiosarcoma	7	56	1	64	2
Fibrosarcoma	110	439	61	610	21
Leiomyosarcoma	2	105	25	132	5
Liposarcoma	135	436	107	678	23
Fibrous Histiocytoma	—	— —	—	— —	—
Neurofibrosarcoma	47	77	9	133	5
Rhabdomyosarcoma	161	181	82	424	14
Synovial Sarcoma	104	77	12	193	7
Undifferentiated Sarcoma	200	—	59	259	9
Other	7	400	16	423	14
Total	773	1771	372	2916	

for this cooperation became even more apparent when two large groups decided to share a common arm in their current ongoing study. The manner in which these two studies have been designed should allow for the evaluation of five treatment arms simultaneously by the two groups. Because it is of utmost importance to be certain that each group is treating the same population of patients, pathology review is mandated.

Histological review is but one facet of the contribution pathologists can make to the investigation of disseminated sarcomas. As Cooperative Groups begin to move into treatment protocols that incorporate surgical debulking in patients who have achieved only partial response, there will be an opportunity to examine carefully the effect of the various anticancer agents on metastatic tumor.

GUIDELINES OF SOFT TISSUE SARCOMA STUDY CRITERIA

Cooperative Group and institutional trials in the past have sometimes differed in criteria as to what constitutes a partial response and what constitutes an evaluable patient. These differences may have resulted in discrepancies in response rates, duration of response, and duration of survival. Since common treatment arms are now shared by some Cooperative Group protocols for advanced soft tissue sarcomas some codification is required.

Discussion of common criteria for patient selection, eligible patho-logical diagnoses, and measurement of response to therapy were ini-tiated in the Spring of 1977 at a meeting of clinicians and pathologists from each of the Cooperative Groups. Common guidelines were accepted by each Cooperative Group and have been submitted for publication.

In advanced disease, general agreement has existed that an objective response constitutes a 50 percent or greater decrease in the sum of the products of the measured lesions lasting at least four weeks. This criterion has been validated by a Cooperative Group study of simulated masses.[80] An effort is being made in surgical adjuvant studies to utilize common criteria for follow-up examinations, confirmation of treatment failure, and definition of disease-free intervals and survival. Three denominators will be used in reporting therapy responses: 1) all entered patients; 2) all patients who receive any protocol therapy including those who were lost-to-followup, refused further therapy, in whom a major protocol treatment violation occurred, or who died before the completion of the defined minimum adequate trial; and 3) those patients who received an adequate treatment trial as defined in the protocol.

By the adoption of these standard study criteria, the Intergroup Soft Tissue Sarcoma Committee and all Cooperative Groups have made a major contribution to the elimination of ambiguities in major clinical investigations. The suggested criteria are easily adaptable to other disease types and should provide a framework by which other solid tumor clinical investigators can make the design, conduct, analysis and reporting of their trials more consistent and comparable.

1. Gehan EA, Sutow WW, Uribe-Botero G, Romsdahl M, and Smith TL: Osteosarcoma. The M.D. Anderson Experience, 1950-1974. In Immunotherapy of Cancer: Present Status of Trials in Man, WD Terry and D Windhorst, eds. New York: Raven Press, pp. 271-282, 1978.

2. Mike V, Marcove RC: Osteogenic sarcoma under the age of 21: Experience at Memorial Sloan-Kettering Cancer Center. In Immunotherapy of Cancer: Present Status of Trials in Man, WD Terry and D Windhorst eds. New York: Raven Press, pp. 283-292, 1978.

3. Frei E, Jaffe N, Gero M, Skipper H, Watts H: Adjuvant chemotherapy of osteogenic sarcoma: Progress and perspectives. J Nat Cancer Inst 60:3-10, 1978.

4. Cortes EP, Holland JF, Glidewell O: Amputation and adriamycin in primary osteosarcoma: A 5-year report. Cancer Treat Rep 62:271-277, 1978.

5. Jaffe N, Traggis D, Cohen D, Watts H, Frei E, Cassady JR: The impact of high-dose methotrexate on the current management of osteogenic sarcoma (In Press).

6. Rosen G: The development of an adjuvant chemotherapy program for the treatment of osteogenic sarcoma. Front Radiat Therap Oncol 10:115-133, 1975.

7. Rosen G, Marcove RC, Caparros B, Nirenberg A, Kosloff C, Huvos AG: Primary osteogenic sarcoma: The rationale for preoperative chemotherapy and delayed surgery (In press).

8. Sutow WW, Vietti TJ, Fernbach DJ, Lane DM, Donaldson MH, Lonsdale D: Evaluation of chemotherapy in children with metastatic Ewing's sarcoma and osteogenic sarcoma. Cancer Chemother Rep 55:67-78, 1971.

9. Friedman MA, Carter SK: The therapy of osteogenic sarcoma: Current status and thoughts for the future. J Surg Oncol 4:482-510, 1972.

10. Evans AE: Mitomycin-C. Cancer Chemother Rep 14:1-9, 1961.

11. Sullivan MP, Sutow WW, Taylor G: L-phenylalanine mustard as a treatment for metastatic osteogenic sarcoma in children. J Pediatr 63:227-237, 1963.

12. Sutow WW, Sullivan MP, Wilbur JR, Vietti TJ, Kaizer H, Nagamoto A: L-phenylalanine mustard administration in osteogenic sarcoma: An evaluation of dosage schedules. Cancer Chemother Rep 55:151-157, 1971.

13. Sutow WW, Wilbur JR, Vietti TJ, Vuthibhagdee P, Fujimoto T, Watanabe A: Evaluation of dosage schedules of mitomycin-C in children. Cancer Chemother Rep 55:285-289, 1971.

14. Sutow WW, Sullivan MP, Wilbur JR, Cangir A: Study of adjuvant chemotherapy in osteogenic sarcoma. J Clin Pharmacol 15:530-533, 1975.

15. Sutow WW: Chemotherapeutic management of childhood rhabdomyosarcoma. Neoplasia in Childhood. Chicago: Year Book Medical Publishers, pp. 201-208, 1969.

16. Finklestein JZ, Hittle RE, Hammond GD: Evaluation of a high dose cyclophosphamide regimen in childhood tumors. Cancer 23:1239-1242, 1969.

17. Cortes EP, Holland JF, Wang JJ, Sinks LF: Doxorubicin in disseminated osteosarcoma. JAMA 221:1132-1138, 1972.

18. Gottlieb JA, Baker LH, O'Bryan RM, Sinkovics JG, Hoogstraten B, Quagliana JM, Rivkin SE, Bodey GP, Rodriguez VT, Blumenschein GR, Saiki JH, Coltman C, Burgess MA, Sullivan P, Thigpen T, Bottomley R, Balcerzak S, Moon TE: Adriamycin used alone and in combination for soft tissue and bony sarcomas. Cancer Chemother Rep 6:271-282, 1975.

19. Sutow WW, Sullivan MP, Fernbach DJ: Adjuvant chemotherapy in primary treatment of osteogenic sarcoma. ASCO 15:20, 1974.

20. Sutow WW: Combination chemotherapy with adriamycin in primary treatment of osteogenic sarcoma. Cancer Chemother Rep 6:315-317, 1975.

21. Sutow WW, Sullivan MP, Fernbach DJ, Cangir A, George SL: Adjuvant chemotherapy in primary treatment of osteogenic sarcoma. A Southwest Oncology Group Study. Cancer 36:1598-1602, 1975.

22. Sutow WW, Romsdahl MM, Dyment PG, Frias AE: Long-term follow-up evaluation of CONPADRI-I adjuvant chemotherapy in osteosarcoma. ASCO 18:127, 1977.

23. Cortes EP, Holland JF, Wang JJ, Glidewell O: Adriamycin and amputation in primary osteogenic sarcoma. ASCO 15:170, 1974.

24. Cortes EP, Holland JF, Wang JJ, Sinks LF, Bloom J, Senn H, Bank A, Glidewell O: Amputation and adriamycin in primary osteosarcoma. N Eng J Med 291:998-1000, 1974.

25. Cortes EP, Holland JF, Wang JJ: Adriamycin (ADM) in primary osteosarcoma (OS). AACR 16:241, 1975.

26. Cortes EP, Holland JF, Wang JJ, Glidewell O: Adriamycin in 87 patients with osteosarcoma. Cancer Chemother Rep 6:305-313, 1975.

27. Cortes EP, Holland JF, Wang JJ, Glidewell O: Amputation and adriamycin (ADM) in primary osteosarcoma (OS): 5-year report. ASCO 18:297, 1977.

28. Sutow WW, Gehan EA, Vietti TJ, Frias AE, Dyment PG: Further experience with multidrug chemotherapy in primary treatment of osteogenic sarcoma. AACR 15:232, 1975.

29. Sutow WW, Gehan EA, Vietti TJ, Frias AE, Dyment PG: Multidrug chemotherapy in primary treatment of osteosarcoma. J Bone & Joint Surg 58-A:629-633, 1976.

30. Sutow WW, Gehan EA, Dyment PG, Vietti T, Miale T: Multidrug adjuvant chemotherapy for osteosarcoma: Interim report of the Southwest Oncology Group Studies. Cancer Treat Rep 62:265-269, 1978.

31. Sutow WW: Late metastases in osteosarcoma. Lancet 1:856, 1976.

32. Jaffe N, Frei E, Traggis D, Watts H: Weekly high-dose methotrexate-citrovorum factor in osteogenic sarcoma. Presurgical treatment of primary tumor and of overt pulmonary metastases. Cancer 39:45-50, 1977.

33. Gottlieb JA, Baker LH, Quagliana JM, Luce JK, Whitecar JP, Sinkovics JG, Rivkin SE, Brownlee R, Frei E: Chemotherapy of sarcomas with a combination of adriamycin and dimethyl triazeno imidazole carboxamide. Cancer 30:1632-1638, 1972.

34. Gottlieb JA, Baker LH, O'Bryan RM, Luce JK, Sinkovics JG, Quagliana JM: Chemotherapy of metastatic sarcoma using combinations with adriamycin. Biochem Pharmacol Supp 2:183-192, 1974.

35. Gottlieb JA, Baker LH, Burgess MA, Sinkovics JG, Moon T, Bodey GP, Rodriguez V, Rivkin SE, Saiki J, O'Bryan RM: Sarcoma chemotherapy. In Cancer Chemotherapy Fundamental Concepts and Recent Advances. Chicago: Year Book Medical Publishers, Inc., pp. 445-454, 1975.

36. Rosen G, Murphy ML, Huvos AG, Gutierrez M, Marcove RC: Chemotherapy, en bloc resection, and prosthetic bone replacement in the treatment of osteogenic sarcoma. Cancer 37:1-11, 1976.

37. Jaffe N, Watts H, Fellows KE, Vawter G: Local en bloc resection for limb preservation. Cancer Treat Rep 62:217-223, 1978.

38. Rab GT, Ivins JC, Childs DS, Cupps RE, Pritchard DJ: Elective whole lung irradiation in the treatment of osteogenic sarcoma. Cancer 38:939-942, 1976.

39. Taylor WF, Ivins JC, Dahlin DC, Edmonson JH, Pritchard DJ: Trends and variability in survival from osteosarcoma. Mayo Clin Proc 53:695-700, 1978.

40. Taylor WF, Ivins JC, Dahlin DC, Pritchard DJ: Osteogenic sarcoma experience at the Mayo Clinic, 1963-1974. In Immunotherapy of Cancer: Present Status of Trials in Man, WD Terry and D Windhorst, eds. New York: Raven Press, pp. 257-269, 1978.

41. Perez C, Razek A, Tefft M, Nesbit M, Burgert O, Kissane J, Vietti T, Gehan E: Analysis of local tumor control in Ewing's sarcoma. Preliminary results of a cooperative intergroup study. Cancer 40:2864-2874, 1977.

42. Burgert O, Gehan EA, Nesbit ME: Prognostic factors in Ewing's sarcoma. ASCO 19:413, 1978.

43. Nesbit M, Vietti T, Burgert O, Tefft M, Gehan E, Perez C, Razek A, Kissane J: Intergroup Ewing's sarcoma study (IESS): Results of three different treatment regimens. AACR 19:81, 1978.

44. Marcove RC, Mike V, Hajek JV, Levin AG, Hutter RVP: Osteogenic sarcoma under the age of twenty one - a review of one hundred and forty-five operative cases. J of Bone and Joint Surg 52A:411-423, 1970.

45. Sweetnam R, Knowleden J, Jedden H: Bone sarcoma: Treatment by irradiation, amputation, or a combination of two. Brit Med J 3:363-367, 1971.

46. Uribe-Botero G, Russel WO, Sutow WW, Martin RG: Primary osteosarcoma of bone - a clinico-pathological investigation of 243 cases with necropsy studies in 54. Am J of Clin Pathol 67:427-435, 1977.

47. Martini N, Huvos AG, Mike V, Marcove RC, Beattie EJ: Multiple pulmonary resections in the treatment of osteogenic sarcoma. Ann of Thoracic Surg 12:271-297, 1971.

48. Joseph WL, Morton DL, Adkins P: Prognostic significance of tumor doubling time in evaluating operability in pulmonary metastatic disease. J of Thoracic and Cardiovascular Surg 61:23-32, 1971.

49. Beattie EJ, Martini M, Rosen G: The management of pulmonary metastases in children with osteogenic sarcoma with surgical resection combined with chemotherapy. Cancer 35:618-621, 1975.

50. O'Bryan RM, Luce JK, Talley RW, Gottlieb JA, Baker LH, Bonnadonna G: Phase II evaluation of adriamycin in human neoplasia. Cancer 32:1-8, 1973.

51. Weiss AJ, Metter GE, Fletcher WS, Wilson WL, Grage TB, Ramirez G: Studies on adriamycin using a weekly regimen demonstrating its clinical effectiveness and lack of cardiac toxicity. Cancer Treat Rep 60:813-822, 1976.

52. Jaffe N: The potential of combined modality approaches for the treatment of malignant bone tumors in children. Cancer Treat Rep 2:33-53, 1975.

53. Sutow WW, Gehan EA, Dyment PG, Vietti T, Miale T: Mutlidrug adjuvant chemotherapy for osteosarcoma: Interim report of the Southwest Oncology Group Studies. Cancer Treat Rep 62:265-269, 1978.

54. Sutow WW, Sullivan MP, Wilbur JR, Vietti TJ, Kaizer H, Nagamoto A: L-phenylalanine mustard administration in osteosarcoma; an evaluation of dosage schedules. Cancer Chemother Rep 55:151-157, 1971.

55. Sutow WW, Vietti TJ, Fernbach DJ, Lane DM, Donaldson MH, Lonsdale D: Evaluation of chemotherapy in children with metastatic Ewing's sarcoma and osteogenic sarcoma. Cancer Chemother Rep 55:67-78, 1971.

56. Evans AE, Heyn RM, Nesbit ME, Hartmann JR: Evaluation of mitomycin-C in the treatment of metastatic osteogenic sarcoma. Cancer Chemother Rep 53:297-298, 1969.

57. Baum E, Greenberg L, Gaynon P, Krivit W, Hammond D: Use of cis-platinum diammine dichloride in osteogenic sarcoma in children. ASCO 19:385, 1978.

58. Ochs JJ, Freeman AI, Douglass HO Jr, Higby DS, Mindell ER, Sinks LF: Cis-dichlorodiammineplatinum (II) in advanced osteosarcoma. Cancer Treat Rep 62:239-245, 1978.

59. Gottlieb JA, Baker LH, O'Bryan RM, Sinkovics JG, Hoogstraten B, Quagliana JM, et al: Adriamycin used alone and in combination for soft tissue and bony sarcomas. Cancer Chemother Rep 6:271-282, 1975.

60. Benjamin RS, Baker LH, O'Bryan RM, Moon TE, Gottlieb JA: Chemotherapy for metastatic osteosarcoma - studies by the M.D. Anderson Hospital and Southwest Oncology Group. Cancer Treat Rep 62:237-238, 1978.

61. Henderson ED, Dahlin DC: Chondrosarcoma of bone - A study of two hundred and eighty-eight cases. J of Bone and Joint Surg 45A:1450-1458, 1963.

62. Marcove RC, Mike V, Hutter RVP, Huvos AG, Shoji H, Miller TR, Kosloff R: Chondrosarcoma of the pelvis and upper end of the femur. An analysis of factors influencing survival time in one hundred and thirteen cases. J of Bone and Joint Surg 5A:561-572, 1972.

63. Spjut HJ: Cartilagenous malignant tumors arising in the skeleton. Proceedings Seventh National Cancer Conference Philadelphia: J.P. Lippincott, pp. 921-924, 1973.

64. Strander H, Cantell K, Ingimarsson S, Jakobsson PA, Nilsonne U, Soderberg G: Interferon treatment of osteogenic sarcoma: A clinical trial in modulation of host immune resistance in the prevention or treatment of induced neoplasias. M. Chiriges, ed. Washington, D.C.: DHEW (NIH 77-893), pp. 377-382, 1974.

65. Cadman NL, Soule EH, Kelly PJ: Synovial sarcoma. Cancer 18:613-627, 1965.

66. Gerner RE, Moore GE: Synovial sarcoma. Ann Surg 181:22-25, 1975.

67. Hajdu S, Shiu M, Fortner JG: Tenosynovial sarcoma. Cancer 39:1201-1217, 1977.

68. Enterline HT, Culberson JD, Rochlin DB, Brady LW: Liposarcoma. Cancer 13:932-950, 1960.

69. Martin RG, Butler JJ, Albores-Saavedra J: Soft tissue tumors: Surgical treatment and results. In Tumors of Bone and Soft Tissue. Chicago: Year Book Medical Publishers, Inc., pp. 333-347, 1965.

70. Russell WO, Cohen J, Enzinger F, Hadju SI, Heise H, Martin RG, Meissner W, Miller WT, Schmitz RL, Suit WD: A clinical and pathological staging system for soft tissue sarcomas. Cancer 40:1562-1570, 1977.

71. Lindberg RT, Murphy WK, Benjamin RS, et al: Adjuvant chemotherapy in the treatment of primary soft tissue sarcomas: A preliminary report. In Management of Primary Bone and Soft Tissue Tumors. Chicago: Yearbook Medical Publishers, pp. 343-352, 1977.

72. Mauer HM, Moon T, Donaldson M, et al: Intergroup rhabdomyosarcoma study. A preliminary report. Cancer 40:2015-2026, 1977.

73. Ratzer ER, Pool JL, Melamed MR: Pleural mesotheliomas: Clinical experiences with thirty-seven patients. Am J Roentgenol 99:863-880, 1967.

74. Moertel CG: Peritoneal mesothelioma. Gastroenterology 63:346-350, 1972.

75. Legha SS, Muggia FM: Therapeutic approaches in malignant mesothelioma. Cancer Treat Rev 4:13-23, 1977.

76. O'Bryan RM, Luce JR, Talley RW, Gottlieb JA, Baker LH, Bonnadonna G: Phase II evaluation of adriamycin in human neoplasia. Cancer 32:1-8, 1973.

77. Rosenbaum C, Schoenfeld D: Treatment of advanced soft tissue sarcoma. ASCO 18:287, 1977.

78. Lowenbraun S, Moffitt S, Smalley R, Presant C: Combination chemotherapy with adriamycin, cyclophosphamide and methotrexate in metastatic sarcomas. ASCO 18:286, 1977.

79. Gottlieb JA, Benjamin RS, Baker LH, O'Bryan RM, Sinkovics JG, Hoogstraten B, Quagliana JM, Rivkin SE et al: The role of DIC in the chemotherapy of sarcoma. Cancer Treat Rep 60:199-203, 1976.

80. Moertel CG, Hanley JA: The effect of measuring error on the results of therapeutic trials in advanced cancer. Cancer 38:388-394, 1976.

14

Drug evaluation

Rose Ruth Ellison

INTRODUCTION

Phase I Studies

Phase I studies have traditionally been performed by single institutions each undertaking its own developmental studies aimed at defining toxicity, tolerated drug dose, and suitable routes and schedules for administration. Less often these studies have been undertaken by two or three institutions working together closely. The need for clinical pharmacologic studies, including the determination of drug levels in blood, urine and other fluids as well as the requirement for close day-to-day monitoring of such studies, makes it more difficult to perform them within the Cooperative Group framework. This has been done, however, with some compounds and in some groups.

Under the guidance of the Division of Cancer Treatment, new agents are now flowing rapidly from animal studies to Phase I contractors and then to Phase II disease-oriented studies. Cooperative Groups have representatives attending the Phase I-II drug liaison meetings sponsored by the Investigational Drug Branch (IDB) and are establishing contacts with drug houses. At Group meetings the representatives present pertinent material concerning "Group A" and "Group B" drugs. While the use of Group A drugs is limited to the Phase I-II working group contractors, up-to-date information about these substances allows Group members to plan ahead for the time when such agents are transferred to Group B status. It also permits Groups to devise suitable broad and specific Phase II protocols.

Phase II Studies

Cooperative Groups have played an extensive role in Phase II drug studies in the past and continue to do so. The potential scope of such studies involves the definition of several needs and problems.

In the past, the Groups frequently conducted broad-based single-drug studies. Determination of the effectiveness of new drugs in numerous diseases, rare or common, was the goal of such studies. Recently, the Groups have begun to focus upon single diseases. Such focus has allowed rapid accrual of information on tumor types with relatively low incidence. Thus, renal cancer has been studied using four drugs on a randomized basis in one Group. This study compared the use of megace, cyclophosphamide, VP-16, and galactitol. Another Group completed a pilot study of piperazinedione in renal cancer. Pediatric intergroup studies have allowed the investigation of a number of tumors not apt to be seen in any large number by individual institutions or by a single Group.

Phase II studies done within a Group also permit rapid completion of studies of new agents in common tumors. The use of master protocols for common diseases, with additions of specific information concerning the drug to be tested and specific directions concerning dose modifications, etc., has helped to provide an organized approach.[1] In some instances, these single-drug studies have stipulated randomization among several drugs to avoid bias in choice. Phase II studies in the various Cooperative Groups usually stipulate the accumulation of 20 to 40 adequately treated patients in each desired tumor category. In general, patients who are eligible for these protocols will already have received conventional or combination therapy and have measurable disease. In diseases where no effective chemotherapy exists or where the objective response rate with conventional agents is less than 15 percent, the introduction of Group B agents appears reasonable and rational in previously untreated patients with generalized disease. In some instance the number of patients to be entered into a study is not fixed in advance but results from an ongoing decision-making process. For example, if a response is observed in the first 20 patients, then 5 additional patients are allocated to a particular therapy arm, up to a maximum of 40 patients (i.e., 4 or more responses).

NECESSARY APPROACHES IN THE FUTURE

The emphasis in new drug studies must be on logical planning. Studies of single drugs in specific diseases must be devised to provide adequate exploration of drug dose and schedule. The study of combinations of drugs and of the variety of possible doses and schedules is equally important. Here, studies must be innovative as well as logical. Pilot studies are necessary to determine the tolerability of combinations before broad trials of efficacy are undertaken and before these are included in Phase III comparative studies. Pilot studies are also indicated in planning multimodal approaches for treatment of evident disease and for adjuvant management of situations with poor prognosis. In all instances, the patient tolerance for the particular treatments to be undertaken must be verified before the efficacy is studied in depth and certainly before initiating controlled trials.

Thus, there is a need for a mechanism for handling such Phase II studies in signal tumors and, ultimately, in rarer tumors. This necessitates availability of suitable patients. Patients to be included in such studies must not be in the terminal stages of their disease but must be defined to include those who at least have a chance of responding. The quality controls essential for these studies have been developed or are developing in the various Groups. The patient population and referral patterns have already become known. The ability of Group members to follow protocol stipulations and report information in standard fashion is apparent. The involvement of a Group helps to eliminate bias in selection of patients for study and bias in evaluation of results.

Although the Cooperative Groups cannot claim to be unique in having studied new agents from early Phase I trials through Phase II and into Phase III, significant contributions have been made by both broad Phase II and disease specific Phase II studies. As an exercise in historical perspectives, one can examine the life history of several drugs and assess the role played by Cooperative Groups in the development of these agents through various human clinical trials. Brief overviews of some of these agents follow.

Fluorinated Pyrimidines

Initial studies on 5-Fluorouracil and 5-fluorodeoxyuridine were conducted at the University of Wisconsin. These led to the use of 5-FU as a 4 or 5-day course given at monthly intervals. Numerous investigations followed, studying the use of 5-FU by continuous intravenous, intraarterial and oral administration. Over the next 7 years, reports emanating from individual institutions proliferated rapidly. At the same time, however, Cooperative Group studies were also undertaken. A Phase I-II study of 5-FU compared three dose levels of 5-FU given daily intravenously for 14 to 42 days as well as a 5-day oral course.[2] Patients developed toxicity sufficient to require discontinuation of the drug if it was given daily at doses of 6 mg/kg per day or greater. Less toxicity appeared when the drug was given orally. A low rate of objective responses was seen, with transient responses occurring at levels of mild toxicity. A pilot study undertaken by Khung and Hall tested the use of 5-day courses of fluorouracil orally, given in capsules or in solution to 75 patients.[3] The use of 5-FU in solution provided more consistent results. The predominant toxicity was gastrointestinal. This was a Phase I-II study in which some objective regressions were seen, but the data were insufficient to judge the response rate.

A large Phase II study of FUDR was completed in 288 patients, 229 of whom were evaluated. The drug was given as a 5-day course intravenously and a 24 percent complete plus partial response rate was reported.[4]

Further investigation of the role of weekly treatment with 5-FU was undertaken under Group auspices. Evaluation of 359 patients (out of 548 treated weekly with 15 mg/kg but no loading dose) indicated 28 percent CR plus PR, with the therapeutic effect evident by the sixth week.[5] This Phase I-II study was followed by a Phase III comparative trial of weekly intravenous and oral 5-FU.[6] This indicated no significant difference between oral and IV drug, other than somewhat more gastrointestinal toxicity in those receiving the drug orally. The response rate was poor, 13 percent with oral and 9 percent with intravenous drug among those patients who received at least one dose of 5-FU.

The use of 5-FU given intravenously was also investigated at weekly intervals and at 3 different dose levels. Twenty mg/kg per week caused intolerable toxicity. Smaller doses (7.5 and 15 mg/kg) were tolerable and the 15 mg/kg dose resulted in 20 percent responses. It was felt that this was a useful outpatient regimen. A nongroup study again reported favorably on the use of Fluorouracil orally,[7] postulating the particular value of this regimen in patients with liver metastasis because of direct delivery of drugs through the portal system to the liver. Studies were undertaken to investigate the use of high-dose continuous intravenous 5-FU at four different doses given for 48 hours in 26 patients.[8] Toxicity was found to be dose related with severe toxicity at the highest level used. No complete or partial response was seen in the 13 patients with measurable disease but it was felt that this was a feasible means of drug administration.

Cytosine Arabinoside

Initial work on the clinical pharmacology of ara-C was not performed as a Group study. Subsequent evaluation of the effects of continuous infusion of ara-C was undertaken in adult acute leukemia.[9] A Phase I-II study was instituted to define the effect of dose and schedule of ara-C on the normal bone marrow function and kinetics in man.[10] The steep dose-response curve with respect to marrow depression resulting from 48 to 96 hour infusions and the lack of myelosuppressive or antitumor effects after large single doses led the authors to suggest the use of continuous infusion or of 24-hour infusions at intervals less than 2 weeks. Continuous infusion for 24 hours also produced more marrow suppression, with doses up to 1,200 mg/M^2, but without further marrow suppression after still further increase in dose. Responses were seen in 15 percent of those treated and were more frequent with longer treatment at higher doses.

Further investigation included the use of a prolonged administration of cytosine arabinoside.[11] The drug was given subcutaneously every 8 hours for a total of 10 days to 85 patients with metastatic cancer. While tolerable hematologic toxicity was consistently produced, tumor regression of metastatic carcinoma of the colon, breast, or malignant melanoma was transient and occurred in less than 10 percent of the cases.

Further study of the toxicity and antitumor activity of ara-C in solid tumors was undertaken in a Phase I-II study.[12] After initial dose-finding studies in which the drug was given either daily for 10 days or at a higher dose for the first 3 days of each week, the Phase II study was limited to 3.5 mg/kg daily with 10 days, given to 225 evaluable patients. Toxicity occurred at all dose levels. Responses were seen in fewer than 10 percent of the evaluable patients. The responses were brief and rarely of clinical benefit, with the most responsive tumors being breast, gastrointestinal, adenocarcinoma, and soft tissue and bone sarcomas. Even in these tumors fewer than 15 percent responses were seen.

Purine Analogs

The initial investigations of purine analogs including 8-Azaguanine, 6-mercaptopurine, 6-thioguanine, and chloropurine were undertaken prior to the institution of Cooperative Groups. As derivatives of these agents appeared and as intravenous preparations became available, some studies were undertaken within Cooperative Groups but most of the efforts were either at individual institutions and not clearly group-oriented, or were undertaken as part of Phase III studies.

There were several reports of the use of imidazolyl thioguanine including one in which a pilot study of weekly oral administration was undertaken by Selawry in patients with advanced cancer. Although several patients had brief tumor regression, it was associated with major toxicity and this drug too was not used further in Group studies. An exploratory trial of 9-ethyl-6-mercaptopurine was undertaken in a limited number of patients with chronic or acute granulocytic leukemia.[13]   While effects were seen in patients with CML, these did not appear to be different from those to be obtained from 6-MP.

In a Phase I-II study of 6-MP patients received the drug intravenously daily for 7 days or once a week.[14]   The daily schedule was toxic.   The Phase II study, therefore, compared 2 dose levels given weekly.   No therapeutic effects were seen despite toxic effects in three-quarters of the 69 patients.   A concurrent study of large doses of 6-mercaptopurine given intravenously once and twice weekly in adults with acute leukemia, indicated prohibitive toxicity at 40 mg/kg given twice weekly, but no improvement in remission response when compared historically to daily oral 6-MP.[15]

A Phase I trial of intravenously administered thioguanine was undertaken because of the known erratic absorption of this drug when given orally.[16]   The drug was given either once or twice weekly, with dose escalation in those patients not developing toxicity.   After three weeks a moderate, severe or life-threatening marrow suppression developed in 40 to 50 percent of patients on both regimens, with more frequent severe toxicity in those receiving drugs twice weekly despite the fact that less drug was given.   Although this was considered a Phase I trial, responses were seen in one-fifth of the patients (all with solid tumors) evaluable for responses.

Hexamethylmelamine (NSC-13875) (HXM)

Hexamethylmelamine (HXM) is an alkylating agent resembling triethylenemelamine.   It has moderate activity in animals (Walker carcinosarcoma 256 in rats, sarcoma 180 and adenocarcinoma 755 in mice). Chronic toxicity studies in dogs and monkeys were performed with doses from 21 to 85 mg/kg/day.   The first Phase I study was done by member institutions of a Cooperative Group and reported 5 years after the compound completed animal toxicity testing.[17]   Significant weight loss and severe gastrointestinal toxicity occurred at a daily dose of 15 mg/kg and the recommended Phase II dosage was 12 mg/kg/day po.

The majority of the Phase II studies on HXM were conducted by Cooperative Group members.   The results in a study of 256 patients were published four years after the original Phase I study.[18]   The dosage was 12 mg/kg/day po for 21 consecutive days.   The major side effect was GI intolerance (nausea and vomiting), resulting in 10 percent of patients voluntarily dropping from the program.   A better than 20 percent response was reported in lung, ovarian, uterine and testicular cancers, with statistically significant numbers in lung and ovary only. No hematologic diseases were studied.   Despite the large number of case accessions this broad Phase II study (typical of the first generation of Phase II single agent programs) provided useful information on only these two tumor types.

Over 600 patients with lung cancer have been studied but not exclusively by Cooperative Group programs. Small cell cancers have a higher response rate (30 percent) than adenocarcinoma of the lung (20 percent) with epidermoid the lowest (about 10 percent).[19]

With evidence that in ovarian cancer HXM had activity approximately equal to that of alkylating agents, the agent was combined with 5-FU, cytoxan, and methotrexate (HEXA-CAF) (NCI) and with cyclophosphamide, adriamycin and cis-platinum (CHAD-an ECOG pilot). The latter two programs have had significantly higher response rates (60 to 80 percent) with a moderate number of complete remissions reported. One Group studied 21 patients with cervical cancer and found 8 partial responses.[20]

A major Phase II study was carried out comparing HXM to bleomycin.[21] Although an initial dosage of 300 mg/M^2/day for 60 days was recommended, only 22 of 36 evaluable patients with lymphoma tolerated the full dosage. Responses were noted in approximately 30 percent of patients, with rare complete remissions in patients with histiocytic lymphoma. This response rate is very significant considering that patients had been treated extensively, including alkylating agents.

Despite these favorable results HXM remains a rarely used drug in large part as a result of its significant GI toxicity.

CCNU (1-2-Chloroethyl -3-cyclohexyl-1-nitrosourea, NSC-79037)

In contrast to BCNU, CCNU is of particular interest because of its ease of administration (po) and higher lipid solubility. Two large broad Phase II studies were carried out by the Cooperative Groups. In one study of 329 patients 4 complete responses were noted (ovary, lung, melanoma).[22] The dose was 130 mg/M^2 every 6 weeks. A sufficient number of patients was accrued in head and neck, colorectal, lung, melanoma, breast, ovary, kidney cancers and lymphomas to assess response rates. Bone marrow toxicity was delayed (6 to 7 weeks) and moderate. Response rates of greater than 15 percent were noted in all but breast and renal cancers. It is of interest that a 16 percent response rate in bowel cancer was thought "to have no place in the treatment of gastrointestinal adenocarcinoma", although the overall effect of 5-FU is in the same range of activity.

A Phase II-III study comparing CCNU with methyl CCNU at approximately equitoxic doses was undertaken in Hodgkin's disease and non-

Hodgkin's lymphomas.[23]   The remission induction frequency was identical for the 2 drugs, when used in advanced previously treated non-Hodgkin's lymphomas (19 percent and 17 percent CR + PR), but a higher response frequency was found for CCNU (52 percent CR + PR) (14 of 27) than for methyl CCNU (26 percent) (5 of 19) in Hodgkin's disease, with comparable hematologic toxicity.

A broad Phase II study of 298 patients yielded a 16 percent response rate in primary brain tumors and showed 3 of 11 with oat cell lung cancer responding. Impressive results were observed in lymphomas with 4 of 8 responses in Hodgkin's disease and 3 responses of 9 evaluable patients with non-Hodgkin's lymphomas. Few responses were observed in both melanoma and breast cancer.[24]

One Group compared the relative efficacy of CCNU and BCNU in patients with advanced Hodgkin's disease, finding a 73 percent response rate for CCNU (16 of 22) and 26 percent for BCNU (5 of 19).[25] Based on this observation, the group then studied MOPP versus CCNU + velban + procarbazine + prednisone (CVPP) versus CCNU + Oncovin + procarbazine + prednisone (COPP) and demonstrated equal remission induction but less toxicity and a longer remission duration with CVPP program.[26]

In lung cancer, CCNU is equal in effectiveness to cyclophosphamide. The combination of CCNU and cytoxan produces a consistent response rate of approximately 40 percent in small cell lung cancer[27] and this combination (cytoxan: 700 mg/M^2 + CCNU 70 mg/M^2 q 4 weeks) has become the standard arm of all Phase III studies in one Group. Of interest was the failure to demonstrate an advantage of the combination in nonoat cell cancer.[28]

The clinical use of CCNU has been very extensive, with studies in virtually all of the so-called "signal tumors". Comparisons with other nitrosoureas, BCNU and methyl CCNU have been done as well. Significant activity has been demonstrated in Hodgkin's disease, brain tumors and small cell lung cancer; the Cooperative Groups playing a major role in these studies. The integration of CCNU into both combination chemotherapy protocols and combined modality studies (adjuvant programs in Stage I small cell lung cancer adjuvant treatment in nonsmall cell lung cancer treatment programs in localized and disseminated small cell lung cancer and a pilot combination study in advanced nonsmall cell lung cancer) should clarify better the role of this agent in the management of patients with cancer.

1. Bennett JM, Zelen M: Pilot studies and new agents programs of the Eastern Cooperative Oncology Group. Submitted to Cancer Treat Rep, 1980.
2. Gold GL, Hall TC, Shnider BI, Selawry O, Colsky J, Owens AH, Dederick MM, Holland JF, Brindley CO, Jones R: A clinical study of 5-Fluorouracil. Cancer Research, 19:935-939, 1959.
3. Khung CL, Hall TC, Piro AJ, Dederick MM: A clinical trial of oral 5-Fluorouracil. J Clinical Pharmacol & Ther, 7:527-533, 1966.
4. Wilson WL, Biesel H, Krementz ET, Lien RC, Prohaska JV: Further clinical evaluation of 2'-deoxy-5-fluorouradine. Cancer Chemother Rep, 51:85-90, 1967.
5. Jacobs EM, Reeves WJ, Wood DA, Pugh R, Braunwald J, Bateman JR: Treatment of cancer with weekly intravenous 5-Fluorouracil. Cancer, 27:1302-1305, 1971.
6. Bateman JR, Pugh RP, Cassidy FR, Marshall GJ, Irwin LE: 5-Fluorouracil given once weekly: comparison of intravenous and oral administration. Cancer, 28:907-913, 1971.
7. Lahiri SR, Boileau G, Hall TC: Treatment of metastatic colorectal carcinoma with 5-Fluorouracil by mouth. Cancer, 28:902-906, 1971.
8. Hill GJ, Grage TB, Wilson WL, Ansfield FJ: 5-Fluorouracil intravenous infusion for 48 hours, repeated every two weeks. J of Surg Oncol, 4:60-70, 1972.
9. Ellison RR, Carey RW, Holland JF: Pharmacologic study of continuous intravenous infusions of cytosine arabinoside in patients with neoplastic disease. J Clinical Pharmacol & Ther, 8:800-809, 1976.
10. Frei E, Bickers JN, Hewlett JS, Lane M, Leary WV, Talley RW: Dose schedule and antitumor studies of arabinosyl cytosine. Cancer Res, 29:1325-1332, 1969.
11. Burke PJ, Owens AH, Colsky J, Shnider BI, Edmonson JH, Schilling A, Brodovsky HS, Wallace HJ, Hall TC: A clinical evaluation of a prolonged schedule of cytosine arabinoside. Cancer Res, 30:1512-1515, 1970.
12. Davis HL, Rochlin DB, Weiss AJ, Wilson WL, Andrews NC, Maddon RE, Sedransk N: Cytosine arabinoside toxicity and antitumor activity in human solid tumors. Oncology, 29:190-200, 1974.
13. Johnson CB, Frommeyer WB, Hammack WJ, Butterworth CE: 9-ethyl-6-mercaptopurine: Preliminary clinical observations. Cancer Chemother Rep, 20:137-141, 1962.
14. Regelson W, Holland J, Gold G, Lynch J, Olson K, Horton J, Hall T, Krant M, Colsky J, Miller SP, Owens A: 6-mercaptopurine given intravenously at weekly intervals to patients with advanced cancer. Cancer Chemother Rep, 51:277-282, 1967.
15. Ellison RR, Hoogstraten B, et al: Intermittent therapy with 6-mercaptopurine and methotrexate given intravenously to adults with acute leukemia. Cancer Chemother Rep, 56:535-542, 1972.
16. Padilla F, Vietti T, Lehane D, Whitecar J, Coltman CA: Phase I trial of intravenous thioguanine. Submitted to Cancer Chemother Rep, 1976.
17. Wilson WL, de la Garza JG: Phase I studies of hexamethylmelamine. Cancer Chemother Rep, 48:49-52, 1965.
18. Wilson WL, Schroeder JM, Bisel HF, Mrazek R, Hummel RP: Phase II study of hexamethylmelamine. Cancer, 23:132-136, 1969.
19. Stolinsky DC, Bogdon DL, Solomon J, Bateman JR: Hexamethylmelamine alone and in combination with DTIC in the treatment of advanced cancer. Cancer, 30:654-659, 1972.
20. Stolinsky DC, Bateman JR: Further experience with hexamethylmelamine in the treatment of carcinoma of the cervix. Cancer Chemother Rep, 57:497-499, 1973.
21. Bennett JM, Lenhard RE, Ezdinli E, Carbone PP, Pocock SJ, Johnson GJ: Chemotherapy of non-Hodgkin's lymphomas: The ECOG experience. Cancer Treat Rep, 61:1079-1083, 1977.
22. Cruz AB, Metter G, Armstrong DM, Aust JB, Fletcher WS, Wilson WL, Richardson JD: Treatment of advanced malignancy with CCNU. Cancer, 38:1069-1076, 1976.
23. Maurice P, Glidewell O, Jacquillat C, Silver RT, Carey R, Ten Pas A, Cornell CJ, Burningham RA, Nissen NI, Holland JF: Comparison of methyl CCNU and CCNU in patients with advanced forms of Hodgkin's disease, lymphosarcoma and reticulum cell sarcoma. Cancer, 41:1658-1663, 1978.
24. Hoogstraten B, Haas CD, Haut A, Talley RW, Rivkin S, Isaacs BL: CCNU and bleomycin in the treatment of cancer. Med & Pediatr Oncol, 1:95-106, 1975.
25. Selawry OS, Hansen HH: Superiority of CCNU over BCNU in treatment of advanced Hodgkin's disease. AACR 13:46, 1972.
26. Cooper MR, Spurr CL, Glidewell O, Holland JF: The superiority of a nitrosourea (CCNU) containing four-drug combination over MOPP in the treatment of Stage III and IV Hodgkin's disease. AACR, 16:111, 1975.
27. Edmonson JH, et al: Cyclophosphamide and CCNU in the treatment of inoperable small cell carcinoma and adenocarcinoma of the lung. Cancer Treat Rep, 60:925-932, 1976.
28. Edmonson JH, et al: Mechlorethamine plus CCNU in the treatment of inoperable squamous and large cell carcinoma of the lung. Cancer Treat Rep, 60:625-628, 1976.

15

Biostatistics

Marvin Zelen, Edmund Gehan, and Oliver Glidewell

Preface

"From here on, as far ahead as one can see, medicine must be building as a central part of its scientific base a solid underpinning of biostatistical and epidemiological knowledge. Hunches and intuitive impressions are essential for getting the work started, but it is only through the quality of numbers at the end that the truth can be told."

Lew Thomas, M.D.
Science 198 (1977)

INTRODUCTION

Controlled experimentation is now regarded as the principal way to generate scientific data on the value of medical treatments. Ex-cathedra judgements by medical doyens no longer dominate the practice of therapeutic medicine. The clinical trial is reserved for this type of prospective controlled experimentation and has become one of the most important methodologic advances associated with the scientific basis of therapeutics. Essentially clinical trials are a post World War II advance. They received much impetus from studies carried out under the auspices of the Medical Research Council (MRC) in the United Kingdom during the late 1940's. The success of these early MRC clinical trials was due in large part to the role of the medical statistician, Sir Bradford Hill. It was his influence that made scientific studies out of these investigations.

Today a nearly parallel situation exists with regard to multiinstitutional cancer clinical trials. The medical specialists are essentially carrying out their specialties. That is the medical oncologists, radiotherapists, and surgeons are treating patients; the pathologists are evaluating their slides. What draws these efforts together into a scientific study is the cooperation of the various specialties to pool their contributions towards common goals and the role of the biostatistician. The biostatisticians' role in drawing upon statistical and computer methodology for the study design, data collection, data management, and analysis is fundamental for turning good clinical practice into good clinical scientific investigation. Of course even with the best methodology, the outcome of a clinical trial can be disappointing due to the initial selection of therapies having little a priori promise of having therapeutic value. The need for innovative and well run pilot studies, carried out by skilled investigators, is as important as ever.

EARLY HISTORY AND THE CHANGING ROLE OF STATISTICAL CENTERS

The history of the development of Statistical Centers as a part of the Clinical Cooperative Group Program began in 1955 with the organization of the Cooperative Groups. It was recognized at the outset that a Statistical Center was an integral component of a Clinical Cooperative Group so that groups of clinicians and several Statistical Centers were recruited at the same time to form the nucleus of each Cooperative Group. The individuals at the National Cancer Institute mainly responsible for the organization of the Statistical Centers were Dr. Kenneth Endicott (Head, Cancer Chemotherapy National Service Center), Dr. Marvin Schneiderman (Chief, Biometrics Section, CCNSC), and Dr. Gordon Zubrod (Clinical Director, National Cancer Institute). Drs. Endicott and Schneiderman traveled around the United States contacting key individuals in clinical cancer research and biostatistics to be part of the original Clinical Cooperative Groups Program.

Two points can be made in this initial phase of development: (1) there was recognition that Statistical Centers are essential resources for a Clinical Cooperative Group; and (2) biostatisticians should be equal collaborators with research oriented clinicians and have a major responsibility in the design, analysis, and interpretation of cancer clinical studies.

The Clinical Cooperative Groups organized in the first few years of the program are listed in Table 1 along with the chairmen and responsible biostatisticians. The Cooperative Cancer Study Groups were originally organized on a geographical basis. The present structure of the

TABLE 1
Early Clinical Cooperative Cancer Study Groups,
Chairmen and Biostatisticians

Clinical Cooperative Groups	Chairmen	Biostatisticians
Acute Leukemia Group A (Subsequently, Children's Cancer Study Group)	J. Burchenal and L. Murphy (Sloan Kettering Institute)	I. Bross (Cornell University Medical College)
Acute Leukemia Group B (Subsequently, Cancer and Leukemia Group B)	E. Frei, III (National Cancer Institute)	M. Schneiderman (National Cancer Institute)
Eastern Cooperative Group (Subsequently, Eastern Cooperative Oncology Group)	G. Zubrod (National Cancer Institute)	M. Schneiderman (National Cancer Institute)
Southeastern Group	W. Rundles (Duke University)	B. Greenberg and E. Gehan (University of North Carolina)
Southwest Cancer Chemotherapy Study Group (Subsequently, Southwest Oncology Group)	G. Taylor (M.D. Anderson Hospital)	E. MacDonald (M.D. Anderson Hospital)
Western Cooperative Group	C. Finch (University of Washington) and M. Wintrobe (University of Utah	No well-defined center
University Group Prostate Studies		D. Mainland (New York University)

Cooperative Groups has resulted from attrition, reorganization, and consolidation. The original Statistical Centers were part of university departments of biostatistics (University of North Carolina, New York University), at cancer research centers (M.D. Anderson Hospital, Cornell Medical College), and at the National Cancer Institute. Today, the Statistical Centers for the Cooperative Groups are found at universities and centers for cancer research. The NCI and private industry serve as Statistical Centers for the contract supported Cooperative Groups.

The Cooperative Groups were initially engaged in short-term chemotherapy studies. Patients entered studies with advanced disease; the major end-point was tumor response. Survival was relatively short and were not considered a significant end-point. Follow-up of patients rarely exceeded a few months or was not even carried out. Patient records only spanned a few weeks or months.

The staff of these early Statistical Centers consisted of one or more part-time biostatisticians and a statistical clerk. The statistical clerk assisted with the statistical calculations using a desk top calculator, and was often expected to act as a secretary as well. There was no computer orientation nor capability as this development was still in its incubation stage. Clinical data were often collected on a single all-purpose form which was used for all studies. Some groups did not have forms and abstracted relevant information from hospital records after a decision was made to write a study. There was no capability for interim analyses. Most of these intitial studies were randomized using sealed envelopes containing treatment assignments that were mailed to each cooperating institution. Sometimes the reasons for carrying out a randomized study were not well understood by the participants. (An apocryphal story is told where an investigator complained about the change of the paper quality of the randomization envelopes. He found it more difficult to determine the treatment assignment by holding the envelope against a window.) Quality control was usually carried out by a final review of case records by a study chairman and discussions of individual cases by investigators at Group meetings.

From these crude beginnings many of the Statistical Centers have evolved into relatively complex organizations carrying on a great many expanded responsibilities and activities. This has enabled the Groups to conduct a larger number of studies and to adopt more complex treatment programs. The statistical analyses of these trials have changed from a naive tabulation of results to the use of modern statistical tools for modeling and analyses. Nearly all the Groups are conducting adjuvant studies as well as protocols requiring earlier staged disease. Patient followup and surveillance span periods of years rather than months as in the past.

Associated with the expanding activities of the Cooperative Groups has been a general scientific upgrading and broadening of functions within the Statistical Centers. There is greater emphasis on data monitoring and improving the quality of the clinical data submitted to the Center. "Second Party" review of clinical data invariably raises the quality of the data. Interim analyses of all studies are routinely presented at Group meetings. Study chairmen and investigators routinely visit the Statistical Centers to collaborate on record reviews. Most Statistical Centers annually review the participation of each institution for the timeliness and quality of data submission. A Cooperative Group having a poorly functioning Statistical Center may be in great difficulty.

Many of the Cooperative Group Statistical Centers are so complex that a move because of the election of a new Group Chairman is out of the question. It takes several years for a Center to recruit and train supporting staff to enable it to operate smoothly. A free-standing Statistical Center allows an investigator to assume the position of Group Chairman without being bogged down attempting to transfer or start a major department. Several of the current multisite/protocol Statistical Centers should be regarded as national resources.

THE EVOLUTION OF STATISTICAL CENTERS

The evolution of Statistical Centers from the early beginnings in the 1950's to the present can be traced to three major developments:

1) Development of new statistical methodology created to meet the special needs of clinical trials.
2) Widespread access to computers.
3) Recognition of the need for data managers.

There have been enormous advances made during the past ten years in the creation of new statistical methodology which specifically meets the needs for clinical trials. These new techniques have affected both the planning and analyses of clinical trials. Amongst the leaders in developing these new statistical methodologies are the biostatisticians associated with the Cooperative Clinical Cancer Program. The bibliography contains the methodologic papers published in the period 1970 to 1979.

These new techniques have led to ways of modeling the prognostic factors (e.g., anatomic and histologic staging, demographic factors, performance status, extra disease symptoms, etc.) affecting major endpoints. This has allowed simultaneous evaluation of all variables without the requirement to analyze data "piecemeal" category by category. The "piecemeal" analysis requires large numbers of patients or "thins" the data to such a degree that the analysis has little sensitivity to detect real differences.

The availability of new statistical modeling techniques has served as a stimulus for many investigations among disease sites characterizing the effect of prognostic factors on disease-free interval, survival, and tumor response. The bibliography contains many such papers.

These new methods of statistical analyses require substantial use of computers. The calculations are too difficult to be done without one. Fortunately, the advances in statistical methodology coincided with the growing access of high speed computers in Statistical Centers. By the mid-sixties nearly every university or research center had computing access. The widespread access to computers has had a profound effect on the operations and capabilities of Statistical Centers.

There was an early recognition in the Cooperative Group Program of the potential for using computers for statistical analyses. The Cancer Chemotherapy National Service Center initially funded the BMD software development of UCLA. (This was the first integrated collection of statistical programs aimed at the needs of biomedical investigations.) However, it was not until the early seventies that computers began to play a significant role in the processing, management, and retrieval of the data in the Cancer Cooperative Group Program. All Statistical Centers now have computer capabilities. These capabilities range from being able to automate routine checking and editing procedures on the data to the use of rather complicated data file systems which allow complex manipulations and retrieval of data sets. Several of the Statistical Centers have developed unique expertise in software systems which are at the forefront of the applications of computers to the processing of clinical trial data.

All Statistical Centers are still in the phase of more effectively utilizing high speed computers. The recent developments in computer hardware have made interactive computing available to all Centers. Interactive computing allows the statistician to better analyze the data as now the data analytic process can be iterative and evolving. "Turn around" times with batch processing range from hours to days compared to seconds with interactive computing. During the next several years the trend to cheaper hardware will continue. The main technical problem will continue to be the development of integrated software which can be used in a routine environment by all levels of computer users.

The third phase in the evaluation of the present day Statistical Centers was the recognition in the early seventies of the inadequacy of clerk/secretaries to process clinical data. The clerk/secretary has been replaced by the present day "data manager". These individuals have substantial knowledge of cancer, knowledge of procedures to be followed in the conduct of protocol studies, and possess computer capability. The recruitment and training of data managers has significantly enhanced the quality of the data. The decision to replace clerk/ secretaries in the data management process was first made in the Statistical Centers of the Clinical Cancer Cooperative Group Program. Even the designation "data manager" was chosen to imply that the position was an important one. Today, the data manager position is commonly used wherever clinical trials are conducted.

THE STRATEGY OF CLINICAL CANCER TRIALS

Background

Good strategy in cancer clinical trials has two goals:
1)   Maximize the number of true positive treatments found.
2)   Minimize the number of false positive treatments found.

The attainment of these goals, in large measure, depends on the number of patients in a clinical trial. The statistical assessment of the data fixes the probability of finding a false positive treatment and maximizes the probability of finding true positive treatments. Generally the probability of finding a false positive (significance level) is fixed at 0.05. When there are small numbers of patients in a trial the sensitivity of being able to find effective treatments is low.

To illustrate the problems of small patient numbers, suppose one considers a trial for comparing the proportion of responses amongst two treatments. Furthermore let us consider the effect of sample size on two distinct situations--detecting a difference between two treatments with response probabilities: 0.2 versus 0.4 and 0.4 versus 0.8. Table 2 summarizes the probabilities of detecting a difference between the treatments as a function of varying sample size. For example if 38 patients are used in each of two treatment groups to total 76 patients, there is a probability of 0.50 of detecting a difference between two treatments when one treatment has a 20 percent chance for response and the other a 40 percent chance for response.

TABLE 2
Effect of Sample Size on Sensitivity: Comparison of Proportions

(Level of Significance is 0.05, Two Sided Test)

Sensitivity*:	0.40	.50	.60	.70	.80	.90	.95
Sample Size**: (.2 vs. .4)	58	76	98	124	156	210	308
Sample Size**: (.4 vs. .8)	14	20	24	30	40	52	76

*   Sensitivity refers to power of the test (probability of finding a true positive).

** Sample size refers to total number of patients in both groups. Half the indicated sample size is the number of patients required in each treatment group.

We shall investigate a similar problem when the endpoint is a time metric such as survival or disease-free survival. Suppose one is comparing two treatments where the better treatment has a 50 percent larger median survival time. For example, one might compare a median of 2 years versus a median of 3 years. Table 3 summarizes the probability of finding a better treatment as a function of sample size. For comparison, Table 3 also contains the calculations for detecting a doubling of a median. Note that if 50 patients are in a clinical trial, then the probability is 0.30 of detecting a 50 percent increase in the median. The calculations in Table 3 assume that no observations are incomplete (censored). If observations are censored, then more patients would be required.

TABLE 3
Effect of Sample Size on Sensitivity: Survival

Level of Significance is .05, Two Sided Test)

Sensitivity*:	.30	.40	.50	.60	.70	.80	.90
Sample Size**: (50% increase in median)	50	70	94	120	150	190	256
Sample Size**: (100% increase in median)	18	24	32	42	52	66	88

*   Sensitivity refers to power of the test (probability of finding a true positive) assuming exponential distributions.

**   Sample size refers to total number of patients in both groups. Half the indicated sample size is the number of patients required in each treatment group.

Tables 2 and 3 show the effect of different sample sizes on the sensitivity of a statistical test.   These calculations are based on idealized conditions where one is assuming that the two treatment groups are composed of homogeneous patients with respect to the ability to respond to therapy.   On the other hand, if the differential effects of the treatments depend on prognostic factors, the required sample sizes may be larger.

SAMPLE SIZES OF CURRENT CLINICAL TRIALS

A survey was made on the results of clinical trials published in Cancer during the period 1977 to 1979. Phase I and retrospective studies were omitted from the survey. Twelve monthly issues of the Journal were surveyed and contained 54 prospective clinical trials. The trials were both randomized and nonrandomized.   Table 4 summarizes the frequency distribution of the number of patients in these trials.   The median sample size was 50 patients.

TABLE 4
Results of a Survey of Number of Patients in Published Clinical Trials
Appearing in Cancer 1977-79*

Number of Patients	Number of Trials**
10 - 20	9
21 - 40	14
41 - 60	8 (median = 50)
61 - 80	5
81 - 100	2
101 - 200	8
201 - 400	4
401 ------	4
Total	54

*   Omitting Phase I and retrospective studies
** Based on sampling 12 issues of Cancer for 1977-79

There is no reason to believe that the sample sizes of these clinical trials are atypical of current clinical cancer research. Note that 16 trials contained more than 100 patients. (These large studies were mainly from Cooperative Groups or foreign programs.) Thus a "typical trial" is conducted on 50 patients and has a probability less than .40 for detecting a change from 0.2 to 0.4 when comparing response proportions; the sensitivity is 0.30 in detecting a 50 percent change in median survival.

Good scientific planning requires that the sensitivity of an experiment should be relatively high-- in the neighborhood of 0.80 or higher. Many past and current trials fail to achieve this goal. It is only when several institutions cooperate and pool their resources can this goal be achieved.

Our small survey of recently published clinical trials included both nonrandomized and randomized studies, studies from single institutions as well as those involving several cooperating institutions. We must recognize that published positive results appearing in leading journals are often adopted uncritically by practicing oncologists. As a result, it is important to consider the effect in clinical practice of trials having relatively small patient numbers on the number of false positive and true positive treatments. Alternatively one could pose the question--is it better to have a large number of small trials or a small number of large trials?

To answer the question we shall calculate the ratio of the expected number of false positive therapies to the expected number of true positive therapies under various conditions, i.e.,

$$R \; = \; \frac{\text{Expected number of false positive therapies}}{\text{Expected number of true positive therapies}}$$

For this purpose define:

θ =   A priori probability that clinical trial will result in a significant advance,

α =   Probability of reporting a false positive result,

β =   Probability of detecting a true positive result.

The triple (θ, α, β) are the parameters which enable one to calculate the ratio, R, of false to true positives.

The parameter θ refers to the proportion of trials which are true positives. It reflects the level of basic science and clinical innovation which can produce positive therapies.

The parameter α is the probability of finding false positives. Technically it is the significance level of a statistical test and is often taken to be .05.

The quantity β refers to the power or sensitivity of a test. That is, it is the probability of being able to detect a real difference between treatments. It depends on the actual magnitude of the true difference, the false positive rate, and the sample size.

The ratio of false positive to true positive results can easily be calculated by noting that:

$$R \; = \; \frac{\text{Expected number of false positive treatments}}{\text{Expected number of true positive treatments}} = \frac{(1-\theta)\,\alpha}{}$$

If the values θ = .10, α = .05, and β = .30 are adopted, then

$$R \; = \; \frac{(1-.10)\,(.05)}{(.10)\,(.30)} \; = \; 1.5$$

This means that there would be 1.5 false positive treatments for every true positive treatment. Note that the value of β = .30 corresponds to the power of a statistical test if one wishes to detect a 50 percent increase in survival with a trial having a total sample size of 50 patients. This is our "typical" sample size for trials reported in the referred literature.

One can vary the parameters (θ, α, β) to determine the range of values for R. Table 5 summarizes these calculations for $\theta = (.05, .10, .20)$ and $\beta = (.3, .5, .9, 1.0)$ with $\alpha = .05$. Note that the range of false positives to true positives for $\beta = .30$ (corresponding to detecting a 50 percent increase in survival with a total sample size of 50) varies from .67 to 3.2 depending on the value of θ. This means that the proportion of false positive therapies (possibly) being used in practice, based on clinical trials of sample size 50, may vary from 40 percent to 76 percent. If one were to take the other extreme and take $\beta = 1$ (corresponding to sample sizes over 400) we have the ratio of false positives to true positive treatments range from 0.20 to 0.95; or expressed as the proportion of false positive therapies used in the clinic the range is 17 percent to 49 percent. Whichever way one perturbs the parameters θ and β, all indications are that the proportion of false positive therapies in use in the clinic may be alarmingly high.

TABLE 5
Summary of Ratio of False Positive to True Positive Treatments Over a Range of Parameters

(False Positive Rate is 5%)

		θ		
		.05	.10	.20
	.3	3.2	1.5	.67
β	.5	1.9	.9	.40
	.9	1.0	.5	.25
	1.0	0.95	.45	.20

θ = A priori probability that clinical trial will result in a significant advance

β = Probability of detecting a true positive treatment

The only way to reduce the number of false positives is to adopt a smaller false positive error rate. However, doing this lowers the power of the statistical test and thus results in failing to find true positives. The power of the test can be raised by having larger sample sizes. To illustrate the problem, Table 6 summarizes the calculations of the ratio of false positives to true positives as a function of sample size and power where the proportion of false positives is taken as $\alpha = .01$.

Note that if $\alpha = .05$, the smallest value of the R-ratio is .20; i.e., one false positive for every five true positive therapies. This may be an unacceptably high figure. On the other hand, if $\theta = .10$ or .20, then

TABLE 6
Summary of Ratio of False Positive to True Positive Treatments Over a
Range of Parameters

(False Positive Rate is 1%)

		θ		
		.05	.10	.20
	100	.66	.31	.14
	200	.31	.15	.06
Sample	300	.23	.11	.05
Size*	400	.20	.10	.04
	500	.20	.09	.04

θ = A priori probability that clinical trial will result in a
significant advance

* Sample size refers to total sample size of trial. Each
treatment group contains half of total number of patients.

the ratio of false positive to true positive treatments may be less than
one in ten provided that the sample size of a trial is between 200-400
patients.

Thus our main conclusions from this study of the strategy of clinical
trials are:

1) Do not initiate a clinical trial in a disease site unless there is
reasonable a priori probability better than .05 that a true
difference exists.

2) Comparative clinical trials should be planned with 200-400
patients (100-200 patients per treatment).

3) Trials based on small numbers of patients are likely to
produce more false positive results than true positive results.

To these three conclusions we can add a fourth:

All positive results on therapies should be independently
confirmed. This will both lower the false positive rate and
raise the true positive rate.

RESOURCE NEEDS AND EVALUATION OF STATISTICAL CENTERS

Review Period

Currently many major clinical trials started by a Cooperative Group will take at least five years to complete. However, the Groups and their Statistical Centers are reviewed for funding recommendations every three years. A Longer term for funding would enable the Statistical Centers to make long-term plans for both personnel and equipment. It is strongly recommended that Statistical Centers be reviewed for funding every five years. (This is especially important in academic institutions where a minimum appointment is generally three years).

Support for Computing

The increased complexity of the data structure of clinical trials and the more complicated high dimensional statistical analyses have made access to a well run computational facility essential to Group Statistical Centers. Each Center should receive adequate support so that modern computing is available as needed. This includes interactive computing and graphics. A study should be made as to how this can be accomplished on a Program level.

Personnel Requirements

Since the inception of the Cooperative Group Program, the funding of personnel has been done without any study of the requirements for Statistical Centers.

Statistical Centers generally have four kinds of personnel designated by function: statistical and computer scientists, data management personnel and administrative personnel. The statistical scientists are generally at the Ph.D. level. Computer scientists have a range of formal training up to a doctorate. The data management staff usually consists of individuals with varying backgrounds (R.N., B.A., or M.A.) who have been trained on the job.

STATISTICAL PERSONNEL

Biostatisticians should devote approximately 20 percent of their time to methodologic research relating to the planning and analysis of clinical trials. Such developments have the potential for significantly raising the quality level of clinical trials and enhancing the uses of the data. Furthermore, without involvement in methodological research, the statistician may not be current with the latest statistical developments which may affect both the planning and analyses of ongoing clinical studies.

Failure to provide opportunities for pursuing methodological research will result in not attracting promising young statisticians to the clinical cancer program. This is especially true in the universities where promotion will depend in large measure on published methodological research. Statisticians in the Cooperative Group program tend to gravitate away in order to take advantage of opportunities for carrying out methodological research.

The protocol workload of a statistician may be highly variable. However, one can make average assessments of demands on time. Effort is expanded on interim reports, final data analyses, preparing reports for scientific publication, planning of studies and associated committee work. Table 7 gives average effort expenditures per activity.

TABLE 7
Average Measures of Activity and Effort for Statisticians

Activity	Effort	Effort per Year
Interim Analyses	.5-1.5 weeks/study	2%-6% (2 reports/yr)
Final Analyses	4-10 weeks/study	8%-19%
Planning Studies	.5-2 weeks/study	1%-4%
Committee and Administration	25% year	25%
Special Reports and Scientific Publications	2-4 weeks/ manuscript	4%-8%/ manuscript

Consequently, if 20 percent of time is reserved for methodological research, 25 percent effort is allocated for committee and related administrative matters, and 5 percent for planning studies, one has 50 percent time to carry out the data analyses for interim and final reports as well as collaborate on manuscripts for publication.

Table 8 displays various combinations of activities on interim and final reports which the statistician could undertake with 50 percent effort.

A typical responsibility would entail a statistician being responsible for seven ongoing studies and two final reports per year.

TABLE 8
Distribution of Interim and Final Reports Per Statistician

Number of Interim Studies	Number of Final Reports
12-16	0
8-11	1
4-7	2
1-3	3
0	4

A Cooperative Group, in a steady state situation, will terminate one-third to one-sixth of its studies every year. This figure includes studies which take 3 to 6 years to meet their objectives. Thus for every ten ongoing studies there will be 1.7 to 3.3 studies requiring a final analysis. On the basis of units of ten ongoing studies, a Cooperative Group requires on the average 1.5 Full-Time Equivalent statistical effort to carry out the necessary interim and final analyses of studies. Table 9 shows these requirements as a function of different numbers of ongoing studies.

TABLE 9
Average Statistical Effort as a Function of Ongoing Studies

Number of Ongoing Studies	Statistical Effort (FTE)
10	1.5
25	3.75
35	5.25
50	7.50

Of course the tables cited present average figures and are subject to changes to suit individual circumstances. Also the figures are based on a steady state situation in which there is no accumulation of final reports.

If a Statistical Center is funded much below this figure, there are serious reservations about the Center's ability to mount a high quality scientific effort.

DATA MANAGEMENT PERSONNEL

Data management requires individuals with varied kinds of talents depending on how the Statistical Center carries out its data processing responsibilities. Individuals may be data managers having responsibility for the data editing and possible file organizations. Some may have a combination of responsibilities requiring programming and computing experience. More advanced computer file management systems require data base administrators who are responsible for overall management of file handling software such as data dictionary, automatic editing procedures, etc. They also have the responsibility for forms design.

All of these responsibilities reflect new ways of carrying out clinical data management and processing. It is only in recent years that the data management responsibility has been accepted as a professional responsibility which should be staffed with professionals rather than clerks or secretaries. Training for these positions is usually acquired on the job.

In this section we will only discuss the staffing needs for data managers. The data manager's duties require interacting with investigators and study chairmen, giving workshops to train institutional data managers as well as carrying out the actual data management on the records coming into the Statistical Center.

A study of the data processing system for cancer clinical trials shows that:

1) For every patient entered, there are 2.8 patients in followup entered in previous years as well as off study patients still having information to be completed.

2) There are on the average 19.6 subsequent record updates or correction events for every patient entered.

3) Each patient generates on the average six forms. The average number of data items (processed) per form is 60. Hence each patient generates 360 data items (on the average) which is processed by a data manager.

Synthesizing the above figures, it is estimated that an ideal goal for data managers is to be responsible for processing 2,500 forms per year. This corresponds to 416 patients per year; or in other measures of information it corresponds to 150,000 data items. In addition there will be updating and correction for 8,100 additional events. (Missing data arriving late or corrections require inordinate amounts of time.) One data correction or updating is approximately equivalent to five routine data processing items. Hence the 8,000 data corrections are equal to 40,000 routine data items. Thus the base load of a data manager should be 190,000 items/year.

We can now estimate how data management workloads change as a function of number of long-term studies. Long-term studies require two follow-up forms per year averaging 80 items of information. It should be understood that the follow-up effort of a data manager exceeds the actual patient follow-up time as the data manager is often requesting and receiving information after the patient is off study. An average figure is that there is an additional year required to complete a patient's file and have a study chairman review after a patient is terminated from a study.

One can now assess how the changing nature of studies affects the data manager's work load. Suppose one has two kinds of studies--those having an average follow-up time of one year and others having an average follow-up time of four years. During the first year of a study, a patient may generate an average of 280 items of information. Subsequent follow-up years generate 80 items per year. Therefore, a one-year patient plus one year of data management followup generates 360 data items. A three-year patient plus one year of data management follow-up generates 360 data items. A patient on study for three years plus one year of follow-up generates 280 + 4 (80) = 600 data items. Hence a longer term patient generates 600/360 = 1.67 times more data than a shorter term patient.

Table 10 shows the data manager work load for 1,000 patients as a function of the proportion of longer term patients.

TABLE 10
Data Management Requirements (Per 1,000 Patients) as a Function of Changing Population

Percent (%) of Long-Term Patients	Total Data Items/Year	Required Number of Data Managers
0	457,200	2.4
5%	472, 516	2.5
10%	487,832	2.6
20%	518,465	2.7
30%	549,097	2.9

This table is only an average allocation. Data management requirements will vary depending on: 1) number of items managed and
processed; 2) actual proportions of short- and long-term patients; and
3) the quality of the personnel and the data processing system. In
addition, one requires a supervisory senior data manager (or data base
administrator) for every three data managers. This supervisory person
is generally responsible for training data managers as well as general
supervision. Thus the data management activities of a Group require
approximately 3.2 to 3.9 data managers and supervisory personnel per
1,000 patients.

OVERVIEW

The preceding section on personnel resources are the requirements if
the Cooperative Group Program desires to have statistical collaboration
and data management activities at a good scientific level. The
statistician's responsibility for a clinical trial requires that he or she be
well-trained in statistics and computing, is knowledgeable about cancer,
keeps up with the current literature on cancer therapy, is capable of
interacting with study chairmen and investigators, and possesses the
administrative ability to use computer scientists, data managers, and
other supporting personnel to maximum advantage. The statistician's
responsibility in a clinical trial is a continuing collaboration from start
to finish.

The NCI Cooperative Group Program must decide if there is a need for
high quality statistical collaboration. If the answer is in the affirma-
tive then resources must be provided to meet current clinical trial
obligations or the number of current trials should be reduced to match
capabilities. Alternatively, if the Program only wishes to have a
"statistical service", then many of the talented biostatisticians currently participating in the Program will depart. The NCI will then have
to turn to commercial firms or attempt to recruit individuals with less
training to the Program.

REFERENCES 309

1. Armitage P, and Gehan EA: Statistical methods for the identification and use of prognostic factors. International Journal of Cancer 13:16-36, 1974.

2. Bartolucci AA: A Bayesian plotting solution to the problem of analyzing survival data modeled by the Weibull distribution. Biometrie-Praximetrie XV:137-144, 1975.

3. Bartolucci AA, and Dickey JM: Comparative Bayesian and traditional inference for gamma-modeled survival data. Biometrics 33:343-354, 1977.

4. Bartolucci AA, and Fraser MD: Comparative step-up and composite tests for selecting prognostic indicators with survival. Biom Zeit 19:437-448, 1977.

5. Begg, CB, and Mehta CR: Sequential analysis of comparative clinical trials. Biometrika #69, 1979.

6. Benedetti JK, and Brown MB: Strategies for the selection of log-linear models. Biometrics 34:680-686, 1978.

7. Bernstein D, and Lagakos SW: Sample size determination for stratified clinical trials. J Stat Comp Sim 8:65-73, 1978.

8. Breslow NE: Analysis of survival data under the proportional hazards model. Rev Int Stat 43:45-58, 1975.

9. Breslow N, and Powers W: Are there two logistic regressions for retrospective studies? Biometrics 34:100-105, 1978.

10. Breslow N: Contribution to the discussion on the paper by D.R. Cox, Regression models and life table. J Roy Statist Soc (B) 34:216-217, 1972.

11. Breslow N: Covariance analysis of censored survival data. Biometrics 30:89-100, 1974.

12. Breslow N: A generalized Kruskal-Wallis test for comparing K samples subject to unequal patterns of censorship. Biometrika 57:579-584, 1970.

13. Breslow N: On large sample sequential analysis with applications to survivorship data. J Appl Prob 6:261-274, 1969.

14. Breslow N, and Crowley J: A large sample study of the life table and product limit estimates under random censorship. Ann Stat 2:437-453, 1974.

15. Breslow N, and Zandstra R (for Children's Cancer Study Group A): A note on the relationship between bone marrow lymphocytosis and remission duration in acute leukemia. Blood 36:246-249, 1970.

16. Breslow N: Perspectives on the statistician's role in cooperative clinical research. Cancer 41:326-332, 1978.

17. Breslow N, Palmer NF, Hill LR, Buring J, and D'Angio GJ: Wilms' tumor: Prognostic factors for patients without metastases at diagnosis. Cancer 41:1577-1589, 1978.

18. Breslow N: The proportional hazards model: Applications in epidemiology. Commun Statist-Theor Meth A7(4):315-332, 1978.

19. Breslow N: Regression analysis of the log odds ratio: A method for retrospective studies. Biometrics 32:409-416, 1976.

20. Breslow N, and Haug C: Sequential comparison of exponential survival curves. J Amer Stat Assoc 67:691-697, 1972.

21. Breslow N: Sequential modification of the UMP test for binomial probabilities. J Amer Stat Assoc 65:639-648, 1970.

22. Breslow N: Statistical analysis of survival data under the proportional hazards model (synopsis). Proceedings of the 8th Biometrics Conference, 1974, Editura Academiei Republicii Socialiste Romania 1976: 229-236, 1974.

23. Breslow N, and McCann B: Statistical estimation of prognosis for children with neuroblastoma. Cancer Research 31:2098-2103, 1971.

24. Brown BW Jr: Designing for cancer clinical trials: Selection of prognostic factors. Cancer Treat Rep, 1978.

25. Burdette WJ, and Gehan EA: Planning and Analysis of Clinical Studies. Charles C, Thomas Publishing Co., Chicago, IL, 1970.

26. Byar DP, Huse RB, Bailar JC III, and the Veterans Administration Cooperative Urological Research Group: An exponential model relating censored survival data and concomitant information for prostatic cancer patients. J National Cancer Institute 52:321-326, 1974.

27. Byar DP, and Corle DK: Selecting optimal treatment in clinical trials using covariate information. J Chron Dis 30:445-459, 1977.

28. Crowley J, and Breslow N: Remarks on the conservatism of sigma (o-E) squared/E in survival data. Biometrics 31:957-961, 1975.

29. Efron B: Bootstrap methods: Another look at the jackknife. Ann Stat 7, 1979.

30. Efron B, and Hinkley DV: Conditional variance of the maximum likelihood estimator. Biometrika 65:457-483, 1978.

31. Efron B: The efficiency of Cox's likelihood function for censored data. J Amer Stat Assoc 72:557-565, 1977.

32. Efron B: Regression and anova with zero-one data: Measures of residual variation. J Amer Stat Assoc 73:113-121, 1978.

33. Freireich EJ, and Gehan EA: The limitations of the randomized clinical trial. Methods in Cancer Research: Cancer Drug Development 17, ed. Busch and DeVita, Academic Press, New York, 1978.

34. Gail M: The determination of sample sizes for trials involving several independent 2x2 tables. J Chron Dis 26:669-673, 1973.

35. Gail M, Williams R, Byar DP, and Brown C: How many controls? J Chron Dis 29:723-731, 1976.

36. Gail M: A review and critique of some models used in competing risk analysis. Biometrics 31:209-222, 1975.

37. Gehan EA: Adjustment for prognostic factors in the analysis of clinical studies. In Methods and Impact of Controlled Therapeutic Trials in Cancer, Part I. UICC Technical Report Series, Geneva, 36:35-74, 1978.

38. Gehan EA: Biostatistical contributions to clinical trials. In Oncology 1979, being the Proceedings of the Tenth International Cancer Congress, 2, Experimental Cancer Therapy ed. Clark, Cumley, McKay and Copeland, 1971.

39. Gehan EA: Clinical trials in cancer research. To appear in NIH Journal of Environmental Health Perspectives, 1979.

40. Gehan EA: Comparative clinical trials with historical controls: A statistician's view. Biomedicine 28:13-19, 1978.

41. Gehan EA: Design and evaluation of Phase II studies. To appear in Cancer Treat Rep, 1978.

42. Gehan EA, and Schneiderman MA: Experimental design of clinical trials. Cancer Medicine, ed. J Holland and E Frei, Lea and Febiger, Philadelphia, 2nd edition, 1979.

43. Gehan EA, and Freireich EJ: Nonrandomized controls in cancer clinical trials. New Engl J Med 290:198-203, 1974.

44. Gehan EA, Smith TL, et al: Prognostic factors in acute leukemia. Seminiars in Oncology 3:271-282, 1976.

45. Gehan EA, Glover FN, et al: Prognostic factors in children with rhabdomyosarcoma. To appear in J National Cancer Institute, 1979.

46. Gehan EA, Nesbit M, et al: Prognostic factors in children with Ewing's Sarcoma. To appear in J National Cancer Institute, 1979.

47. Gehan EA, and Walker M: Prognostic factors for patients with brain tumors. NCI Monograph No 46: Modern Concepts in Brain Tumor Therapy: Laboratory and Clinical Investigations 189-195, 1978.

48. Gehan EA, and Siddique MM: Simple regression methods for survival time studies. J Amer Stat Assoc 68:848-856, 1973.

49. Gehan EA: Statistical methods for survival time studies. Cancer Therapy: Prognostic Factors & Criteria of Response, ed., MJ Staquet, Raven Press, New York, 1975.

50. Gehan EA, Smith TL, and Buzdar AU: Use of prognostic factors in analysis of historical control studies. To appear in Cancer Treat Rep, 1979.

51. George SL, and Fernbach DJ, et al: Factors influencing survival in pediatric acute leukemia: The SWOG experience. Cancer 32:1542-1553, 1973.

52. George SL, and Desu MM: Planning the size and duration of a clinical trial designed to study the time to some critical event. J Chron Dis 27:15-24, 1974.

53. Green SB, and Byar DP: The effect of stratified randomization on size and power of statistical tests in clinical trials. J Chron Dis 31:445-454, 1977.

54. Greenberg RA, Bayard S, and Byar DP: Selecting concomitant variables using a likelihood-radio step-down procedure and a method of testing goodness of fit in an exponential survival model. Biometrics 30:601-608, 1974.

55. Hanley JA: A language for computer generation of medical data forms. Biometrics 34:288-298, 1978.

56. Herson J: Evaluation of toxicity: Statistical considerations. To appear in Cancer Treat Rep, 1978.

57. Hovsepian JA, Byar DP, and The Veterans Administration Cooperative Urological Research Group: Carcinoma of the prostate: Correlation between radiologic quantitation of metastases and patient survival. Urology VI:11-16, 1975.

58. Hutchison GB: Anatomic patterns by histologic type of localized Hodgkin's disease of the upper torso. Lymphology 5:1-14, 1972.

59. Hutchison GB: Criteria of cure: Statistical considerations. International Symposium on Hodgkin's Disease 561-565, 1972.

60. Kalbfleisch JD, and Prentice RL: Marginal likelihoods based on Cox's regression and life model. Biometrika 60:267-278, 1973.

61. Kalbfleisch JD: Some efficiency calculations for survival distribution. Biometrika 61:31-38, 1974.

62. Klotz JH: Maximum entropy constrained balance randomization for clinical trials. Biometrics 34:209-222, 1978.

63. Klotz J: Truncated geometric response-duration of response models for clinical trials. J Amer Stat Assoc 71:331-334, 1976.

64. Krall JM, Uthoff VA, and Harley JB: A step-up procedure for selecting variables associated with survival. Biometrics 31:49-58, 1975.

65. Lagakos SW: A covariate model for partially censored data subject to competing causes of failure. J Roy Stat Soc C 27, 1978.

66. Lagakos SW: General right censoring and its impact on the analysis of survival data. Biometrics 35, 1979.

67. Lagakos SW: Interpretations of survival-type data arising from clinical trials. Seminars in Oncology 1, 1974.

68. Lagakos SW, and Kuhns MH: Maximum likelihood estimation for censored exponential survival data with covariates. J Roy Stat Soc C 27:190-197, 1978.

69. Lagakos SW, and Williams JS: Models for censored survival analysis: A cone class of variable-sum models. Biometrika 65:181-190, 1978.

70. Lagakos SW, Sommer CJ, and Zelen M: Semi-Markov models for partially censored data. Biometrika 65:311-318, 1978.

71. Lagakos SW: A Stochastic model for censored-survival data in the presence of an auxillary variable. Biometrics 32:551-560, 1976.

72. Lagakos SW: Using auxillary variables for improved estimates of survival time. Biometrics, 33:399-403, 1977.

73. Lee ET, Desu MM, and Gehan EA: A Monte Carlo study of the power of some two-sample tests. Biometrika 62:425-432, 1975.

74. Livingston R, Gehan EA, and Freireich EJ: Design and conduct of clinical trials. Cancer Patient Care at M.D. Anderson Hospital and Tumor Institute, ed. RL Clark and CD Howe, Yearbook Medical Publishers Inc., Chicago, IL., 269-646, 1976.

75. Miller D, Leikin S, Albo V, Vitale L, Sather H, Coccia P, Nesbit M, Karon M, and Hammond D: The use of prognostic factors in improving the design and efficiency of clinical trials in childhood leukemia. Cancer Treat Rep, In Press, 1979.

76. Moertel CG, and Hanley JA: The effect of measuring error on the results of therapeutic trials in advanced cancer. Cancer 38:388-394, 1976.

77. Muenz LR, Green SB, and Byar DP: Applications of the Mantel-Haenszel statistic to the comparison of survival distributions. Biometrics 33:617-626, 1977.

78. O'Fallon JR, et al: Should there be statistical guidelines for medical research papers? Biometrics 34:687-695, 1978.

79. Pocock SJ: The combination of randomized and historical controls in clinical trials. J Chron Dis 20:175-188, 1976.

80. Pocock SJ: Daily variations in sickness absence. J Roy Stat Soc C 22:375-391, 1973.

81. Pocock SJ: Group sequential methods in the design and analysis of clinical trials. Biometrika 64:191-200, 1977.

82. Pocock SJ, and Simon R: Sequential treatment assignment with balancing for prognostic factors in the controlled clinical trial. Biometrics 31:103-116, 1975.

83. Prentice RL: Exponential survivals with censoring and explanatory variables. Biometrika 60:279-288, 1973.

84. Prentice RL: A log gamma model and its maximum likelihood estimation. Biometrika 61:539-544, 1974.

85. Sather H, Coccia P, Nesbit M, Level C, and Hammond D: Disappearance of the predictive value of prognostic variables in childhood acute lymphoblastic/undifferentiated leukemia. Cancer, In Press, 1979.

86. Schoenfeld DA: Asymptotic properties of tests based on linear combinations of orthogonal components of the Cramer-von Mises statistic. Ann Stat 5:1011-1026, 1977.

87. Schoenfeld D, and Gelber R: Designing and analyzing clinical trials which allow institutions to randomize patients to a subset of the treatment under study. To be published in Biometrics, 1979.

88. Schoenfeld D: Tests based on the orthogonal components of the Cramer-von Mises statistic when parameters are estimated. To be published in Ann Stat, 1979.

89. Schotz WE: The continuous labelling indices. J Theor Biol 34:29-65, 1972.

90. Schotz WE: Double label estimation of the mean duration of the S-Phase. J Theor Biol 46:353-368, 1974.

91. Schotz WE: Double label indices. J Theor Biol 36:397-412, 1972.

92. Simon RH: Adaptive treatment assignment methods in clinical trials. Biometrics 33:743-749, 1977.

93. Simon R, Weiss GH, and Hoel DG: Sequential analysis of binomial clinical trials. Biometrika 62:195-200, 1975.

94. Susarla V, and Van Ryzin J: Nonparametric Bayesian estimation of survival curves from incomplete observations. J Amer Stat Assoc 71:897-902, 1976.

95. Temkin NR: An analysis for transient states with application to tumor shrinkage. Biometrics 34:571-580, 1978.

96. The Veterans Administration Cooperative Urological Research Group: Factors in the prognosis of carcinoma of the prostate: A cooperative study. J Urol 100:59-65, 1968.

97. Williams JS: Efficient analysis of Weibull survival data from experiments on heterogenous patient populations. Biometrics 34:209-222, 1978.

98. Williams JS: Lower bounds on convergence rates of weighted least squares to best linear unbiased estimates. A Survey of Statistical Design and Linear Models, Elsevier. 555-570, 1975.

99. Williams JS, and Lagokos SW: Models for censored-survival analysis: Constant-sum and variable-sum models. Biometrika 64:215-224, 1977.

100. Zelen M: The analysis of several 2x2 contingency tables. Biometrika 57:129-138, 1970.

101. Zelen M: Aspects of the planning of clinical trials in cancer. A Survey of Statistical Design and Linear Models, Elsevier, 629-646, 1975.

102. Zelen M: Data analysis methods for inferring the natural history of chronic diseases. Prediction of Response, NCI Monograph, 275-282, 1972.

103. Zelen M: Exact significance tests for contingency tables embedded in a 2 to the nth classification. Proceedings of the Sixth Berkeley Symposium I:737-757, 1972.

104. Zelen M: The importance of prognostic factors in planning therapeutic trials. Cancer Therapy: Prognostic Factors and Criteria of Response, Raven, 1-6, 1975.

105. Zelen M: Keynote address on biostatistics and data retrieval. Cancer Chemother Rep 4:31-41, 1973.

106. Zelen M: Problems in cell kinetics and the early detection of disease. Reliability and Biometry, Society of Industrial and Applied Mathematics, Philadelphia, 701-726, 1974.

107. Zelen M: Problems in the early detection of disease and the finding of faults. Bulletin of the International Statistical Institute: 38th Session 1:649-661, 1971.

REFERENCES

108. Zelen M: The randomization and stratification of patients to clinical trials. <u>J Chron Dis</u> 27:365-375, 1974.

109. Zelen M: Statistical options in clinical trials. <u>Seminars in Oncology</u> 4:441-446, 1977.

110. Zelen M: Theory of early detection of breast cancer in the general population. <u>Breast Cancer: Trends in Research and Treatment</u> (edited by Heuson, Mattheim, and Rozencweig), Raven Press, 1976.

16

Immunotherapy

Brigid G. Leventhal, Albert F. LoBuglio, and Larry Nathanson

INTRODUCTION

There are a number of reasons why immunotherapy has theoretical advantages in the treatment of malignant disease. In the first place, one might hope that it would be possible to stimulate effective specific antitumor immunity in those tumors where appropriate antigens have been identified. In the second place it would seem reasonable to expect that patients might benefit from the nonspecific stimulation of the immune system leading to the killing of tumor cells as innocent bystanders and/or to reversal of the immunosuppression that is produced in the patients both by the presence of an extensive tumor and by the drug treatments employed. Finally, other potentially beneficial side effects with adjuvants have been seen in animals, for example, an increase in hematopoietic colony-forming units in the bone marrow.

This report will deal with the immunotherapy studies that have been conducted by the Cooperative Groups. In addition to the results obtained we will try to address ourselves to the rationale for the individual studies and point out where possible the benefits in having such a tumor studied on a groupwide basis. The only references cited will be either direct reports of Group activities or those which can be considered "Group associated" e.g., reviews of immunotherapy by Group Immunotherapy chairmen or reports of immune evaluation on a segment of patients on a groupwide study. These reports are selected and not comprehensive.

SOLID TUMORS

MELANOMA

The earliest solid tumor to be studied by the Cooperative Groups was
malignant melanoma. Clinical observation of spontaneous regression
and a variety of in vivo and in vitro assays which indicate that
melanoma patients do, in fact, have identifiable immunity against
tumor associated or even tumor specific transplantation type antigens
have supported the view that host defense may play an important role
in the natural history of malignant melanoma.[1] Beginning in about
1967 Morton and other investigators in single institutions began to
report regression of intradermal melanoma lesions when directly
injected with BCG.[2] In the course of these studies it was noted that
about 10 percent of patients showed regression of uninjected nodules as
well, and in several studies where it was measured, the ability of PPD
negative patients to convert to PPD positivity following BCG immunotherapy seemed to correlate with response.[3] These observations are
consistent with the notion that regression of a tumor may, in fact have
an immunologic basis and have sustained the interest in the possible
systemic adjuvant effect of BCG in melanoma.

Single institution studies using historical controls tended to suggest that
BCG was of benefit in Stage I (Clark level 3-5) and Stage II melanoma;
however a study by Cunningham et al[4], and one other nongroup trial
with prospective, randomized controls failed to demonstrate benefit of
BCG when compared to no therapy in Stage I and II melanoma.

The use of chemoimmunotherapy, primarily in patients with late stage
melanoma has accounted for the largest single group of immunotherapy
trials. The use of DTIC and BCG compared to BCG alone was not
associated with any superiority of disease-free interval or survival in
Stage III patients.[4] A randomized controlled trial was conducted in
which patients with disseminated melanoma were treated with DTIC
combined with BCG or with a triple drug regimen (DTIC, hydroxyurea,
BCNU) with and without BCG.[5] Another Group employed MER with
and without chemotherapy in Stage IV melanoma.[6] In neither of these
studies was there significant benefit with the addition of immunotherapy. Toxicity in general was limited to inflammatory reactions,
principally at the injection site and was more severe for the MER which
was injected intradermally than for the BCG which was applied more
superficially, by scarification. DTIC plus cytoxan was studied with or
without the addition of Corynebacterium parvum vaccine in patients
with metastatic malignant melanoma.[7] This study was also based on
several single institution studies which suggested both therapeutic

efficacy and diminution of hematologic toxicity in patients receiving C parvum. At the end of the study the authors concluded that C parvum failed to modify the therapeutic effect or the hematologic toxicity of chemotherapy patients with metastatic malignant melanoma.

Thus, the pattern in melanoma has been that of suggestive preliminary results from single institutions, usually with historical or selected controls. But when the agents were used in a Cooperative Group setting in prospectively randomized, controlled clinical trials, no significant benefit has been seen with the addition of immunotherapy to chemotherapy or surgery in melanoma. These trials have been in patients with a large tumor burden as well as those with a small tumor burden.

LYMPHOMA

The rationale for Group studies in Lymphoma was that these disorders have been characterized as having cellular immunodeficiency at onset and persistent immunodeficiency following successful therapy, even after several years of unmaintained remission. Further, despite a high incidence of complete remission on combination chemotherapy, about half of Hodgkin's patients ultimately relapse and this failure rate has not been affected by maintenance drug therapy. Similarly, patients with non-Hodgkin's lymphoma achieve a 55 percent complete remission rate and these patients for the most part proceed to relapse. Thus, both groups are characterized by effective tumor reduction therapy but ultimately fail with regrowth of tumor cells. It appeared tenable to examine whether immunotherapy might alter the relapse rate in patients with lymphoma. No controlled trials of this therapy with reasonable patient numbers exist in the literature and considerable concern exists regarding the safety of immunotherapy in immuno-compromised patients, that of systemic BCG disease.

The first study, initiated in Hodgkin's disease, examined two different drug regimens, MOPP and BCVPP, for induction of complete remission.[8] The patients were then randomized to receive one of three maintenance programs: 1) No therapy; 2) BCG (2×10^6 viable organisms) ID at months 1, 2, 4, 6 and then every three months; or 3) Chemotherapy with BCVPP for six additional months. The BCG was well tolerated without excessive serious toxicity. This study has not had final evaluation but to date, the two-year remission durations are similar in all three limbs. Of the 124 patients who have been entered in the maintenance phase of the study, only 10 percent have died so that the efficacy results will require further followup. This Group has proceeded to its next study in Hodgkin's disease which includes a maintenance therapy study in which one-half of the patients receive a more intensive BCG regimen since the preceding modest dose regimen was well tolerated. These studies will allow analysis of the potential efficacy of low-dose and high-dose BCG on maintenance treatment in Hodgkin's disease.

A second Cooperative Group has examined immunotherapy in non-Hodgkin's lymphoma. The strategy in this study was two-fold: first, to determine if BCG altered the induction chemotherapy response rate and, secondly, to determine if BCG caused a beneficial effect as a maintenance regimen compared to no therapy. In this study, BCG was given in high dose (6×10^8 viable organisms) by scarification on day 8 and 15 of each 21-day cycle (induction regimen) and monthly x 18 for maintenance.[9] The BCG was found to be well tolerated with no life-threatening complications. This study had an accrual of 755 patients which enabled analysis by histologic cell type in regards to response rate and maintenance. Chemoimmunotherapy produced a somewhat higher response rate (75 percent) compared to chemotherapy alone (71 percent and 67 percent) in patients with nodular lymphomas, but these differences are not significant. BCG did not influence remission duration. Survival with CHOP + BCG is better than with CHOP + bleomycin, but longer followup is necessary to see whether this holds up. The current study in non-Hodgkin's lymphoma is examining the effect of levamisole (immunopotentiator) alone or in combination with BCG on induction response rate with CHOP. The maintenance aspect of the study is comparing no therapy versus levamisole maintenance treatment. Thus, these two studies will be able to identify potential benefits of BCG or levamisole on both initial response rate and maintenance, as well as the effect of combined immunotherapy with both agents on initial remission rate.

In brief, the efficacy of BCG administration by selected dose regimens will have had a reasonable trial for impact on response and survival in both major types of malignant lymphoma. In addition, levamisole will have had a trial in non-Hodgkin's lymphoma. These studies have adequate patient numbers and expert histopathology panel review to allow careful analysis of response by histologic subtype and to deter-mine the effects of immunotherapy as an independent variable. This type of analysis could not have been done at any single institution and is a good example of patient accrual and careful analysis of Cooperative Group efforts.

OVARIAN CARCINOMA

This tumor, which generally presents in a disseminated state can now be studied in standard animal models and appears to be responsive to both specific (antibody) and nonspecific (adjuvant) immunotherapy in these model systems. This tumor is being evaluated in an ongoing study that deserves mention. Patients with ovarian carcinoma with bulky measurable disease have been randomized to receive adriamycin and cytoxan (AC) with or without BCG.[10] Current results are as follows:

	AC + BCG	AC
Number	57	61
CR*	7 (12%)	1 (2%)
PR	23 (40%)	21 (34%)
Expired	22 (39%)	33 (54%)

* laparotomy proven

These results significantly favor the BCG regimen. Although there is no difference in remission duration, the survival duration of the BCG treated patients (median 23.5 months) is significantly longer than that of patients receiving AC alone (median 13 months).

CONCLUSIONS

At the time the early Group immunotherapy trials were instituted around 1972, most clinicians had little or no experience with the use of biologic products as therapeutic agents. It seems logical that they would wish to begin their experimentation with these agents in patients with advanced disease where greater risks may be justified. However, the animal models for immunotherapy suggest that adjuvants should be given at a time when body burden of tumor is minimal and ideally should be given in direct contact with the tumor.[2] As the Groups have progressed in their experience, adjuvant trials for solid tumor patients with resection of bulk disease have been designed and are currently underway. The disease-free interval expected for many of these patients with conventional therapy alone is several years, and therefore some time will elapse before the effect of immunotherapy can be evaluated. These ongoing studies will not be discussed further.

Single institutions which see a positive effect of immunotherapy have criticized Group studies for using adjuvants such as BCG in doses which are too low. This criticism is likely to be answered soon, since as the Groups have gained experience in tumors such as lymphoma, they have been willing to escalate the doses employed for study.

ACUTE LEUKEMIA

Acute leukemia was selected for study by the Groups because of the identification of tumor specific or tumor associated antigens as well as immune reactivity to these antigens. Interest was quickly stimulated by early promising results in pilot studies from several countries.

ACUTE LYMPHATIC LEUKEMIA (ALL)

The initial report of successful immunotherapy in ALL was that of Mathe et al in 1969 using tumor cell vaccine with BCG and other adjuvants for remission maintenance.[2] This report stimulated the to design of a trial in which patients with ALL were placed into remission with chemotherapy and then were randomized after 2 and 10 months of complete remission to no further therapy, BCG, or continued chemotherapy. This was an attempt to give immunotherapy to a patient population with minimal leukemic cell load. The results reported in 1975 show that BCG and no therapy gave comparable remission durations, while the group receiving continued chemotherapy at each randomization was superior.[11] Later data in AML suggested that although BCG did not always prolong remission duration in adult patients, there might be significant prolongation of survival. Dr. Heyn and her colleagues, therefore went back and reanalyzed their sequential treatment data in this group of patients. They found that during the follow-up period of 5 years in this study, there appeared to be no favorable effect of BCG on second remission duration or survival.[12] During this same period of time a number of nongroup studies had also cast doubt on the contribution of BCG to remission duration or cure in ALL. At the present time, to our knowledge there are no United States Group studies in progress on immunotherapy in ALL.

ACUTE MYELOGENOUS LEUKEMIA (AML)

Early uncontrolled single institution data in AML suggested that BCG given alone or with tumor cells might have a therapeutic effect in this tumor as well. The first Group study in AML was that reported by Vogler and Chan.[13] These authors also realized that animal models required that if immunotherapy was to be effective it must be given at a time when tumor burden was low. They therefore designed a study in which immunotherapy was instituted after intensive consolidation treatment. Of 372 patients initially entered in this study, because of deaths, failures to achieve remission, and early relapses, as well as a percentage of inevaluable cases, only 61 patients were randomized to the maintenance program which is the point at which immunotherapy was given. The data indicate a significant prolongation of remission with the addition of immunotherapy. Median duration of survival was 93.2 weeks in the BCG-MTX groups and 78.1 weeks in the MTX group (p < 0.10). A significantly greater proportion of the BCG group survived the first 20 months although 4-year survival was similar in the two groups. These authors feel that immunotherapy does represent a significant advance in the management of patients with acute myeloblastic leukemia.[14] They emphasize the large number of patients that had to be entered into the study before the selected group for whom immunotherapy was of benefit could be identified. This Group has recently completed a second protocol in AML.[15] On this study, after intensive induction and consolidation, patients were randomized for maintenance to receive no further therapy, BCG or chemotherapy. This time there was no difference in remission duration in the three arms, but the survival in the BCG arm (101 weeks) was significantly better than the chemotherapy and no further therapy arms.

The reasons for this improvement in survival must be due to variables that have not yet been identified and the final analysis of this protocol is not yet complete; however, the Group has recently activated a protocol in which induction therapy is followed by intensive consolidation with chemotherapy. Patients are then randomized for maintenance to receive chemotherapy alone, BCG alone or chemotherapy plus BCG. It will be of great interest if it were possible to retain the antitumor effect of chemotherapy and counteract its immunosuppressive effect simultaneously with the BCG. It is important to note that these second and third line protocols are direct outgrowths of the logical progression of the Group's own studies.

Another Group has also investigated the effect of BCG in AML.[16] Of the 479 patients initially entered in this CIAL (chemoimmunotherapy of acute leukemia) study, 55 percent achieved a complete remission. The median duration of remission for patients on OAP maintenance was 75 weeks versus 81 weeks on OAP + BCG (p = .88). Survival also was not significantly different, (p = 0.60).

Based on their own and other pilot data, a third Group elected to investigate the effect of the methanol extraction residue of BCG (MER) in acute myelogenous leukemia.[17] This study was designed so that some of the patients received MER during induction as well as during maintenance.[18] At the time the study was reviewed there were 553 patients evaluable. There was a 46 percent CR rate in patients receiving chemotherapy alone and a 53 percent CR rate in those who received MER and chemotherapy. There is no apparent effect of MER in remission induction.

In an earlier study this Group had examined the possible immuno-therapeutic effect of Poly I:C, an interferon inducer, given after 90 days of remission duration in AML.[19] No clinical effect of the drug was seen, but the Group was able to collect the evaluation specimens to prove that interferon levels were significantly affected by the dose of Poly I:C given.

The Group studying only children initiated a study of chemoimmuno-therapy in childhood AML in 1975. Patients on this study received initial chemotherapy for remission induction and then were randomized to receive chemotherapy with or without BCG plus allogeneic tumor cells during remission and maintenance.[20] This study represented a monumental technical effort since patients from around the country had to have cells collected which were shipped to a central repository and stored in viable condition until they were needed as an immune reagent for therapy by another institution. An aliquot of the cells was HL-A typed and serums of immunized patients are being collected to be studied for the presence of antibody to the specific HL-A type used in immunization. This allogeneic cell study failed to show enhanced therapeutic benefit.

In summary then, the initial study in ALL failed to show an effect of BCG nonspecific immunotherapy. Other studies have since confirmed this negative result. Group studies of nonspecific immunotherapy in adult AML have tended to show mixed results on remission duration and/or survival when BCG was given after remission induction was complete. Because AML responds relatively poorly to induction ther-apy, large numbers of patients have had to be entered initially before sufficient numbers were available to ask a question concerning mainte-nance therapy. It is unlikely that these numbers could be achieved within a single institution and therefore, the Group mechanism is the only one by which this type of question can be asked in a controlled fashion. In addition, two negative studies, one of Poly I:C and one of allogeneic cells plus BCG, which failed to demonstrate an immuno-therapeutic effect, had their value greatly enhanced by the fact that relatively sophisticated correlates of treatment (interferon production in the one case and HL-A antibody production in the other) are being measured on a groupwide basis.

IMMUNE EVALUATION STUDIES

The Groups individually and to a certain extent collectively via interim meetings of the Immunotherapy chairmen, have given a great deal of thought as to how methods can be standardized among the various participating institutions. Wet workshops have been held by many of the Groups to demonstrate laboratory methods. With standard methods available, for example, it has been possible to report for groupwide studies the incidence of T cell leukemias in the patient population.[21] Working against a background of information provided by a group of patients well studied in a standard fashion one Group has established a more sophisticated analysis of patients entered into protocol in which terminal transferase, membrane receptors, membrane antigens and histochemistry are being correlated with morphology and response.[22] This Group has also initiated studies to examine the newly identified B cell differentiation antigens on leukemic and lymphoid tumors.[23] Surface markers have been analyzed as well as several other factors, such as circulating immunoglobulin levels at the time of diagnosis which might reflect the functional subcategory of tumor lymphocytes;[24] however, Lapes et al were unable to correlate immune reactivity in NHL with histologic subtype.[25]

One most interesting study is the determination of immunocompetence after therapy of successfully treated lymphoma patients.[26] Over 100 patients have been studied who have been off therapy for periods ranging from 3 to 186 months. It was found that about two-thirds of these patients have a unique immune deficit of impaired response to neoantigen challenge (development of skin test reactivity to KLH and DNCB) despite normal lymphocyte count, normal recall skin test response and normal DRH skin test response. This was true regardless of the nature of the initial diagnosis or therapy and persisted up to three years off therapy. This analysis established the existence of a long standing immune deficit in lymphoma despite successful therapy which may play a role in recurrent infectious or malignant complications.

These few examples demonstrate that certain types of immune analysis can be done in Cooperative Group settings, although basic immunology research is usually restricted to individual laboratories. However, the protocols of the Groups lead to patient populations which can be studied carefully for specific immune mechanisms or deficits. In general the regimentation of therapy should not inhibit creativity and once new methods are developed the investigator will, ideally, have a group of patients studied and treated in a standard fashion as a resource in which to test his new observations.

In order to assure this sort of quality control, another problem which the Groups have solved to some extent in the course of these studies is the development of new record keeping formats for laboratory as well as clinical data since toxic reactions to immunotherapy, for example, tend to take a different form from that to other agents.

SUMMARY

Immunotherapy is a relatively new (or newly rediscovered) means of treating cancer patients. In general the pattern of Group immuno-therapy studies in the first few years, 1972 to 1975, was that early promising results from single institutions were not confirmed when they were repeated by a Group on a controlled, randomized basis. These studies probably prevented many patients from being placed on inef-fective therapy; however, they were performed in patients with advanced disease where immunotherapy would not be expected to be the most efficacious. These results should not therefore discourage further exploration of the potential for this mode of therapy. In addition, as the early studies were performed, the Groups gained experience with the use of immunotherapy. In a conscious effort to educate themselves properly about the problems presented when entering into a new area, at least two Groups limited their initial studies to single agents. Most Groups are now in a position to design studies which are based on their own prior data or on pilot data from their own member institutions rather than design purely derivative studies. For example, the ovarian carcinoma protocol, which may well show that this tumor is responsive to immunotherapy, was designed completely within the Group.

Immune evaluation and correlation is being done in an increasingly sophisticated fashion by all the Groups. The identification of a syndrome such as the persistent immunosuppression of patients up to three years off therapy for malignant lymphoma is highly significant. The ability to collect adequate numbers of tumor cells, store them and redistribute them to the members for use as a vaccine is heartening when one considers the possible use of specific immunotherapy at a future date.

The principal difference between Cooperative Group studies and indi-vidual institution studies is in numbers. The most obvious numerical difference is in patient accrual. In view of the fact that many of the tumors which are currently considered one pathological entity are likely to turn out to be heterogenous, as is becoming increasingly true for non-Hodgkin's lymphomas for example, large numbers of patients in any one study may be needed to identify the subgroup of patients that truly benefit from a particular therapeutic maneuver. Having a large group also prevents the type of bias which may occur in a single institution study where one type of patient may be overrepresented. The large number of investigators who address themselves simultaneously to a particular clinical problem, should also provide the Groups with an advantage. This can be seen particularly in the immune evaluation studies where individual investigators have made techniques available for the study of larger numbers of patients than they could accrue on their own.

The need for collection of information at a central repository can have the effect of more formal recording of patient data, which can make effective retrospective analysis possible, as was done by Dr. Heyn and her co-workers in the ALL-BCG study. The Groups have been an important force for standardization of diagnostic techniques particularly in histopathology by their use of lymphoma panels or central reference pathologists in childhood solid tumors as well as in cell marker techniques with wet workshops and central reference labs for participating institutions. These would not have taken place without the backbone of the Group structure holding the institutions together.

As a final evidence of the possible positive "spinoffs" from having an established group of investigators in an ongoing relationship with one another, we could cite a study done by Group investigators in 1966.[27] They elected to perform a cooperative study of Imuran in "autoimmune" disease. They were able to use this drug effectively because of their experience in cancer chemotherapy and, in fact, noted improvement in 16 patients with a variety of diagnoses.

REFERENCES

1. Nathanson L: Spontaneous regression of malignant melanoma, a review of the literature on incidence, clinical features and possible mechanisms. Natl Cancer Inst Monogr 44:67-76, 1976.

2. Levanthal BG, Konior GS: Immunologic treatment of neoplasms. In Man in Mechanisms of Tumor Immunity, I Green, S Cohen, RT McCluskey, eds. Johns Wiley and Sons, Inc., pp. 408-427, 1977.

3. Sarraf AM, Costanzi JJ: The value of cellular mediating immunity in patients with disseminated melanoma treated with chemoimmunotherapy. AACR 19:13, 1978.

4. Cunningham TJ, Shoenfeld D, Nathanson L, Wolter J, Patterson WB, Cohen MH: A controlled study of adjuvant therapy in patients with Stage I and II malignant melanoma. In Immunotherapy of Cancer: Present Status of Trials in Man, WD Terry, D Windhorst, eds. New York: Raven Press, pp. 19-26, 1978.

5. Costanzi JJ: Chemotherapy and BCG in the treatment of disseminated malignant melanoma. In Immunotherapy of Cancer: Present Status of Trials in Man, WD Terry, D Windhorst, eds. New York: Raven Press, pp. 87-93, 1978.

6. Kostinas JE, Leone LA, Rege VB: Procarbazine, vinblastine and dactinomycin in Stage III and IV melanoma with or without MER. ASCO 19:355, 1978.

7. Presant CA, Bartolucci AA, Smalley RV, Vogler WR: Effect of Corynebacterium parvum on combination chemotherapy of disseminated malignant melanoma. In Immunotherapy of Cancer: Present Status of Trials in Man, WD Terry, D Windhorst, eds. New York: Raven Press, p. 113, 1978.

8. Bakemeier RF, Costello W, Horton J, DeVita VT: BCG immunotherapy following chemotherapy induced remissions of Stage III and IV Hodgkin's disease. In Immunotherapy of Cancer: Present Status of Trials in Man, WD Terry, D Windhorst, eds. New York: Raven Press, pp. 513-517, 1978.

9. Jones SE, Salmon SE, Fisher R: Adjuvant immunotherapy with BCG in non-Hodgkin's lymphoma: A Southwest Oncology Group controlled clinical trial. In Adjuvant Therapy of Cancer II, SE Jones, SE Salmon, eds. New York: Grune & Stratton, pp. 163-171, 1979.

10. Alberts D, Moon T, O'Toole R, Neff J, Thigpen JT, Blessing J: BCG as an adjuvant to adriamycin-cyclophosphamide in the treatment of advanced ovarian carcinomas: Ongoing analysis of a Southwest Oncology Group Study. In Adjuvant Therapy of Cancer II, SE Jones, SE Salmon, eds. New York: Grune & Stratton, pp. 483-494, 1979.

11. Heyn RM, Joo P, Karon M, Nesbit M, Shore N, Breslow N, Weiner J, Reed A, Hammond D: BCG in the treatment of acute lymphocytic leukemia. Blood 46:431-442, 1975.

12. Heyn R, Joo P, Karon M, Nesbit M, Shore N, Breslow N, Weiner J, Reed A, Staher H, Hammond D: BCG in the treatment of acute lymphocytic leukemia. In Immunotherapy of Cancer: Present Status of Trials in Man, WD Terry, D Windhorst, eds. New York: Raven Press, 1978.

13. Vogler WR, Chan YK: Prolonging remission in myeloblastic leukemia by tice strain Bacillus Calmette-Guerin. Lancet ii: 128-131, 1974.

14. Vogler WR, Bartolucci AA, Omura GA, Miller D, Smalley RV, Knospe WH, Goldsmith AS: In Immunotherapy of Cancer: Present Status of Trials in Man, WD Terry, D Windhorst, eds. New York: Raven Press, pp. 365-373, 1978.

15. Omura GA, Vogler WR, Lynn MJ: A controlled trial of chemotherapy versus BCG immunotherapy versus no further therapy in remission maintenance of acute myelogenous leukemia (AML). ASCO 18:272, 1977.

16. Murphy S, Hewlett J, Balcerzak S, Gutterman J, Freireich E, Gehan E: Chemotherapy versus chemoimmunotherapy remission maintenance for acute leukemia. ASCO 19:385, 1978.

17. Cuttner J, Holland JF, Bekesi JG, Ramachandar K, Donovan P: Chemoimmunotherapy of acute myelocytic leukemia. ASCO 16:264, 1975.

18. Cuttner J, Glidewell O, Holland JF, Bekesi JG: Chemoimmunotherapy of acute myelocytic leukemia with MER. In Immunotherapy of Cancer: Present Status of Trials in Man, WD Terry, D Windhorst, eds. New York: Raven Press, pp. 405-413, 1978.

19. McIntyre OR, Rai K, Glidewell O, Holland JF: Polyriboinosinic: Polyribodytidylic acid as an adjunct to remission maintenance therapy in acute myelogeneous leukemia. In Immunotherapy of Cancer: Present Status of Trials in Man, WD Terry, D Windhorst, eds. New York: Raven Press, pp. 423-431, 1978.

20. Baehner RL, Bernstein ID, Higgins, G, McCredie S, Chard RL, Hammond D: Improved induction remission response in children with acute nonlymphocytic leukemia treated with daunomycin, 5-azacytidine (D-ZAPO). ASCO 18:349, 1977.

21. Humphrey GB, Falletta J, Crist W, Ragab A: Laboratory and clinical characteristics of T cell leukemia and null cell leukemia. AACR 19:220, 1978.

22. Gordon D, Hutton J, Meyer LM, Metzgar R: Terminal transferase, membrane markers and leukemic antigens in adult acute leukemia. AACR 18:59, 1977.

23. Balch CM, Vogler LB, Dougherty PA: Distribution and immunochemical properties of a unique B cell differentiation antigen on human leukemia lymphocytes. AACR 19:119, 1978.

24. Miller D, Leikin S, Albo V, Vitale L, Coccia P, Sather H, Karon M, Hammond D: The use of prognostic factors in improving the design and efficiency of clinical trials in childhood cancer. Cancer Chemother Rep In Press.

25. Lapes M, Rosenzweig M, Barbieri B, Joseph RR, Smalley RV: Cellular and humoral immunity in non-Hodgkin's lymphoma. Correlation of immunodeficiencies with clinicopathologic factors. <u>Am J Clin Path</u> 67:347-350, 1977.

26. King GW, Grozea P, LoBuglio AF: Neoantigen response in successfully treated lymphoma patients. AACR 19:91, 1978.

27. Corley CC, Lessner HE, Larsen WE: Azathioprine therapy of "autoimmune" diseases. <u>Am J Med</u> 41:404-412, 1966.

17

Pathology

Robert McDivitt, James Butler, Edwin R. Fisher, Mary Matthews, and
Raymond Yesner

The Pathology Task Force of the Cooperative Groups reviewed the recently completed DCT Ad Hoc Pathology Working Group Report and endorsed its statement of the pathology discipline's scientific contributions to clinical trials, and recommendations to facilitate these accomplishments. This summary of the pathology discipline's past and current interaction with Groups conducting clinical trials is prefaced to the Working Group Report in the interest of providing added perspective on the remarks contained in it. The information contained in the following paragraphs was obtained from pathology representatives of Groups conducting DCT sponsored clinical trials.

For purposes of discussion, the Task Force has listed Groups conducting clinical trials in one of two categories depending on whether the group engages in clinical trials in one (SGL) or multiple (MLT) disease or organ specific areas. By doing so, it becomes apparent that although the pathology discipline's association with SGL groups in all instances dates back for more than five years; the discipline's association with MLT groups is more recent, in most instances for less than two years.

Although the pathology discipline's association with various MLT Groups has been brief, its organization and integration into Group administrative affairs has proceeded rapidly. In all seven MLT Groups, Pathology Discipline Committees have been established, Pathology Discipline Chairmen elected, and various appropriate Pathology Disease/Organ

TABLE 1
DCT Sponsored Cooperative Oncology Groups Surveyed in
Preparation of Pathology Task Force Report

Single Disease/Organ System Study Groups	Date Pathology Organized
Brain Tumor Study Group	1972
Gynecology Oncology Group	1971
Polycythemia Vera Study Group	1968
Primary Breast Cancer Therapy Group	1971
Radiation Therapy Hodgkin's Group	1967
Uro-Oncology Research Group	-
V.A. Lung Group	1957
V.A. Surgical Adjuvant Group	1973
Wilms' Tumor Study Group	1969

Multiple Disease/Organ System Study Groups	
Cancer & Leukemia Group B	1976
Childrens Cancer Study Group	1965
Eastern Cooperative Oncology Group	1977
Northern California Oncology Group	1976
Radiation Therapy Oncology Group	1977
Southeast Oncology Group	1978
Southwest Oncology Group	1976

Specific Review Committees organized. In addition, most MLT Groups appear to have tried to integrate the pathology discipline into the Groups' administrative affairs, since in five of seven of these Groups, pathologists now sit on the Executive Committee. Pathology is represented on six of nine SLG Group Executive Committees; however, in two of three that do not have pathology representation, there is only one pathologist of record within the Group.

The current level of pathology participation in educational and scientific affairs appears to vary somewhat according to Group size and duration of the pathology discipline's association with the Group. However, pathology programs that have multidisciplinary scientific interest have been conducted at Group meetings in all but one Group. Since this activity has been well received, most Pathology Discipline Committees plan to expand it in the future.

The current level of pathology review activity also varies somewhat from group to group, and appears proportional to adequacy of funding.

Eight of nine SGL Groups report that pathology review is being conducted for all active protocols, and most representatives believe that the pathology discipline has made significant scientific contributions to these protocol designs.   However, the number of active protocols in each SGL Group tends to be relatively small, as compared with MLT Groups. (In five SGL Groups there are fewer than six active protocols for which pathology review is being conducted; in only two SGL Groups are there between 11 and 25.) By comparison, current pathology review activity in MLT Groups is less complete. However, as judged by the number of protocols for which pathology review is being conducted in each MLT Group, the level of pathology review activity is higher.   In four of seven MLT Groups, pathology review is being conducted for between 11 and 25 protocols each; in only one MLT Group is pathology review being conducted for less than six active protocols. Pathology representatives from not all MLT Groups are satisfied with their current level of involvement in protocol design, however, and attribute this to the newness of the discipline within their Groups, and the absence of effective mechanisms for channeling protocol proposals to appropriate pathology discipline committees for their input before implementation.

Pathology representatives also were asked to list publications of clinical trial results to which, in their opinion, pathologists had made a significant contribution. A total of 181 were listed. The majority (151) of these were derived from trials conducted by SGL Groups, as is to be expected, in view of their longer pathology discipline association.   In reviewing these various publications, the Pathology Task Force realized that it would be difficult to summarize the pathology discipline's contribution to each, without engaging in a lengthy and somewhat inappropriate narrative of the experimental design and objectives of each trial in which the pathology discipline had been involved. As an alternative, the Task Force has chosen to append to this document a selected bibliography which contains a few representative publications derived from trials in which the pathology discipline has contributed significantly. We have done so for the interest of those who might wish to pursue in greater depth the mechanism by which pathologists are able to make significant contributions to patient stratification using their own specialized techniques.

During the course of our survey, we also asked about adequacy of current pathology funding.   All MLT Groups and most SGL Groups appear to have funds available to permit pathologists to attend Group meetings. In addition, some pathologists have received supplemental funds to support separate meetings held for purposes of slide review. However, in most Groups funds have not been made available to reimburse pathologists who submit cases for review, even though many pathologists consider this an important factor in the discipline's continued participation in clinical trial activities. Only one MLT Group and two SGL Groups are able to provide this type of reimbursement, the amount per case submitted varying between $15 and $35. Only one (SGL) Group currently provides cost reimbursement for autopsies of clinical trial patients, even though autopsy information is important in evaluating therapeutic response, and in monitoring therapeutic complications.

Pathology representatives from all MLT Groups consider their discipline less than adequately funded; however, most indicate that they receive limited funds which permit the discipline to participate on a somewhat restricted basis. In contrast, pathologists from most SGL Groups are satisfied with their current level of funding. Undoubtedly many factors contribute to this difference in attitude. Among those of importance may be the newness of pathology's association with MLT Groups, differences in size, the amount of funds required, and the degree to which other disciplines understand and support pathology's contribution to the science of clinical trial activity.

PATHOLOGY AD HOC WORKING GROUP

BACKGROUND

Although selected pathology participation in Division of Cancer Treatment contracts and specialized review panels dates back many years, only more recently has an attempt been made to incorporate the pathology discipline into major Cooperative Oncology Group activities. Each Group has tried to do so in accordance with its own standards and needs, which often have differed considerably. This has led to some confusion concerning pathology's prerequisites and responsibilities, which in some instances has been reflected in inadequate discipline representation and funding. In an attempt to respond to problems that have arisen, an eight man ad hoc Pathology Working Group was appointed to study the relationship of the pathology discipline to DCT-sponsored clinical trial activities and to recommend subsequently how this relationship could be improved.

During the first meeting of this Working Group in November, 1977, it was decided that the most effective way to conduct such a study would be to meet with pathology representatives from major DCT-sponsored Cooperative Groups and contracts in order to review conjointly the various organizational activities that had taken place and problems that had arisen. A two-day meeting of this type was held in June, 1978. The Pathology Working Group has met subsequently to review these discussions and submits this summary and recommendations based on the above described activities.

PATHOLOGY DISCIPLINE'S SCIENTIFIC CONTRIBUTION TO CLINICAL TRIALS

The Pathology Working Group suggests that the process of conducting pathology review on cases accessioned into clinical trials for the purpose of confirmation of diagnosis, subclassification, grading, pathological staging, and estimating adequacy of therapy comprises its major scientific contribution. Without this activity, there is no sound basis for patient stratification, weakening other observations that might be derived from the trial. In view of the importance of pathology's contribution to the science of the clinical trials, the Working Group suggests that one pathologist from each member institution be designated Co-Principal Investigator on future institutional clinical trial grant requests.

Fundamental to the concept of this type of retrospective pathology review is the hope and expectation that more precise and meaningful diagnostic criteria will emerge as a result of this activity. Pursuant to this goal, refined diagnostic criteria are often employed. It is to be expected, therefore, that at times differences will exist between submitting and review diagnoses. Should this occur, the Working Group recommends that the contributing pathologist be notified promptly and directly of the difference in diagnostic opinion. The Working Group would emphasize, however, that pathology review of this type must not be misconstrued as pathology consultation since it differs significantly in mechanics, setting, and purpose from the private practice of pathology.

Alternately, it does not appear appropriate to the Pathology Working Group to suggest that the DCT fund, through the clinical trial mechanism, laboratory investigation in pathology unless such investigation appears directly related to the therapeutic response being studied in the trial. Pathologists who seek funding for unrelated investigative activity should do so through the ordinary competitive grant or contract mechanisms.

The Working Group further recommends that, in order for pathology to accomplish its scientific goals, it must be given an opportunity to participate in clinical trial protocol design during the developmental stages. At present it would appear that in some instances pathology review criteria are being inserted into protocols by coordinators without their having consulted the pathologists who are expected to accomplish the enumerated tasks. In order to obviate practices of this type, the Pathology Working Group recommends that pathology input be part of all clinical trial protocol development and design, and that the portion of protocols dealing with pathology be reviewed and approved prior to protocol activation by the appropriate pathology disease/organ specific committee.

The Pathology Working Group also recommends that pathology's contributions to clinical trial protocols should be given greater visibility by means of a separately designated pathology section in each clinical trial protocol. In these sections pathologists should indicate specific hypotheses to be tested which require the use of pathology techniques enumerated previously, as well as others such as electron microscopy, histochemistry, biochemical markers, etc. The Working Group also suggests that clinical trial results not be presented or published until that portion of their contents pertaining to pathology review and clinical pathological correlations have been reviewed and approved by pathologists involved in the clinical trials.

SELECTION OF CLINICAL TRIALS FOR WHICH PATHOLOGY REVIEW IS TO BE CONDUCTED

At times demands for conducting pathology review for clinical trials may exceed the resources available to the pathology discipline of the group proposing the trial. In this event, establishment of priority for conducting pathology review must be the prerogative of the pathology discipline. Factors that will influence this decision include potential scientific accomplishment, availability of pathology expertise, availability of funding, and the potential impact of therapeutic decisions which are implemented or revised as a result of pathology review.

Occasionally clinical trial protocols may be proposed in which significant variance between the submitting and review diagnoses is anticipated, and significant differences in therapy to be administered during the trial are predicated on the pathologic diagnosis. In such instances consideration may be given to conducting pathology review before cases are entered on protocol. In evaluating the desirability of implementing this type of procedure, the Pathology Working Group suggests that numerous factors must be weighed, including availability of pathology expertise at participating institutions, and mechanical problems of conducting a prestudy review dictated by the number of participating institutions. The Pathology Working Group suggests that certain trials of this type may be more appropriately conducted by a single or a few selected participating institutions, rather than by large Cooperative Groups.

INCENTIVES FOR PATHOLOGY DISCIPLINE PARTICIPATION IN CLINICAL TRIALS

In the opinion of the Pathology Working Group, organizations conducting cooperative clinical trials should not expect practicing pathologists to contribute pathologic materials and records for study without compensation. As a minimum, practicing pathologists should be reimbursed for expenses incurred in providing such materials. However, simple financial reimbursement in itself provides limited incentive for the pathologist's continued cooperation, particularly since in recent years the number of requests for material seems to have expanded considerably as the number of clinical trial programs has increased.

The Pathology Working Group suggests that the practicing pathologist's cooperation with the clinical trials programs is best assured by developing mechanisms to involve them in these programs. Among proposed mechanisms are: 1) greater involvement in Cooperative Group administrative affairs, 2) participation in pathology review committees, 3) periodic presentation of clinical trial results, and 4) participation in workshops that illustrate and discuss pathology review criteria.

334 REFERENCES

1. Beckwith J, Palmer N: Histopathology of Wilms' tumor. Cancer 41:1937-1948, 1978.
2. Creasman WT, Boronow R, Marrow CP, DeSaia PJ, Blessing J: Adenocarcinoma of the endometrium: Its metastatic lymph node potential. Gynec Oncol 4:239-243, 1976.
3. Ezdinli E, Costello W, Wasser LP, Lenhard RE, Berard CW, Hartsock R, Bennett JM, Carbone PP: The Eastern Cooperative Oncology Group Experience with the Rappaport classification of non-Hodgkin's lymphomas. Cancer 43:544-550, 1979.
4. Fischer ER, Gregorio R, Redmond C, Vallios F, Sommers SC, Fisher B: Pathologic findings from the National Surgical Adjuvant Breast Cancer Project (Protocol No. 4) 1. Observations concerning the multicentricity of mammary cancer. Cancer 35: 247-254, 1975.
5. Fischer ER, Palekar A, Rockette H, Redmond C, Fisher B: Pathological findings from the National Surgical Adjuvant Breast Project. (Protocol No. 4) V. Significance of axillary nodal micro- and macro metastases. Cancer 42:2032-2038, 1978.
6. Matthews MJ, Kanhouwa S, Pickren J, Robinette D: Frequency of residual and metastatic tumor in patients undergoing curative surgical resection for lung cancer. Cancer Chemother Rep 4:63-67, 1973.
7. Mahaley MS, et al: Neuropathology of tissues from patients treated by the Brain Tumor Study Group. Natl Cancer Inst Monograph No. 46, 77-82, 1976.
8. McGowan L, Bunnag B: The evaluation of therapy for ovarian cancer. Gynecol Oncol 4:375-383, 1976.
9. Newton W, Hamoudi A: Histiocytosis: A histological classification with clinical correlation. In Perspectives in Pediatric Pathology, HS Rosenburg, RP Bolande, eds. Chicago: Yearbook Publishers, pp. 251-283, 1973.
10. Sharp HL, Nesbit ME, White JG, Krivit W: Renal and hepatic pathology following remission of acute leukemia induced by prednisone. Cancer 20:1395-1402, 1967.
11. Slayton RE, Hreshchyshyn MM, Silverberg SG, Shingleton HM, Park RC, DiSai PJ, Blessing JA: Treatment of malignant ovarian germ cell tumors. Cancer 42:390-398, 1978.
12. Soule EH, Newton WA: Intergroup rhabdomyosarcoma study. Identification of a histological subgroup: Questionable Ewing's tumor of soft tissues. ASCO 17:301, 1976.
13. Yesner R, Amatruda TT, Rich BL, Gallagher W, Goodman A: Histological type and endocrine manifestations of lung cancer. Clin Res 11:213, 1963.
14. Yesner R, Gelfman NA, Feinstein AR: Correlation of histopathology with manifestations and outcome of lung cancer. JAMA 211:2081-2086, 1970.

18

Radiation therapy

Simon Kramer, Carlos A. Perez, R.D.T. Jenkin, and James D. Cox

INTRODUCTION

Radiation therapy continues to be one of the major modalities in cure and palliation of locoregional cancer. It has been demonstrated that roughly one-half of all cancer patients are referred for radiation therapy sometime during the course of their disease. Of the referred patients one-half are potentially curable, the other half are treated for palliation. Of those referred for curative radiation therapy, one-half are, indeed, cured (representing one-third of all cured patients in the United States); one-third of those patients suffer locoregional failure and about 17 percent die of distant metastasis.

As palliative treatment for symptomatic local disease, radiation therapy continues to excel in the relief of pain, hemorrhage, obstructive and compressive symptoms, malignant ulceration, and in the repair of weight-bearing structures.

Data on the current practice of radiation therapy has become available. Of 339,262 patients treated in 1977 two-thirds were treated in community hospitals, 19 percent in university hospitals, 12 percent in freestanding facilities, and a few patients in federal facilities. Of 2,278 radiation therapists practicing in 1977, 1,355 were full-time and 923 were part-time. The full-time therapists dealt with 87 percent of the patients, and 13 percent were treated by part-time radiation therapists.

PAST ACHIEVEMENTS OF RADIATION THERAPY

Radiation therapy has always been intensely involved in clinical research. As a discipline, radiotherapists were the first to insist on
complete follow-up data and to press for multidisciplinary management.
Prior to 1950 such clinical research took place primarily abroad: In the
British Isles, Sweden, France and Canada. It consisted largely of
sequential studies, with historic controls, and took place in large
radiotherapy centers. After 1950, when such centers became available
in the United States, much of the clinical research was done in this
country. Again, the majority of studies were both retrospective and
prospective, but employed historic controls. A striking improvement in
the five-year survival rate occurred between 1955 and 1970 (Table 1).

Cooperative clinical trials, with emphasis on radiation therapy, were
commenced in the 1960's (preoperative lung irradiation, 1963; V.A.
studies on lung cancer, 1963; radiotherapy for Stage I & II Hodgkin's
Disease, 1967; radiation therapy in carcinoma of the prostate, 1968;
adjuvant chemotherapy in advanced head and neck cancer, 1968). The
Committee for Radiation Therapy Studies (CRTS) was largely responsible for initiating these studies. Again, with the help of the CRTS, the
Radiation Therapy Oncology Group (RTOG) was formed in 1971 and has
since undertaken a variety of studies which consist primarily of Phase
III protocols in potentially curable patients with cancer of the head and
neck, lung, and brain, and Phase III protocols in patients with metastatic brain and bone tumors. More recently a number of Phase I and II
studies have been undertaken involving the hypoxic cell sensitizer
Misonidazole and Phase I studies for the adjuvant use of hyperthermia
as well as Phase II studies in combination chemotherapy/radiotherapy
for advanced head and neck tumors. The large multimodality Groups
are also undertaking studies involving radiation therapy and here
radiation therapy has been used primarily in an adjunctive mode.
Radiation therapy has played a major role in the studies performed in

TABLE 1
Improvement in 5-Year Survival Rates

Site	Kilovoltage (1955)	Megavoltage (1970)
Hodgkin's	30%	75%
Prostate	10%	55%
Cervix	30%	60%
Nasopharynx	20%	40%
Bladder	5%	25%
Ovary	15%	50%
Tonsil	25%	45%

pediatric tumors. These will be described separately under the heading of pediatrics.

RADIATION THERAPY ACHIEVEMENTS IN COOPERATIVE GROUP RESEARCH

The achievements in Cooperative Group research have been summarized in Table 2. A Master Plan for radiation therapy research was developed approximately two years ago, which deals with the major areas of radiation therapy research and sets priorities in this area. This plan has already been widely utilized by the Division of Cancer Treatment in setting operational priorities for radiation therapy, through the mechanism of its Radiation Oncology Coordination Subcommittee.

The Radiologic Physics Center was initially developed and funded through two of the radiation therapy studies, in conjunction with the American Association of Physicists in Medicine. The Radiologic

TABLE 2
Radiation Therapy Achievements in Cooperative Group Research

- Priorities for radiation therapy research (CROS Research Plan)
- Radiologic Physics Center
- Leadership in radiation oncology community
- Focus on radiation therapy questions in clinical trials
- Uniform techniques in radiation therapy
- Optimal radiation therapy procedures
- Focus on potentially curable patients
- Multidisciplinary protocols in radiation therapy impact areas
- Registry for base line of total practice of members
- Communication of findings to radiation therapy community
- Involvement of community hospital in trials
- Biologic advances in clinical trials:

    Sensitizers
    Hyperthermia
    Particle radiations

- Quality control procedures

Physics Center now acts as a resource to all Cooperative Group studies involving radiation therapy.

The radiation therapists in the Cooperative Groups have assumed a role of leadership in the radiation oncology community by emphasizing the areas of research and by communicating their findings. The need for specific modern radiation therapy techniques and the need for detailed dosimetry requirements and radiation therapy procedures have been emphasized through workshops and publications. Their efforts have focused on radiation therapy questions in clinical trials. From the beginning, special stress has been placed on studies in potentially curable patients. Radiation therapy has had long standing cooperation with the surgical disciplines and this led to development of multidisciplinary protocols in those areas where radiation therapy has a primary impact.

Through the mechanism of the outreach program, a large number of community hospitals have been involved in protocols, either in randomized studies or by accepting the best current practice control arm. This has led to considerable upgrading, not only in the practice of radiation therapy at the community hospitals by adherence to appropriate treatment planning, dosimetry and treatment techniques, but also to an improved multidisciplinary approach to cancer patients.

As biologic advances have been made, particularly in overcoming the problem of the hypoxic cell element in tumors, these advances have been translated into appropriate clinical trials. For example, Phase I studies on Misonidazole have now been completed and Phase II trials are

TABLE 3
Mechanisms of Quality Control in Radiation Therapy

1. Review of protocols, particularly standardization of radiation therapy techniques

2. Design of reliable and practical radiation therapy and treatment planning techniques

3. Review of individual patient radiation therapy factors:
    a) Polaroid picture of ports with patient in treatment positions
    b) Localization of portal films
    c) Recalculation of doses from daily dose sheets
    d) Review of isodose distribution computations

4. Total evaluation and determination of evaluability of patients on study

in progress.   The value of local hyperthermia is being established in Phase I studies. The overall management of the national clinical trials in particle radiation has been undertaken.   There are currently nine Phase III protocols for neutron beam therapy and over 380 patients have been entered so far. Clinical trials in pi meson therapy and in heavy stripped nuclei therapy have been initiated.   In all these studies common control arms are used.

In the area of quality control, radiation therapists have been preeminent (Table 3). Standard radiation therapy treatment planning techniques and dose/time systems have been adopted. Radiotherapists have developed on-line quality control procedures which involve review of the treatment plans and the dosimetry and localization films are submitted within seven days of a protocol patient being entered. As each patient completes treatment all physical parameters and the total dose delivered are reviewed. These detailed quality control procedures have been found extremely useful for the evaluability and protocol adherence of patients entered into trials and verification of dose delivery.

SPECIAL NEEDS IN RADIATION THERAPY FOR COOPERATIVE GROUP STUDIES

There is a need to develop intergroup agreement on appropriate radiation therapy in studies on patients with essentially similar disease. This is being addressed by the Council of Radiation Oncology Committee Chairpersons in the Cooperative Groups.

Prognostic indicators need to be developed that characterize both disease and patient to define relatively homogeneous patient groups in whom clinical trials can proceed. At present, groups of patients with a specific diagnosis are collectively entered into a study to compare different treatment arms. Yet, the biology of their tumor may be so different that it overwhelms any effect of intervention.

There is need to establish a base line on denominators for normal tissue morbidity of curative radiation therapy. This could best be achieved by appropriate patient registries so that a true incidence of such morbidity can be determined. This is essential to be able to arrive at a judgment in combined modality therapy as to the causation of morbidity by combined modality.

The Karnofsky scale is excellent in assessing the effect of palliative therapy, but in the cured patient it is necessary to establish a scoring system that allows us to distinguish between the effects of the disease and effects of treatment and to measure the quality of life.

A major problem is the statistical methodology for prospective trials. While randomized prospective trials clearly represent an excellent statistical method, it introduces difficulties when one is dealing with potentially curable patients. Rather than seeing the physician, in whom he has placed his trust, make the decision on how he is to be treated, the patient must be told that there may be two or more apparently equally good ways of treating him and that the decision is made by random selection. This is disturbing both to referring physician and patient and leads to a considerable loss of potential participants.

Support is needed for the further development of particle therapy. Neutron beam clinical trials are in progress, but are severely handicapped by inadequate equipment. A number of clinically optimized hospital-based machines are needed to conclude these studies in a reasonable time frame. Continued support is also needed for trials with pi mesons, heavy stripped nuclei and protons.

Research in radiation sensitizers and protectors must be expanded. Better electron affinic and other sensitizers must be developed and toxicology testing done before clinical trials can be initiated. Local hyperthermia holds great promise. There is a pressing need to develop equipment for deep local heating and for thermometry.

Perhaps the greatest need lies in the precise delineation in deep seated tumors. Modern diagnostic technology such as CT scanning, positron emitting computerized tomography and ultrasonography are advancing our capabilities enormously. Their applications to tumor definition, radiation therapy planning and measurements of local control must be evaluated.

SUMMARY

Radiation therapy is a small but well organized oncologic discipline. It treats roughly one-half of all cancer patients either alone or in combination with other disciplines. Eighty-seven percent of all radiation therapy patients are being treated by some 1,350 full-time radiation therapists. The field is progressing rapidly and has in no way reached a plateau. In fact, there are excellent prospects for the increased use of radiation therapy with the development of particle therapy, sensitizers and hyperthermia for locoregional control with the likelihood of an excellent quality of life. There is also the probability that the number of cures will be greatly increased when systemic therapy can take care of systemic micrometastases. At that stage radiation therapy could be employed in two-thirds of all cancer patients with an appreciable salvage of the 100,000 patients presently dying of local and regional failure.

19

Surgery

George A. Higgins, Jr., Bernard Fisher, Daniel M. Hays, George C. Lewis, Jr.,
Arnold Mittelman, George R. Prout, Jr., Thomas W. Shields, and James B. Snow

INTRODUCTION

A case can be made for dating the era of clinical cancer chemotherapy
to early December of 1942 when, under the supervision of Dr. Gustav E.
Lindskog, then assistant professor of surgery at Yale and subsequently
chairman of the department, a patient with radioresistant advanced
lymphosarcoma was treated with the investigational highly toxic chemical warfare agent, nitrogen mustard, with a remarkably dramatic
clinical response. The account of events leading up to this first clinical
trial, which was not immediately publicized because of wartime security measures, can be read in a retrospective review of the event by
Alfred Gilman, the noted pharmacologist who was actively involved in
the study of chemical warfare agents under the auspices of the Office
of Scientific Research and Development.[1] Surgeons other than
Lindskog, namely Coley of New York, with his anticancer toxins, and
Charles Huggins of Chicago, employing endocrine manipulative techniques, had also served to establish a firm priority of interest by
surgeons in cancer chemotherapy.

Over a decade later (1954), the Chemotherapy Committee of the
National Cancer Advisory Council formulated an "Announcement of a
Cooperative Program on Chemotherapy of Cancer," which launched
what has become an extensive program of clinical research in cancer.
A new organizational unit designated the Cancer Chemotherapy
National Service Center was established under the National Cancer
Institute to administer a broad program to develop new drugs and to

organize cooperative clinical trials to test the therapeutic effectiveness and limitations of a broad variety of new pharmacologic substances.   Many leading surgeons, including I. S. Ravdin, William
Longmire, William Holden, Anthony Curreri, George Moore, Rudolph
Noer and others, gave generously of their time and effort to what
promised to be a new era in the treatment of patients with neoplastic
disease.

Shortly before this time another surgeon, Dr. Warren Cole, and his
associates, had reemphasized previous observations that the peripheral
blood stream of patients with cancer may carry cells which closely
resemble the neoplastic cells found in the primary tumor.   They also
demonstrated that during operative manipulation of neoplasms the
number of tumor cells in the peripheral blood was greatly increased
with a preponderance of these cells singly and in clumps in the venous
blood draining the tumor area.   Early adjuvant trials were designed to
attack these cells with cancerocidal drugs given at the end of the
operation and in the immediate postoperative period.   Unfortunately
these great expectations which engendered such wide interest and
enthusiasm did not immediately come to pass and the surgical spotlight
came to focus brightly on the fields of vascular surgery, the technical
achievement of maintaining the patient's viability through mechanical
means during cardiac arrest, and whole organ transplantation from one
individual to the other, diverting most of the surgical investigative
thrust away from the field of oncology.   Nevertheless, this paucity of
positive results in no way lessened the magnitude of the cancer problem
and a small nucleus of surgeons continued their quest to find therapeutic modalities which might significantly improve the long-term
outlook for the patients with major visceral cancer whose hope for
survival still consisted of surgical extirpation of the neoplasm before it
had spread beyond the limited reach of the scalpel.

A resurgence of surgical interest in the problem of cancer has occurred
during recent years and this report will focus on the significant
accomplishments which have resulted from surgical involvement in the
cooperative trials program.   It is important to note that many of these
accomplishments have been of a negative nature, disproving concepts
which had long been accepted as valid or finding that many apparent
logical concepts were of no value or even harmful when placed under
the uncompromising scrutiny of the prospective randomized clinical
trial.

GENERAL ACCOMPLISHMENTS

The major purpose of the adjuvant program launched over two decades ago was to assess the effect of known anticancer chemical agents when administered in conjunction with definitive treatment of cancer at a stage when the neoplasm might be clinically curable.[2] The stated aims of the program were three-fold: 1) to improve the prognosis of the cancer patient; 2) to determine whether chemical agents are curative in human cancer; and 3) to develop workable methods and techniques for therapeutic trials in cancer. To a degree all three have been achieved. The outlook for patients with many neoplastic diseases, particularly those of a hematologic nature and the childhood and soft tissue neoplasms, has improved dramatically as a result of this program, and we now speak in terms of cure for malignancies which were formerly uniformly fatal. Likewise, methods and techniques for sophisticated clinical therapeutic trials with multiple disciplinary and statistical participation have evolved.

Those who first developed the program quickly realized the importance of careful protocol design and the necessity of precise definition and careful followup of patients.[3,4] The importance of a precise definition of operative mortality helped establish the concept of 30-day post-operative mortality, regardless of cause, as a standard which has been adopted quite widely. Careful monitoring of operative mortality rates in the early phases of the first protocols demonstrated a significant increase in postoperative mortality in patients receiving drugs at the time of operating, necessitating a decrease in drug dosage.

As the concept of multimodal therapy has evolved, the surgeon's role as a member of a multidisciplinary team has emerged. The importance of staging not only in determining prognosis but also in dictating treatment is an important part of the surgeon's activities. There may also be an increasing role for the surgeon in the detection of early recurrent lesions and the pattern of recurrence. Surgical resections of metastatic lesions in the lungs and liver have proven highly worthwhile, and it seems likely that socalled debulking procedures to remove as much of the tumor mass as possible will be of value in permitting other therapies to be more effective.

BREAST CANCER

Breast cancer was an obvious challenge to those who planned and formulated strategy in the early days of the cooperative trials endeav-

or. Prior to that time, concepts of treatment were fairly solidified and routine utilization of radical mastectomy for this disease had seldom been questioned, despite evidence that little if any progress was being made in improving survival rates. One of the first large Cooperative Group trials compared the administration of Thio-TEPA at the time of operation and in the immediate postoperative period with radical mastectomy alone.[5] Analysis of the entire study showed no benefit from drug plus operation over operation alone. However, there was a diminished recurrence rate in a subset of premenopausal patients with four or more involved axillary lymph nodes, with a somewhat better survival ten years after primary treatment. Results of this pioneer study stimulated workers in this field to re-examine all previous information and concepts and provided an emphasis for other controlled studies which are beginning to evolve treatment plans that show greatly improved survival prospects for patients afflicted with this disease. A wealth of information has been obtained relative to the natural history of breast cancer, and these findings have resulted in hypotheses which have led to a reassessment of the basis for cancer surgery and to the realization that breast cancer is more often than not a systemic disease requiring the use of systemic therapy.

Many aspects of the natural history, pathology and basic treatment of breast cancer are reviewed in another portion of this document and will not be covered in detail in this section.

At least six drugs, cyclophosphamide, melphalan, methotrexate, 5-Fluorouracil, adriamycin and vincristine, have shown activity in advanced measurable disease. In addition, it was shown that a combination of cyclophosphamide, 5-Fluorouracil, and methotrexate (CMF) caused remission in over 50 percent of patients and was more active than a single agent, melphalan.[6] In the last few years a number of adjuvant chemotherapy or chemoimmunotherapy studies have been initiated in breast cancer. The two largest and best controlled ones with the longest current followup are those by the NSABP in the United States [7,8] and the National Cancer Institute in Milan.[9] Both studies randomized patients to receive chemotherapy after mastectomy or to be treated by mastectomy alone and selection of patients was limited to those with positive axillary nodes. In both studies, premenopausal patients showed a statistically significant improved disease-free interval for those receiving chemotherapy (either melphalan alone or the CMF combination) with strong indication that this will be translated into significantly improved survival rates.

There has been much speculation as to why adjuvant chemotherapy has been effective in premenopausal patients but apparently has not altered the course of the disease in women treated in the postmenopausal age

group.   A large prospective randomized clinical trial showed no
advantage of prophylactic surgical oophorectomy after mastectomy
either in survival or in delay of recurrence rates,[10] making it unlikely
that the chemotherapy effect was due to ovarian suppressive effect of
the drugs.   More recent studies indicate that effectiveness of chemotherapy may be associated with decreased levels of estrogen receptor
proteins, which is the case with premenopausal women.   Currently a
number of clinical trials are in progress to better elucidate the optimal
drug regimen and, in addition, how best to administer the drug or drugs
and for what length of time following operation.

A number of clinical trials have been conducted abroad to evaluate the
acceptability of alternative procedures to the standard radical mastectomy.   After a great deal of planning the NSABP in the United States
initiated a randomized clinical trial to study this problem and the
results are now accumulating.   The specific aims of that study are to
determine in patients with clinically negative axillary nodes whether:
1) total mastectomy (TM) followed by axillary dissection of those
patients who subsequently develop positive nodes is as effective a
therapy as is radical mastectomy (RM), and whether 2) total mastectomy with postoperative regional radiation (TMR) is as effective a
treatment as is radical mastectomy or total mastectomy with post-
ponement of axillary dissection until positive nodes occur.   The primary
aim in patients with clinically positive nodes is to ascertain whether
radical mastectomy and total mastectomy with radiation are equivalent
procedures.   In addition to supplying information relative to the merits
of the various treatments, this investigation also provides data of
biological significance, particularly that which confirms or repudiates
the worth of en bloc dissection in cancer surgery.

Information has been obtained from 1,665 patients entered into a trial
at 34 institutions in Canada and the United States.   Results from that
trial, at present in its eighth year with patients on study for an average
of 66 months, fail to demonstrate an advantage for those who had a
radical mastectomy.   No significant difference in the treatment failure
or survival has as yet been observed in clinically negative node patients
who have been randomly managed by conventional radical mastectomy,
total mastectomy with postoperative regional radiation or total mastectomy followed by axillary dissection of those patients who subsequently develop positive nodes.   Similarly, there presently exists no
difference between patients with clinically positive nodes treated by
radical mastectomy or by total mastectomy followed by radiation.   Of
particular interest is the observation that based upon findings from
radical mastectomy patients, there may be as many as 40 percent of
patients having a total mastectomy who had histologically positive
nodes unremoved, and that to date only 15 percent have developed
positive nodes requiring an axillary dissection.   The persistence of such

a difference in incidence can have profound biological significance. The discovery that leaving behind positive axillary nodes has as yet not been influential in enhancing the incidence of distant metastases of the overall proportion of treatment failures and that a disproportionate number of treatment failures in the total mastectomy group occurred in those patients who subsequently required axillary dissection provides reinforcement to the view that positive axillary lymph nodes are not the predecessor of distant tumor spread but are a manifestation of disseminated disease. The findings, should they persist, also could have a profound clinical importance for all cancer surgery from several aspects. They presently indicate that en bloc dissection with removal of breast, pectoral muscles and axillary nodes in continuity is without special merit. There is thus provided indirect evidence to substantiate the equality of the worth of "modified radical" or more appropriately "modified total" mastectomy and radical mastectomy without the need for a direct comparison (clinical trial) of the two.

Findings from a number of clinical trials have suggested that segmental mastectomy might have a place in the management of certain patients with primary breast cancer. Consequently a three-arm clinical trial is now under way in which patients are treated either by total mastectomy and axillary dissection, segmental mastectomy and axillary dissection, or segmental mastectomy and axillary dissection followed by radiation to the breast. This trial could provide information of the greatest significance regarding the operative management of breast cancer. Aside from the biological importance of the findings, there would be provided to women a viable and meaningful incentive for the earlier identification of breast cancer. Such an event would not only produce a positive gain in terms of cosmesis, but would also provide the proper setting for greater curability, for it is likely that under such circumstances systemic therapy will be most effective. In addition, it may be that patients with a poor prognosis i.e., those with large numbers of positive nodes, may be equally appropriate candidates for segmental mastectomy and radiation since without effective systemic therapy, they are apt to die of their disease regardless of the extent of local operation.

From this brief overview it may be appreciated that clinical trials directed toward resolving the surgical dilemma have far reaching consequences. They may delineate a population of patients who need not have their breasts removed.

CHILDHOOD CANCER

Malignant neoplasms are not common in children; nonetheless the impact is not insignificant in the overall picture since the emotional and long-range implications are quite different from cancer in the aged. At least three major Groups have developed protocols on childhood cancer and there are intergroup studies on Ewing's sarcoma, Rhabdomyosarcoma and Wilms' tumor. With the maturation of pediatric surgery and an increase in the number of surgeons trained in that discipline, pediatric surgeons have assumed a more active role in the affairs of these research groups. Although much remains to be learned, the outlook for the child who develops cancer has improved greatly as a result of the information gathered by the Cooperative Groups and their individual participants.

Studies of multiple factors affecting relapse and survival rates in children with nonmetastatic neuroblastoma have been carried out, on a groupwide basis.[11] This has resulted in the development of a staging classification for this tumor, which has been internationally accepted. Reduction in the intensity or elimination of the use of chemotherapy in localized disease has been established as a rational approach to the management of neuroblastoma. It was demonstrated through Group studies that ancillary chemotherapy has no effect on survival in patients with Stage I tumors and probably not in patients with Stage II (resected) disease. This was an achievement in eliminating chemotherapy (vincristine and cyclophosphamide, primarily) from the standard regimen for localized neuroblastoma which had previously been employed in many institutions in the United States. The incidence of Stage I-II neuroblastoma is low, but the volume of patients supplied by Group studies made this determination possible in two years.

Group studies have suggested that patients with disseminated neuroblastoma (Stage IV) have increased survival when excision of the primary tumor is delayed and carried out only after an intensive chemotherapy regimen.[12] It has also been shown that those patients (Stage IV) with apparent complete responses to chemotherapy regimens, i.e., complete elimination of tumor foci clinically, actually have demonstrable tumor within the abdomen if subjected to a standard laparotomy procedure at specific intervals following diagnosis. "Maturation" of the tumor histology in tissue removed at successive secondary procedures has been repeatedly observed. Recently it has been shown that patients receiving a combination of cancer chemotherapeutic agents (cyclophosphamide, vincristine, and DTIC) have an increased two-year and three-year survival when compared with any prior study of this disease in a large series. An evaluation of known cases of "spontaneous regression" of neuroblastoma was carried out in a review of 22 institutions in a Cooperative Group study.

A number of accomplishments in the management of nephroblastoma (Wilms' tumor) can be attributed to studies carried out by Cooperative Groups.[13] In patients in whom the tumor is resectable, demonstration that following nephrectomy and local radiotherapy, multiple courses of dactinomycin significantly reduce the rate of tumor relapse as opposed to the effect of a single postoperative course of dactinomycin was accomplished in a Group study. The difference in susceptibility to dactinomycin of pulmonary versus nonpulmonary metastatic nephroblastoma was also seen in this study, i.e., pulmonary metastatic lesions (particularly in the single-course group) were largely eliminated by subsequent courses of dactinomycin, while nonpulmonary metastases were less responsive.

Recognition of the paramount importance of histologic type in respect to prognosis in children with nephroblastoma was made possible.[14] Only in Group studies has it become clear that histologic type is the single most important factor in determining clinical outcome. Recognition of the importance of the four types of chemotherapy-resistant nephroblastoma would have required decades to establish through individual institutional studies, because of their relatively low incidence (less than 10 percent of all patients with nephroblastoma). This discovery has led to the concept that this group of patients will require separate (nonanatomic) staging and specific and unique forms of treatment.

Recognition of the fact that survival in patients with Clinical Group I (localized, completely resected) nephroblastoma is not increased by the use of local radiotherapy was accomplished in Group trials.[14,15] This is the type of study that would have been extremely difficult to carry out on an institutional basis, because of the high survival rate of all patients in Clinical Group I. The major significance of this contribution is the elimination of the possible long-range effects of radiotherapy in this group of infants and small children. Prior to this study, essentially all patients with nephroblastoma in the U.S. received local radiotherapy, and had significant postradiation changes in the musculoskeletal system as well as an increased risk of late secondary neoplasia.

The increased effectiveness of two-agent chemotherapy (actinomycin-D and vincristine) as opposed to any single-agent form of therapy in Clinical Group II (tumor extending beyond the kidney capsule) Wilms' tumor, which was suggested in institutional and foreign studies, was confirmed in the National Wilms' Tumor Study.[13] This point was unclear prior to this time, as the study of the Medical Research Council of Great Britain suggested that vincristine was almost as effective alone, as in combination with dactinomycin.

A multivariable analysis of the prognostic factors in nephroblastoma in the National Wilms' Tumor Study suggested that many established principles of surgery therapy are of questionable importance and has prompted a reevaluation of the surgical procedures employed for this tumor nationally. [16]

An analysis of patients with bilateral nephroblastoma has demonstrated that this tumor is susceptible to chemotherapy regimens, and that improved survival rates can be obtained when this form of nephro-blastoma is actively treated by successive surgical procedures combined with multiple-agent chemotherapy regimens.

Treatment of patients with rhabdomyosarcoma has undergone a number of changes. Demonstration of the control of microdissemination or of "microscopic residual" disease by chemotherapy-radiotherapy regimens in patients with grossly resected rhabdomyosarcomas was confirmed in Group studies.

It was established that local radiotherapy does not increase rates of tumor-free survival in patients with localized (Clinical Group I) rhabdo-myosarcoma treated with a standard chemotherapy regimen (VAC), following surgical excision.[17] Recognition of the fact that radiotherapy can be omitted is of particular significance in this age group, as noted in the section on nephroblastoma.

It has been shown that a single year of dactinomycin-vincristine therapy is as effective as a two-year course of standard VAC in the management of patients with rhabdomyosarcoma with Clinical Group II disease ("microscopic residual" tumor, positive lymph nodes or tumor extension into adjacent organs).[18] The elimination of cyclophosphamide from the therapy regimen for these patients will reduce the incidence of the long-range effects on the testes, ovary, bladder and kidney, seen following standard VAC therapy.

The pathology evaluation of tumors in over 500 children has shown that the prognosis in patients with soft tissue, small cell and undif-ferentiated cell sarcomas (without demonstrable rhabdomyoblasts but otherwise similar to rhabdomyosarcomas) is similar to that found in classical rhabdomyosarcomas, and that the response to specific chemo-therapy regimens is the same. The pathology review also revealed that in addition to the classical histologic types of rhabdomyosarcoma, i.e., alveolar, embryonal (including botryoid) and pleomorphic, there are two subtypes resembling Ewing's sarcoma, which have not been previously identified in this situation or described in detail.

In respect to the primary hepatic tumors of childhood (hepatoblastoma, hepatocarcinoma), a response to multiple-agent chemotherapy regimens with increased survival has been demonstrated both in apparently completely resected tumors and in nonresectable tumors. Tumors have become resectable after multiple-agent therapy, with extended survival in this study. The effects of chemotherapy regimens in prolonging survival in patients with Ewing's[19] and osteogenic sarcoma, has been shown in Group studies. The first controlled study of the use of chemotherapy in patients with unilateral retinoblastoma is in progress. Approximately 15 percent of these patients succumb to CNS spread or distant dissemination after initial therapy, and the current randomized Group study will attempt to reduce this incidence with an ancillary chemotherapy regimen.

GASTROINTESTINAL CANCER

Since tumors of the gastrointestinal tract comprise a large segment of visceral cancer, it is quite natural that these neoplasms have received much of the attention of those involved in the cancer chemotherapy effort. Although surgical extirpation essentially offers the only hope of cure for patients with these neoplasms, far too often they experience recurrent or disseminated disease in the remote postoperative period. Data accumulated over the past four decades indicate that improved surgical approaches have had little effect on overall survival.[20] Therefore the concept of a multipronged attack capable of destroying small foci of locally or distally disseminated cells is extremely attractive.

In the early trials on <u>gastric cancer</u>, no benefit from the administration of anticancer drugs in conjunction with surgery could be demonstrated.[21-23] However, a number of interesting and helpful concepts were evolved, especially that of a uniform postoperative mortality figure for comparison between institutions. In addition, it was noted that patients could not tolerate the early drug dosage combined with major surgical procedures, necessitating a decrease in drug dosage. One Group also established in a clinical study with laboratory confirmation that concomitant splenectomy reduced tolerance to cancer chemotherapy drugs. Because of the inexplicable continued decrease in the incidence of gastric cancer, accumulation of large numbers of patients has been limited; however, in recent years there has been a great resurgence of interest in exploring combination drug therapy for its effectiveness in advanced gastric cancer and numerous surgical trials have been under way to test multidrug therapy as an adjuvant. At this time none of these trials have progressed sufficiently with a large number of patients to make any statement.

Surgical studies on <u>large bowel cancer</u> have attracted more interest as significant developments have occurred. The early chemotherapy adjuvant studies failed to demonstrate any drug benefit;[24] however, as other protocols have matured with sufficient numbers of patients, a modest but unquestionably significant increase in survival in patients receiving 5-Fluorouracil in conjection with "curative" surgical excision has been demonstrated[25] and current analyses of other trials are pointing strongly in the same direction.[26-28] Current protocols using drug combinations in the adjuvant setting are in progress and there is hope that as we learn better how to use the current modestly effective drugs and as new and more effective drugs are developed, multimodal therapy will result in an improved five-year survival rate.

The use of radiotherapy in conjunction with surgical operation has also stimulated a great deal of interest and enthusiasm. Controlled studies using preoperative radiotherapy in patients with carcinoma of the rectum have shown modest but unquestionable therapeutic benefit.[29] In particular, reduction of the percentage of patients with positive lymph nodes by the use of preoperative radiotherapy has been shown consistently in numerous studies, and this seems to be dose related. Current efforts are directed not only toward proper selection of patients for adjuvant radiotherapy but also toward techniques of administration, total dosage, and the relationship of radiotherapy to operation (preoperative, postoperative or a combination of the two). With continued trials many of these questions will be answered, and may lead to improved survival for patients with rectal cancer and possibly with other large bowel cancer.

The role of immunotherapy as a surgical adjuvant remains highly experimental but again may ultimately prove to be an important role in adjuvant multimodal therapy. The value of CEA and other biological markers is gradually becoming better understood and these markers appear to have a definite role in the followup of patients for early detection of metastases or recurrence and institution of further therapy, such as additional surgery or systemic therapy. Improved screening methods for the early detection of large bowel cancer are under examination and prospects for earlier diagnosis by utilization of the hematest procedure are encouraging. Development of fiberoptic instruments has made it possible to extend diagnostic potential as well as to remove premalignant and in situ polypoid lesions without a major surgical procedure.

Surgical trials in esophageal, pancreatic, and hepatobiliary cancer have not been extensive. With the increased sophistication of radiotherapists and vastly improved technologic developments, the role of radiotherapy in the management of these lesions should increase and a small number of pilot trials combining multimodal therapy in these organ sites is in progress.

The basic problem in curing gastrointestinal malignancy continues to be that lesions in these areas are not diagnosed until relatively late and that surgical resection, being of a local or regional nature, fails because of dissemination of viable cancer cells beyond the surgical field.

GYNECOLOGIC CANCER

Gynecologic surgery in the course of investigative protocols has served almost entirely to set the stage for some adjuvant procedure involving chemotherapy, irradiation or both. Even at the present time, the most pure surgical protocol in gynecologic oncology is not intended to contrast one surgical procedure versus another, but to utilize surgical procedures to provide information as to the pathophysiology of certain gynecologic malignancies. Thus, it appears that it is more appropriate to use pathology as a basis for improving surgical techniques rather than using the results of randomized clinical trials between surgical procedures.

The earliest purposeful involvement of surgery in gynecologic clinical research occurred between 1963 and 1968. Just over 500 patients were randomized between two therapeutic procedures and two adjuvant methods to determine whether the addition of progesterone to the standard therapy programs for endometrial cancer would improve the results. While the study was not a randomized arrangement between the surgery alone and the radiation plus surgery, it seemed from the examination of the data that the two categories were comparable: the radiation under the circumstances of the study appeared to add nothing to the results achieved by surgery. Possibly the most important aspect of this study was that it did involve gynecologic surgeons in Cooperative Group protocols. It was in a way an initiation process for individuals who had never been involved in clinical investigation.

In 1970, additional gynecologic surgical procedures related to adjuvant chemotherapy, radiation or a combination of both were introduced on a more comprehensive scale. The initial study was that of contrasting surgery alone with surgery plus irradiation or surgery plus chemotherapy for Stage I ovarian adenocarcinoma. The study demonstrated that more adequate surgical techniques were required in order to understand the disease better. Failure initially to have adequate surgical exploration and surgical sampling resulted in an inability to stratify the patients properly and to avoid problems that are encounterable with noncomparable study arms. This particular study extended from 1970 to 1978. The second study involving ovarian carcinoma was also initiated about 1971 and terminated in 1976. In this trial better survival could be demonstrated for advanced ovarian cancer when patients had extensive debulking, leaving lesions less than three centimeters in diameter.

A study of cervical cancer relative to surgical techniques was established in 1970 and terminated in 1976. In this study there was a correlation of surgical findings with pathology findings for cancer of the cervix. Knife cone biopsy and hysterectomy were used to provide tissues which were studied for the patterns of distribution of micro-invasive carcinoma. The surgical findings helped to show that the pathologists did not always consistently call changes in the cervix the same thing. Ultimately the study separated the significant risk patients with carcinoma of the cervix at an early stage of invasion from those who had minimal risk. In two other studies surgeons became involved in pathologic evaluation of lymph nodes, parametrium and lateral pelvic wall tissues, to demonstrate a pattern of spread in carcinoma of the cervix and carcinoma of the endometrium. While early carcinoma of the endometrium was chosen for study, cervical carcinoma of all stages was evaluated. There was also an extensive comparison of patients clinically staged with those surgically staged. Again, this study took in all varieties of patients. The surprising finding was a relatively high number of patients with lymph node metastasis to the region of the aorta. In a more recent study, patients with Stage IIB, IIIB or IVA carcinoma of the cervix have had staging laparotomy in order to determine the extent of disease prior to radiation therapy. It also set the stage for a program in immunotherapy. With a background knowledge of tumor distribution a more specific stratification could be employed. An additional staging study has been established for early carcinoma of the ovary in an attempt to understand more about the spread of ovarian carcinoma underneath the diaphragm and in the lateral abdominal gutters.

Future studies will involve surgical evaluation of patients with more advanced ovarian carcinoma, with an attempt to determine more exactly the benefit of debulking, and studies of sarcoma of the uterus to determine a pattern of spread, possibly relating it to causes of failure. As more information is obtained relative to patterns of spread and behavior of tumor through the surgical findings, protocols involving surgery to a greater extent will be developed.

HEAD AND NECK CANCER

It is generally recognized that early squamous cell carcinomas can be successfully treated with radiation therapy or surgery, while more advanced lesions are managed better by a combination of radiation therapy and surgery. The role of combined radiation therapy and surgery with chemotherapy can only be effectively studied through the Cooperative Group mechanism. One Group has pioneered randomized studies of the preoperative versus postoperative radiation therapy for the treatment of advanced squamous cell carcinomas of the upper respiratory and alimentary tracts as well as the efficacy of combinations of chemotherapy and radiation therapy. There are numerous questions such as that of the value of prolonged cyclic chemotherapy with agents such as cis-platinum following the standard combined radiation therapy and surgery. Questions about the relative value of radical versus limited neck dissections in combination with preoperative or postoperative radiation therapy can be answered by continued cooperative trials of stratified and randomized patients.

LUNG CANCER

Because of the already high and alarmingly increasing rate of lung cancer in the United States, one of the first organ sites chosen for study was carcinoma of the lung. Two large Cooperative Groups were organized and nitrogen mustard was selected for use in conjunction with surgical resection.[30] There were no demonstrable benefits in these two trials and they did not continue with other chemotherapy adjuvant trials. A second trial studied cytoxan as the adjuvant drug.[31] This drug again failed to show any benefit in survival, and indeed there was a suggestion that it might result in a smaller five-year survival than for control patients. As a part of the analysis, however, a small number of patients who underwent resection for oat cell carcinoma showed a substantially better survival when receiving cytoxan than the control patients. In a third trial, cytoxan was used in one arm while a second arm alternated cytoxan with methotrexate, a third arm using surgery alone. The current trial is testing a combination of CCNU and hydroxyurea.

Two Groups also conducted a trial using preoperative radiotherapy for patients with a positive histologic diagnosis.[32] The results indicated that long-term survival was decreased by the use of preoperative radiotherapy.

Review of the extensive data accumulated in these trials has been of value in delineating factors in survival for patients undergoing resection, in further elucidation of the extent of pulmonary resection required for lesions located in various areas, in showing the relationship of cell type and lymph node metastases and the frequency and location of residual and metastatic tumor in patients undergoing surgical resection.[33] Currently, cooperative trials are in progress to study the use of nonspecific immunotherapy in patients undergoing pulmonary resection to test observations that this type of therapy may contribute to long-term survival.

Although progress in the therapy of lung cancer through use of adjuvant therapy has been limited, there have been definite contributions to the management of these patients. Through observations of the Cooperative Groups and individual members, preoperative evaluation and staging of patients have greatly increased our selection of patients for thoracotomy and have resulted in improved methods of postoperative management.

UROLOGIC CANCER

Urological investigators were among the first to organize themselves in a Cooperative Group. In 1957 a group chaired by Dr. Herbert Brendler, studied DES, testosterone and other steroids in the management of patients with prostatic carcinoma.[34] The group was short-lived, because there was lack of consensus between NCI and the Group members as to the kinds of drugs that should be studied. However, it was shown that DES was not superior to a placebo in the treatment of patients with prostatic carcinoma in relapse. This was an important contribution because of the persistent attitude that relapse might be reversed by estrogen. In addition, DES, 5 mg daily, was associated with a marked acceleration in death rate, due, not to carcinoma, but to cardiovascular and thromboembolic disease.[35] DES nor bilateral orchiectomy prolonged life, but were effective in most patients in producing palliation.

The group pathologist provided exceptional guidance in the classification of prostatic carcinoma, especially as the histologic types of carcinoma related to survival. He emphasized that cribriform carcinoma carried a poor prognosis. A number of important biochemical studies were made that, though not fully appreciated, have added to our basic fund of knowledge concerning this disease.

The effect of adjuvant radiotherapy was seen in the surgical management of patients with invasive bladder carcinoma.[36] This study is important because it is the only one that compared a control population not receiving adjuvant radiotherapy to one which did. The following are some of the more important observations made:

1)   Conventional clinical staging in the center of the spectrum of aggressive invasive carcinoma was grossly inaccurate.

2)   4,500 rads was associated with no residual tumor in 34 percent of the patients while 9 percent of the control patients had no tumor in their surgical specimens.

3)   Another third of those receiving radiotherapy experienced detectable downstaging of their local carcinoma.

4)   In spite of these observations it was not clear that radio-therapy was a useful modality except when comparing the no-tumor-in-surgical specimen (PO) to the control group that were P+. Here, a statistically significant difference in survival was evident.

During this time there were also numerous reports of the improvement in survival for patients with invasive carcinoma who had received adjuvant radiotherapy. These reports were based on either no controls or historic ones for comparison.

Recently, the group has made an important contribution by analyzing data in terms of the heterogeneity of invasive carcinoma by separating tumors into papillary and solid carcinomas. Unexpectedly, patients with papillary tumors proved to be the patients most likely to have PO survial specimens and were most likely not to have lymphatic invasion. Further, the survival rate of patients with papillary carcinoma who were radiated and were L- and PO is 90 percent. Solid, L+, P+ tumors carried a survival rate of less than 20 percent. These observations are highly important relative to biological potential of invasive bladder carcinoma.

A Group is presently testing a number of possibilities, including the identification of field changes, tests of cytological techniques, the effectiveness of thio-TEPA,[37] the testing of chemotherapeutic agents, and adjuvant chemotherapy in patients with invasive carcinoma. Because of the breadth and depth of their scientific, multidisciplinary make-up, these studies and others promise to be the most important events conducted by any Cooperative Group studying urological disease.

Possibly the most important product of these Cooperative Groups has been the profound influence each has had on many physicians, totalling in the hundreds, who have contributed and participated over the years. It is difficult to quantify these effects. It is, however, safe to say that scores of urologists now distinguish different types of studies, are much more critical of publications, and appreciate much more fully the difficulty with which accurate clinical data are obtained.

THE SARCOMAS

Cancers arising in the "soft tissues" of the body constitute a wide variety of lesions with a variable gradation of malignancy. Wide en bloc excision including removal of involved muscle bundles and in some instances amputation have been the only definitive treatments available. Through the Cooperative Groups as well as individual studies, the role of radiotherapy and chemotherapy in conjunction with surgery is emerging. Surgery alone should be used for Stage I sarcomas in locations where wide margins beyond the lesion can be shown. Otherwise postoperative radiotherapy should be administered to destroy micro foci of tumor cells. Now under study is the role of preoperative radiotherapy, especially in areas of the body that do not lend themselves to radical surgical excision. The use of chemotherapy again is undergoing careful examination. Adriamycin, DTIC and high dose methotrexate have all shown antitumor activity, although followup is still insufficient to state proper dose regimens and effectiveness. Intraarterial chemotherapy followed by surgical excision has been used effectively for large, high grade tumors of the upper extremities.

OSTEOSARCOMA

In the past, prognosis of the mostly young patients, who develop osteosarcoma, has been poor, with an 80 percent mortality within two years of amputation, clearly a situation of multifocal disseminated disease that should respond to effective systemic therapy. Studies employing adriamycin in patients following amputation and subsequently the use of high-dose methotrexate with citrovorum factor rescue have appeared to result in dramatic short-term, disease-free survival.[38,39] Another trial combining cytoxan, vincristine, melphalan and adriamycin (COMPADRI) has also shown great promise.[40]

Historical experience with patients with osteosarcoma has been used for comparison and there have been suggestions that the characteristic of this disease is changing. Adding further confusion has been the Mayo Clinic experience that amputations alone have shown a steady rise in long-term disease-free survival in the past ten years to levels reported with adjuvant chemotherapy. Nevertheless, there is a strong suggestion of drug benefit, and further followup along with additional studies promise to elucidate the situation.

MELANOMA

The highly variable and often inexplicable course of melanoma has long baffled those interested in this increasingly frequent neoplasm. Surgical studies have played a key role in standardization of staging and in cooperation with the pathologist in determining prognostic implications of the level of invasion and size of local lesions.

An intriguing aspect of melanoma has been the regression and disappearance of tumor following local injection of a nonspecific immunostimulant such as BCG. The chemotherapeutic agents having shown most activity are DTIC and Methyl CCNU. Uncontrolled studies have suggested lower relapse rates in patients treated with BCG although this finding was not confirmed in a randomized trial. An NCI supported WHO trial compares DTIC versus BCG versus DTIC+BCG versus no adjuvant treatment. Preliminary results based on 500 patients entered show a significantly better disease-free survival in all three treatment groups over the no-treatment controls.

Surgical trials have demonstrated that prophylactic node dissection does not improve survival in primary melanomas; however, finding unsuspected involved nodes is a predictor of bad prognosis which may justify rigorous systemic therapy in an effort to improve survival rates.[41]

LEUKEMIAS AND LYMPHOMAS

Vast strides have been made in the management of these neoplasms, although for the most part surgical treatment is not involved. However, it has been shown that splenectomy is highly beneficial in most patients with hairy cell leukemia resulting in increased platelet counts and lower transfusion requirements. The exact role of staging laparotomy usually combined with splenectomy and liver biopsy in the management of patients with lymphoma continues to be somewhat controversial, although this procedure unquestionably represents a solid advance in delineating prognosis and treatment for these patients. Standardization of the staging laparotomy procedure can be implemented through Cooperative Group activities. The value of surgical debulking procedures for advanced non-Hodgkin's lymphoma and possibly in Ewing's tumor is under evaluation at the current time.

1. Gilman A: The initial clinical trial of nitrogen mustard. Am J Surg 105:574, 1963.

2. Shimkin MB, Moore GE: Adjuvant use of chemotherapy in the surgical treatment of cancer. JAMA 167:1710, 1958.

3. Higgins G for the Veterans Administration Surgical Adjuvant Cancer Chemotherapy Group: Evaluation of chemotherapeutic agents as adjuvants to surgery in 22 Veterans Administration hospitals: Experimental design. Cancer Chemother Rep 20:81, 1962.

4. Zubrod CG, Schepartz S, Leiter J, Endicott KM, Carrese LM and Baker CG: The chemotherapy program of the National Cancer Institute: History, analysis, and plans. Cancer Chemother Rep 50:349-382, 1966.

5. Noer RJ, Chairman: Breast adjuvant chemotherapy: Effectiveness of Thio-TEPA (Triethylenethio-phosphoramide) as adjuvant to radical mastectomy for breast cancer. Ann Surg 154:629-647, 1961.

6. Canellos GP, Pocock SJ, Taylor SG, Sears ME, Klaasen DJ, Band PR: Combination chemotherapy for metastatic breast carcinoma. Prospective comparison of multiple drug therapy with L-phenylalanine mustard. Cancer 38:1882-1886, 1976.

7. Fisher B, Slack N, Katrych D, Wolmark N: Ten-year follow-up results of patients with carcinoma of the breast in a cooperative clinical trial evaluating surgical adjuvant chemotherapy. Surg Gynecol Obstet 140:528-534, 1975.

8. Fisher B, Glass A, Redmond C, Fisher ER, Barton R, Such E, Carbone P, Economou S, Foster R, Frelick R, Lerner H, Levitt M, Margolese R, MacFarlane J, Plotkin D, Shibata H, Volk H: L-phenylalanine mustard (L-PAM) in the management of primary breast cancer. Cancer 39:2883-2903, 1977.

9. Bonadonna G, Rossi A, Valagussa P, Banfi A, Veronesi U: The CMF program for operable breast cancer with positive axillary nodes. Cancer 39:2904-2915, 1977.

10. Ravdin RG, Lewison EF, Slack NH, Dao TL, Gardner D, State D, Fisher B: Results of a clinical trial concerning the worth of prophylactic oophorectomy for breast carcinoma. Surg Gynecol Obstet 131:1055-1064, 1970.

11. Evans AE, Albo V, D'Angio GJ, Finklestein JZ, Leiken S, Santulli T, Weiner J, Hammond GD: Factors influencing survival of children with nonmetastatic neuroblastoma. Cancer 38:661-666, 1976.

12. Leikin S, Evans A, Heyn R, Newton W: The impact of chemotherapy on advanced neuroblastoma. Survival of patients diagnosed in 1956, 1962, and 1966-68 in Children's Cancer Study Group A. J of Pediatr 84:131-134, 1973.

13. D'Angio GJ, Evans AE, Breslow N, Beckwith B, Bishop H, Feigl P, Goodwin W, Leape LL, Sinks LF, Sutow W, Tefft M, Wolff J: The treatment of Wilms' tumor. Cancer 38:633-646, 1976.

14. Breslow NE, Palmer NF, Hill LR, Buring J, D'Angio GJ: Wilms' tumor: Prognostic factors for patients without metastases at diagnosis. Cancer 41:1577-1589, 1978.

15. Tefft M, D'Angio GJ, Grant W: Postoperative radiation therapy for residual Wilms' tumor. Cancer 37:2768-2772, 1976.

16. Leape LL, Breslow NE, Bishop HC: The surgical treatment of Wilm's tumor: Results of the National Wilms' tumor study. Ann Surg 187:351, 1978.

17. Heyn R, Holland R, Joo P, Johnson D, Newton W, Tefft M, Breslow N, Hammond D: Treatment of rhabdomyosarcoma in children with surgery, radiotherapy and chemotherapy. Med and Ped Oncol 3:21-32, 1977.

18. Maurer H, Moon T, Donaldson M, Fernandez C, Gehan EA, Hammond D, Hays DM, Lawrence W, Newton W, Ragab A, Raney B, Soule EH, Sutow WW, Tefft M: The intergroup rhabdomyosarcoma study. Cancer 40:2015-2026, 1977.

19. Sutow WW, Vietti TJ, Lonsdale D, Talley RW: Daunomycin in the treatment of metastatic soft tissue sarcoma in children. Cancer 29:1293-1297, 1972.

20. Serlin O, Keehn RJ, Higgins GA, Harrower HW, Mendeloff GL: Factors related to survival following resection for gastric carcinoma: Analysis of 903 cases. Cancer 40:1318-1329, 1977.

21. Longmire WP Jr, Kuzma JW, Dixon WJ: The use of triethylenethiophosphoramide as an adjuvant to the surgical treatment of gastric carcinoma. Ann Surg 167:293, 1968.

22. Serlin O, Wolkoff JS, Amadeo JM, Keehn RJ: The use of 5-fluorodeoxyuridine (FUDR) as an adjuvant to the surgical management of carcinoma of the stomach. Cancer 24:223-228, 1969.

23. Dixon WJ, Longmire WP Jr, Holden WD: Use of triethylenethiophosphoramide as an adjuvant to the surgical treatment of gastric and colorectal carcinoma: Ten-year followup. Ann Surg 173:26, 1971.

24. Holden WD, Dixon WJ, Kuzma JW: The use of triethylenethiophosphoramide as an adjuvant to the surgical treatment of colorectal carcinoma. Ann Surg 165:481, 1967.

25. Moore GE, Bross IDJ, Ausman R, Nadler S, Jones R Jr, Slack N, Rimm AA: Effects of 5-Fluorouracil in 389 patients with cancer. Cancer Chemother Rep 52:641, 1968.

26. Dwight RW, Humphrey EW, Higgins GA, Keehn RJ: FUDR as an adjuvant to surgery in cancer of the large bowel. J Surg Oncol 5:243-249, 1973.

27. Grage TB, Metter GE, Cornell GN, Strawitz JG, Hill GJ, Frelick RW, Moss SE: Adjuvant chemotherapy with 5-Fluorouracil after surgical resection of colorectal carcinoma: A preliminary report. Am J Surg 133:59, 1977.

28. Higgins GA, Lee LE, Dwight RW, Keehn RJ: The case for adjuvant 5-Fluorouracil in colorectal cancer. Cancer Clin Trials 1:35, 1978.

29. Higgins GA, Conn JH, Jordan PH, Humphrey EW, Roswit B, Keehn RJ: Preoperative radiotherapy for colorectal cancer. Ann Surg 18:624-631, 1975.

30. Slack NH: Bronchogenic carcinoma: Nitrogen mustard as a surgical adjuvant and factors influencing survival. Cancer 25:987-1002, 1970.

REFERENCES

31. Higgins GA, Humphrey EW, Hughes FA, Keehn RJ: Cytoxan as an adjuvant to surgery for lung cancer. J Surg Oncol 1:221-228, 1969.
32. Shields TW: Preoperative radiation therapy in the treatment of bronchial carcinoma. Cancer 30:1388-1394, 1972.
33. Matthews MJ, Kanhouwa S, Pickren J, Robinette D: Frequency of residual and metastatic tumor in patients undergoing curative surgical resection for lung cancer. Cancer Chemother Rep 4:63-67, 1973.
34. Brendler H, Prout GR Jr: A cooperative group study of prostatic cancer: Stilbestrol versus placebo in advanced progressive disease. Cancer Chemother Rep 16:1962.
35. Bailar JC and Byar DP: Estrogen treatment for cancer of the prostate: Early results with three doses of diethylstilbestrol and placebo. Cancer 26:257-261, 1970.
36. Prout GR Jr, Slack NH, Bross IDJ: Preoperative irradiation as an adjuvant in the surgical management of invasive bladder carcinoma. J Urol 105:223, 1971.
37. National Bladder Cancer Collaborative Group A: The role of intravesical thiotepa in the management of superficial bladder cancer. Cancer Res 37:2916-2917, 1977.
38. Cortes EP, Holland JF, Glidewell O: Amputation and adriamycin in primary osteosarcoma: A 5-year report. Cancer Treat Rep 62:271-277, 1978.
39. Jaffe N, Frei E, Watts H, Traggis D: High-dose methotrexate in osteogenic sarcoma: A 5-year experience. Cancer Treat Rep 62:259-264, 1978.
40. Sutow WW, Gehan EA, Dyment PG, Vietti T, Miale T: Multidrug adjuvant chemotherapy for osteosarcoma: Interim report of the Southwest Oncology Group studies. Cancer Treat Rep 62:265-269, 1978.
41. Veronesi U, Adamus J, Bandiera DC, Brennhovd IO, Caceres E, Cascinelli N, Claudio F, Ikonopisov RL, Javorskj VV, Kirov S, Kulakowski A, Lacour J, LeJeune F, Mechl Z, Morabito A, Rode I, Sergeev S, Van Slooten E, Szczygiel K, Trapeznikov NN, Wagner RI: Inefficacy of immediate node dissection of Stage I melanoma of the limbs. N Eng J Med 297:627, 1977.

20

Basic research

Frederick Valeriote, Brian Durie, Theodore Phillips, and Lewis M. Schiffer

The Cooperative Groups were not established with the intention of generating any basic research program, therefore, it is not surprising that there is little basic research that has resulted directly from the Cooperative Groups. This is not to say that ideas generated in the discussion of protocols or the interaction of the subcommittees have not generated ideas whose fulfillment would be termed basic research; however, it seems that this should not be credited to Cooperative Groups as it is the regular interplay of scientists at any meeting or discussion group. More disconcerting, however, is the limited impact that basic cancer research has had on the Cooperative Groups. It is more the applied research dealing with the screening programs, pharmacology of anticancer agents, experimental chemotherapy and a few studies dealing with hypoxic sensitizers or hyperthermia and radiation as well as more empirical clinical studies which have led to the new protocols whose testing is the basic raison d'etre of the Cooperative Groups. We believe that this is unfortunate for a number of reasons which are indicated below and suggest that in the future a strong commitment be made to bridge the experimental and clinical disciplines under the Cooperative Program. Most important, however, is the fact that the applied experimental research studies are not closely programmed with the needs of the Cooperative Groups.

Before proceeding, it is necessary to discuss what is meant by basic and applied research since it is to the latter that this analysis will be directed. Understanding the mechanism of enzymatic repair of radiation damage or underlying cellular or biochemical aspects of transformation would be considered as basic research by most scientists.

Analysis of the biochemical action of methotrexate would not be considered as basic research (although, for example, structure modification and affinity to dihydrofolate reductase might be). Combination chemotherapy or combined modality studies certainly are in the realm of applied research as are pharmacokinetics and the vast majority of Division of Cancer Treatment funded research. The Cooperative Group members, as academicians, should be kept up-to-date with the basic science literature and be able to apply such information to the design of new protocols. There is little evidence that this is, indeed the case as most of the protocols generated are derived more from the applied research related to Phase I, II and III clinical studies plus a few studies at the experimental level. There is thus a significant input which would be called "applied" rather than "basic" research.

The integration of the applied component of research into the Cooperative Program is the most important area to stress at present. For example, while some novel combination of agents with different doses or schedules might be proposed by a Cooperative Group protocol, it is often not tested previously in an experimental system, whereas, such testing can be readily done for a number of animal tumors which are closely related to human tumors, one example being myeloma. Some may argue there is input from basic science studies into Cooperative Group protocols with significant examples related to interaction of anticancer agents, be they chemotherapeutic, immunotherapeutic or radiotherapeutic. For example, there are biological rationale for the interaction of two anticancer agents such as one which produces damage at the level of DNA and the second which inhibits repair of such damage, or of radiation induced damage and its repair, or of hypoxic sensitizers dealing with the hypoxic fraction of cells in a tumor during radiation exposure, or of the stimulation of the immune system in a tumor-bearing host to eradicate a proportion of that population. These and a multitude of other examples which we consider applied experimental research have become the basis for original protocols from disease-oriented committees of different Cooperative Groups which have advanced the treatment of those cancers. For example, experimental studies showed that infusion of cytosine arabinoside was more effective than single doses and this was tested in the Cooperative Groups as well as different durations of infusion which significantly affected response rates and survival. An example of a current rationale is late intensification which attempts to eradicate early possible drug-resistant clones. Finally, a number of combinations with synergistic interactions have been demonstrated on a variety of experimental tumor models in major drug screening laboratories such as NCI and Southern Research Institute and these have been the basis for many of the Cooperative Group Phase III protocols.

We suggest that each Group have a subcommittee which not only reviews proposed clinical protocols for their scientific basis but also keeps the different disease-oriented committees up-to-date in terms of experimental studies which might be of interest to them. This committee should have a high proportion of experimental scientists who are actively working with different model systems. For example, the member who also sits on the Myeloma Committee should review periodically the research studies which have been carried out with experimental plasmacytoma models and also his laboratory should examine limited single agents or combinations which the Committee has an interest in and is proposing for clinical protocol development and for which experimental studies are lacking. Feedback from the experimentalists can then define such critical items as dose, schedules, and which agents to combine before a committee commits the patients, which are often a limited resource, to an extensive and expensive clinical protocol. Further, there are new techniques being developed in experimental systems which can have direct applicability to clinical trials; for example, the discovery of receptors in hormone-responsive tumors is being put to use by many groups by defining those populations of patients and their response to different types of treatment for predictive and therapeutic application not only in breast cancer but also in other areas such as prostate and now in the leukemias. Similarly, information from the laboratory in terms of defining different classes of lymphocytes is being applied to the subclassification of leukemias and lymphomas for the purpose of dissecting out those categories which respond best to specific treatments and then building upon these treatments. Finally, flow cytometry techniques are being defined which should allow more sophisticated questions of tumor cell kinetics to be asked, answered, and applied to better scheduling procedures.

The Cooperative Groups are an excellent resource for obtaining large quantities of fluids, tissues and other patient materials to answer important basic questions. This resource has been used only to a limited extent in the past.

In conclusion, we feel that the Cooperative Groups can have a significant impact on the direction and fruitfulness of both basic and applied cancer research. Further we feel that both basic and applied research have not been as optimally interfaced with the Cooperative Groups as is possible and this latter translation should receive top priority in any modification of the Cooperative Groups.

21

Cancer education

Virgil Loeb, Jr., George C. Lewis, Jr., and Joseph Newall

The educational impact of the Cooperative Clinical Cancer Trials Group Program is difficult to define and impossible to quantitate but its scope and magnitude are readily apparent. No reliable figures are available to document the amount of physician participation in the clinical investigation program nor are there meaningful numbers to convey the extent of involvement of clinical scientists, basic scientists, biometricians, nurses, paraprofessionals, medical students, and, certainly not least, patients with cancer. Whether one chooses to regard the scientific quality of the cooperative clinical investigations with enthusiasm or with disdain, there is agreement upon their enormous educational influence. How best to portray this tangible and yet elusive facet of the total program is no simple task. In the absence of criteria with which to validate effectiveness, it is reasonable to highlight in narrative form the educational ramifications of Cooperative Group activities. Judgement as to the importance and significance of this impact is subject to individual interpretation.

For the purpose of this overview, we will assume familiarity with the organization and the operation of the Cooperative Groups as well as with the breadth of their specific and general involvement in cancer treatment research. Basically, the separate Groups represent a consortium of institutions (medical schools, hospitals, clinics, etc.) working together through elected and appointed members to pose and to attempt to solve important clinical therapeutic questions concerning cancer management which presumably cannot be studied better through individual efforts. Goals and constituency vary considerably among the various Groups, some of which confine their studies to those utilizing single therapeutic disciplines or modalities, others to single neoplasms with multimodal treatment approaches, and still others across the board to virtually all types of malignant disease using conjoint therapeutic efforts including surgery, irradiation, chemotherapy, immunotherapy, and the gamut of what is considered to represent optimal supportive medical care. A recent compilation by the National Cancer Institute indicates that the Cooperative Clinical Trials Program currently supports over 130 projects involving surgical therapy, over 200 projects involving radiotherapy, over 200 projects involving chemotherapy, and over 160 projects utilizing immunotherapy.

Common to most, if not all Groups, is a critical mass of participants including clinical physicians ("academic" and "community", "full time" and "part time", with and without remuneration), biometricians, basic scientists from "bridging" fields, oncology nurses, fellows, house staff, medical students, technicians and data managers, not to overlook clergy, social workers, administrators, et al. It goes without saying that in the deliberations and the implementation of such an ecumenical effort, there must be an educational spinoff that may even transcend the new knowledge sought as justification for the Groups' existence in the first place. Sharing of expertise among the many scientific disciplines involved with targeted clinical cancer investigation inevitably provides a learning experience for all contributors and participants.

How then can we portray the educational thrust of this collaborative effort over the past twenty plus years? Tabulation of numbers of involved institutions and individual members is at best inaccurate and fraught with misinterpretation. It would be duplicating other efforts to present a historical summation of the program goals and end results. Whether responding to its original charge in 1955 as the drug-testing arm of the Cancer Chemotherapy National Service Center, or functioning as the clinical trials component of the Cancer Chemotherapy Program in 1966, or as a quasi confederation of independent groups under the Clinical Investigation Branch of the National Cancer Institute Extramural Program in 1968, or whether serving within its current locus as a component of the Division of Cancer Treatment, there has been an inherent educational matrix which has spawned new knowledge, new teachers, new clinicians, and new investigators in a rapidly emerging and expanding field of medical concern. According to figures provided by the Clinical Investigation Branch of the Division of Cancer Treatment, as of November, 1978 there were 658 institutions participating in Cooperative Group activities including most medical schools, all but two comprehensive cancer centers, most other cancer centers, most VA Hospitals, and 41 foreign institutions. The number of affiliated hospitals in 1977 was 493, a number which more than doubled when Cancer Control hospitals joined the Groups. An impressive number of physicians were actively involved in the Group Program in 1977 including 1,611 medical oncologists, 404 pathologists, 289 pediatric oncologists, 721 radiation oncologists, 709 surgical oncologists, 50 statisticians, 227 psychiatrists, and others. Of a total of 75,697 patients on treatment and in follow-up status for all clinical studies in the DCT, 63,498 were patients in grant-funded Cooperative Group trials. The network of Cooperative Groups has an extensive geographic distribution and there is considerable interaction with cancer centers and with community cancer programs. Although initiated and sustained primarily as a clinical research effort, the Cooperative Group Program also provides what should be the best of current medical care to a large number of cancer patients. The program has served as a training resource for young physicians as well as a medium for exchange of information among clinical scientists.

It must be emphasized that the interfaces between the Cooperative Group Program and "academic medicine" on one hand and the community physicians on the other have not always been harmonious. Attitudes with respect to collaborative or interinstitutional clinical therapeutic trials have varied across a wide spectrum. However, the encouraging evidence and demonstration of therapeutic success in several types of malignant disease together with the pragmatic observation that research funding is, in fact, available for such efforts has served to kindle a crescendo of interest by the academic community in cooperative clinical endeavors. Even the emerging emphasis involving interdisciplinary or multimodal strategy is being accepted with increasing enthusiasm and many physicians give credit to the stimulus and demands of the Clinical Trials Program for this major change in academic attitude.

For virtually the first time in medical education the importance of biostatistical methodology and demographic expertise have been given proper visibility and perspective. Furthermore, the implementation of the treatment protocols generated by the Clinical Trials Program at the level of the community physician has provided a new dimension in training opportunities and responsibilities for continuing medical education. This is particularly important when one considers the changing attitudes and increased commitment of medical schools and students with respect to community outreach involvement and improved delivery of medical care. The Cooperative Groups offer a forum for medical institutions with relatively small numbers of clinical cases to learn about current research, to participate in its execution, and to organize studies which can develop meaningful data in a relatively short period of time. This represents a training ground for future clinical oncologists and may be the only place where practical epidemiology and biostatistics are experienced by the student and house staff group.

It has been said that in many respects the academic medical community needs the Cooperative Clinical Trials Program badly, perhaps even more than the Cooperative Groups need the academic community. The conceptualization, the development of an investigative protocol, the essential analysis of the experimental model and the pharmacologic data, the construction of a biostatistical design, the data gathering and data management, the ongoing analysis of the study in progress, and the final analysis and publication - all of these efforts represent learning experiences for those who participate directly in Cooperative Group investigations. For those who may contribute clinical cases but who are less involved with protocol generation, there is opportunity for continuing education with respect to cancer treatment and related research on a broad front.

There are potential counterbalancing features. Some of the Cooperative Groups have become extremely large with the result that a relatively small number of investigators are responsible for protocol development and an increasingly large number of participants simply go along with Group activities in a passive role. In some respects it is reasonable to look upon a majority of Group members as not actively participating in clinical research. This is not to minimize the educational impact, although one might question whether there is inappropriate emphasis and support of this aspect.

There are strong protagonists and antagonists of the role of the Cooperative Group Program in cancer education. Although acknowledging that when there were few trained oncologists and many clinical problems the Cooperative Group system was helpful, there are those who now claim that the Groups have too many trained clinicians and not enough challenging problems for the role that Cooperative Groups play in clinical research. Clinicians have developed a tendency to look upon the protocol not so much as a research device but more as a recipe for cancer management. Criticism has been levied at the Cooperative Group Program from the standpoint of quality of education for students and house officers, citing that trainees are not encouraged to make clinical judgements nor to be imaginative on their own. Counterbalancing these reservations, it is generally agreed that a well designed Cooperative Group protocol can serve as a model for the conduct of clinical investigations. The educational impact on those many scientists and paraprofessionals who are actively involved in the generation and implementation of cooperative research protocols is acknowledged with little contrary opinion. Where the Cooperative Groups serve as a forum for discussion of current and future states of the art and science of cancer management, the educational ramifications are clearly visible and worthwhile.

It is estimated, albeit very roughly, that by 1985 three times the current number of specialists will be needed to satisfy the requirements for adequate delivery of oncologic care in the United States. It is important to acknowledge that the Cooperative Group Program has played and continues to provide an important role in the education of this essential cadre of physicians.

22

Interrelationships: the groups, the NCI and other governmental agencies

Hugh L. Davis, John R. Durant, and James F. Holland

INTRODUCTION

The beginnings of the Cooperative Group Program were first apparent in 1955 when Dr. Sidney Farber, Mrs. Albert Lasker, and others approached Congress with the proposal that it increase support for the chemotherapy of cancer. Congress responded by appropriating 5 million dollars to the National Cancer Institute to establish the Cancer Chemotherapy National Service Center. A Clinical Studies Panel was organized to advise the National Cancer Institute and the scientific community of the progress in cancer treatment and to review the scientific merit of grant submissions. By 1958, 17 Clinical Cooperative Groups were organized under the CCNSC and operated under research grants from the NCI. The CCNSC was in existence until 1966 when the NCI underwent internal reorganization and the Cooperative Group Program was transferred to the Cancer Therapy Evaluation Branch of the Chemotherapy Program. The Cooperative Groups remained there for two years until another NCI reorganization occurred. The Cooperative Groups were then transferred to the Associate Director for Extramural Affairs. The Clinical Investigations Branch was developed as the staff mechanism supporting this program.

The Cooperative Group Program remained in the Extramural Affairs Division until the enactment of the National Cancer Program in 1971. At this time, the Division of Cancer Research Resources and Centers was created, and the Groups with the Clinical Investigations Branch was administratively moved into this newly created Division. At the same time, the Division of Cancer Treatment was created. The mission of the Clinical Cooperative Groups was perceived as closely allied with that of the DCT, and following a conference at the NIH in the fall of 1974 (now known as the Potomac Conference), the administrative responsibility for the Cooperative Groups was transferred to the Division of Cancer Treatment in 1975.

The Cooperative Group Program has since remained in the DCT, along with its peer review committee, the Cancer Clinical Investigations Review Committee (CCIRC). Further organizational changes in July of 1978 resulted in a separation of program and review. The administrative responsibility for the Cooperative Groups remains in the DCT under the Cancer Therapy Evaluation Program and the Clinical Investigation Branch. The Review Committee (CCIRC) was transferred to the Division of Cancer Research Resources, and separation of program and review had been accomplished.

These administrative transpositions have not significantly affected the conduct of Cooperative Group research, which because of its broad base and multiinstitutional nature has a momentum of its own.

Some "science-administration" milestones in the Cooperative Group Program are:

1. The earliest scientific goal of the first two Cooperative Groups was to study treatment for acute leukemia since that represented the major opportunity in cancer therapy in the mid 1950's.

2. Before 1960, as the CCNSC program identified, procured or developed further active chemotherapeutic agents, the activities of the Groups were rapidly expanded to include the study of patients with lymphomas, carcinomas, and sarcomas. Group constitution was diverse with some Groups stressing problems in medical oncology and drug development, and others --pediatric oncology, urologic oncology, radiation oncology, surgical oncology, and even specific organ cancers such as the prostate and breast.

3. In 1968, following the Williamsburg Conference, the Groups were encouraged progressively to develop multidisciplinary programs. The Cooperative Groups were slowly and deliberately restructured toward multidisciplinary Groups by inviting several disciplines to participate.

4. Upon joining the DCT in 1975, the Cooperative Group Program was further restructured to emphasize the following types:

1. Multidisease, multiprotocol Cooperative Groups which were multimodal including:

   A. Cancer and Leukemia Group B
   B. Children's Cancer Study Group
   C. Eastern Cooperative Oncology Group
   D. Southeastern Cancer Study Group
   E. Southwest Oncology Group

2. Specialty Groups:

   A. Hodgkin's Disease Radiotherapy Group
   B. Gynecologic Oncology Group
   C. National Surgical Adjuvant Breast Project
   D. National Wilms' Tumor Study Group
   E. Polycythemia Vera Group
   F. Radiation Therapy Oncology Group

3. Related Resource Groups

   A. Lymphoma Pathology Reference Center
   B. Radiologic Physics Center
   C. Cancer Clinical Investigations Coordinating Center

The Group organization thus has "matured" as the National Cancer Institute has matured, and at this time the taxonomy is well established. During this period, there were many changes in the Cooperative Groups. A number were phased out, and new ones were created. The history of these is best displayed in attachments 1 and 2 which show the life history of the current Cooperative Groups.

GROWTH OF SIZE AND RESOURCES OF THE COOPERATIVE GROUPS

Attachment 2 shows the support of the Cooperative Groups from 1970 to 1977. This amounted to approximately $29 million for fiscal year 1978. The growth was accompanied by a number of changes in the Cooperative Group structures. In the early and mid 1960's, the major thrust of the Cooperative Group Program reflected the state of the art of cancer therapy. Single agents were tested in refractory tumors. When evidence of effectiveness of combination therapy accumulated, combination programs were used for that small subset of tumors which was initially deemed to be responsive. Radiation therapy gradually assumed a prominent role in the multidisciplinary management of cancer, and surgery likewise became an important component in the several studies incorporating adjuvant chemotherapy or radiation therapy. Accordingly, the increased growth and resources expended on the Cooperative Groups were marked by an increasingly complex organizational structure. All the major Groups have several similar characteristics of organizational structure as follows:

1. There is an elected chairman and in some instances an elected co-chairman or vice-chairman.

2. Most of the Groups have an appointed executive officer.

3. There is an elected executive committee to manage the administrative affairs.

4. The principal investigators or full members at each institution constitute the voting membership.

5. The statistician is appointed or elected.

The scientific organization of the Cooperative Groups varies with the mission of each Group, but a typical organization is composed as follows:

1. Modality committees representing the specialties of surgical oncology, radiation oncology, pathology, medical oncology and in some instances, pediatric oncology.

2. Disease committees representing the major classes of human neoplasms such as hematologic, breast, lung, GI, and others.

3. Subcommittees of the disease committees representing particularly important problems within an overall disease structure.

4. Other related areas of interest are just evolving, and these include committees that are dedicated to quality control, data processing, psychosocial issues, toxicity, and other similar areas.

5. The advent of the cancer control programs in several of the Cooperative Groups has led to a substructure generally headed by a cancer control committee. This committee supervises performance of studies at those institutions who are receiving funds for cancer control activities. The cancer control activities may be special such as in the Children's Group where selected protocols are used by institutions designated as cancer control affiliates, or conversely, the remainder of the groups, and principally the ECOG and SWOG have made available to most cancer control affiliates the major Group protocols. These patients are analyzed sepa-

rately as cancer control patients. In this way, it will be possible to demonstrate the impact of technology transfer. This is the transfer of research information into the community noting its comparability and applicability for a wider distribution.

COMMENT

The Cooperative Groups are now large, highly complex organizations. The chairmen and executive committees have many administrative duties in simply running such large machines. A Group may now consist of 30 to 50 institutions, as many as a thousand investigators, and up to 6,000 patients enrolled on study annually. The percentage of time that is committed to running such large structures has been ever increasing. The modalities themselves are defining their own areas of research interest and their place in the overall therapy programs of the Groups, making this generation of studies highly complicated.

A study idea is generally presented to a disease committee by an individual investigator. It is reviewed in its early draft form by the disease and modality committees. There are usually 2 to 3 cycles of review taking from 6 to 12 months. The impact of multidisciplinary participation upon the complexity of Aroup activities has been major. The impact of this complexity on the science of the Groups awaits further definition and the passage of time to determine if the opportunity for further breadth of research is realized, or if the opportunity is outbalanced by the inertia.

COMPETING PROGRAM AREAS

The Cooperative Groups are complex, highly organized research units which are entering approximately 20,000 patients per year on protocol studies. There are approximately 758 U.S. and numerous foreign institutions participating. This program utilizes approximately $30 million a year in government resources. It would be surprising indeed if this had not resulted in aggressive interaction with numerous government agencies, with the Congress, and with the professional and lay public. Some of these areas of interaction influence the Cooperative Group Program.

Prior to the National Cancer Program created in 1971, treatment research was performed in the Cooperative Group Program, the traditional R01 grants program, and selected areas where treatment research contracts were deemed advisable. After the enactment of the National Cancer Program, a number of additional areas were created or expanded which greatly increased the scope of overall clinical activities and, in some instances, led to considerable competition for scarce resources.

THE CANCER CENTERS PROGRAM

There had been categorical and specialized cancer centers existent for decades. The categorical centers are illustrated by Memorial Sloan-Kettering, the M. D. Anderson Hospital and Tumor Institute, and the Roswell Park Memorial Institute. Numerous specialized centers have been created over a number of years. The program, however, was greatly expanded with the National Cancer Plan. At the present time there are 20 comprehensive cancer centers. There are approximately 70 specialized cancer centers. Most of these centers are participants in Cooperative Group research. One of the missions of the cancer centers is to perform treatment research along with delivering the best available treatment to the cancer patients it serves. On occasion this dual responsibility leads to competition within the institution for scarce government resources. For the most part, this has worked out for the larger institutions, but it is clearly a problem in the smaller specialized centers to maintain an active in-house cancer treatment program and also a major Cooperative Group affiliation. In addition, both the centers and Cooperative Groups have competing outreach programs.

THE GROWTH OF ORGAN SITE PROGRAMS

It is of interest that the organ site programs (comprehensive programs to study a particular organ site of cancer) are split between two divisions of the NCI. The Breast Cancer Task Force resides in the Division of Cancer Biology and Diagnosis. The other programs (prostate, bladder, large bowel, pancreas) reside within the Division of Cancer Research Resources and Centers. When clinical trials are performed within these programs, it may require interactions with institutions that also have Cooperative Group affiliations as well as interactions with other divisions of the National Cancer Institute. Specifically, interaction occurs with the Division of Cancer Treatment which is the sponsor of most investigational cancer drugs in the United States. In large bowel, bladder and breast, there have been programs aimed at work similar to the Clinical Cooperative Groups. This was especially marked in surgical adjuvant breast cancer research where the Division of Cancer Treatment was sponsoring adjuvant trials in the Clinical Cooperative Groups and in contract trials with the National Surgical Adjuvant Breast Project as well as in other institutions. The NSABP was jointly funded in two divisions of NCI and by two mechanisms, grant and contract. Clearly, this represents a diffusion of program energy and activity. Only the final outcome of these studies will show whether this administrative adaptation to pursue the scientific goals has been productive.

THE CONTRACT PROGRAM OF THE NCI, SPECIFICALLY THE TREATMENT CONTRACT PROGRAMS

Prior to 1968, most of the Phase I and II trials of relatively new investigational drugs were carried out by the Cooperative Groups and cancer centers. Examples of this were the Eastern Solid Tumor Group and the Clinical Drug Evaluation Program which concentrated heavily on Phase I-II trials. These programs were funded for the most part through research grants. Following 1968, within the Chemotherapy Section of the NCI and the Cancer Therapy Evaluation Branch, there was a gradual emphasis on treatment contract programs, specifically to test new drugs in Phase I and Phase II. When the Cooperative Groups moved to the DCRRC in 1971 and the DCT was created, this contract program expanded greatly. As of 1978, the contract program had approximately $20 million of DCT resources. The contract program is not extensively covered in this review, but its overall scope includes: a) Phase I studies of new agents; b) Phase II, and III studies; and c) specific contract supported disease study groups, e.g., the GI Tumor Study Group, the Lung Cancer Study Group, the Head and Neck Cancer Study Group, the Ovarian Cancer Study Group, etc. Many of the studies performed by contract groups directly compete with the activities of grant supported Cooperative Groups and, at times, were successful. There are, of course, instances where the contract supported groups were able to evaluate drugs and disease-oriented therapies more swiftly than the Cooperative Groups. However, this large contract program, administratively managed by the same Division, results in direct competition for resources within the Division, thus creating its own impedance.

THE DEVELOPMENT OF CANCER CONTROL

The Cancer Control Program was reestablished by the National Cancer Act and funds were specifically targeted by Congress for these activities. The activities of the old Regional Medical Programs were incorporated into the present Cancer Control Program. The mandated mission of the Cancer Control Program is technology transfer, making the "best therapy" available to all cancer patients. To this end, the Cancer Control Program has set up community cancer centers and disease-oriented demonstration projects. The mission of Cancer Control is not research - it is demonstration. Thus, many patients entered on these demonstration protocols are diverted from research programs. Since the best cancer treatment is "investigational", this policy results in competition for scarce patient resources. In 1975 and 1976, "control" activities were expanded to include Cooperative Group participation. A number of contracts were advertised, specifically targeted toward the Cooperative Groups and designed to widen the scope of their activities and to bring the latest in technology and Group protocols to smaller communities. If successful, it seems inevitable that this activity means that fewer patients will be treated at large centers. Early stage cancer, in particular, is primarily handled by affiliate institutions. Although this is potentially very useful and may reduce medical costs, it may interfere with research concerned with the management of this critically important stage of cancer. Further, it must be recognized that with more investigators involved and with wider diffusion of responsibility for addressing and answering critical research questions, the nonresearch posture of cancer control will mean that answers will probably be more difficult to achieve, slower in coming, and less reliable. Furthermore, premature dissemination of preliminary results is inevitable; wide application of unproven treatment may eventually be detrimental (e.g., drug resistance or even second neoplasms which may occur after ineffective adjuvant therapy). Indeed, premature translation has already resulted in a major dispute in regard to mammography.

COMMENT

The Cooperative Groups were the principal resource for the successful study of cancer treatment in the 1950's and early 1960's. As a result of NCI initiative, they are now only a part of a greatly expanded National Cancer Program. At present, this stimulus has resulted in a highly competitive atmosphere involving centers, contract programs, the organ site programs, and cancer control. The merit of this approach needs constant reexamination. At this time, the facts are not in as to whether this ongoing experiment of administrative diversity by the NCI is efficient and productive or wasteful and self-defeating.

An additional result of the expansion of resources resulting from the National Cancer Program is the increasing dependence of academic institutions on federal support. Cancer "care" is thus increasingly subsidized by federal dollars. What will happen to these many programs in a recession? Will local resources be made available for these massive programs or will they simply atrophy?

THE RAPID GROWTH OF ONCOLOGY AS A SPECIALTY

The body of knowledge and practice within the various traditional disciplines have each gradually been recognized as an important sub-specialty.

Medical oncology was not considered a subspecialty of internal medicine prior to 1973. At that time, a subsection of the American Board of Internal Medicine was created, and the first examinations were held. Prior to this time, medical oncology was vaguely described as "clinical oncology", and a heterogenous group of individuals participated. Medical oncology is now one of the fastest growing subspecialties of internal medicine. There is currently a major push to revitalize surgical oncology which all but disappeared in the early 1970's. Surgical oncology had gradually declined as cardiac surgery increased; however, a number of surgeons with distinguished records retain their interest. No separate certifying board exists at this time. Radiation oncology is a recognized specialty, and in the 1960's, there was a great proliferation of training programs to enlarge the pool of professional radiotherapists so as to provide the key personnel for these necessarily highly complex facilities to perform high quality radiotherapy. There is general agreement that this program has been a success.

The impact of the increasing proliferation of specialists devoted to cancer treatment means that more and more cancer patients will be treated in the private practice environment rather than at centers and academic institutions with major Cooperative Group affiliations or other research emphasis. This has already resulted in a subtle change in the type of patient that comes to the large centers, i.e., patients with more advanced disease who have received considerable prior therapy, much of it of high quality. The early patient (where the true promise of the concept of combined modality therapy may be realized) is being increasingly treated in his own community and is not a "study" patient followed by investigators trying further to improve cancer therapeutics. This has exacerbated the competition for scarce research resources. It is not possible to state whether the overall care of the cancer patient nationwide for today's tomorrow has been improved by this proliferation of subspecialists. The figures for survival illustrate that acute lymphocytic leukemia and Hodgkin's disease are improved. However, it will be much more difficult to show this for common adult solid tumors which have been more refractory to systemic treatment. The proliferation of practicing specialists has resulted in expansion of the Groups to include these important resources. The pressure is on for further growth so as to include sufficient physicians to assure adequate patient resources.

ADMINISTRATIVE INTERACTIONS CONFRONTING THE COOPERATIVE GROUP

ADMINISTRATION BY THE NCI

The overall responsibility for the Cooperative Group Program is in the Division of Cancer Treatment. The program responsibility is in the

Cancer Therapy Evaluation Program, and the day-to-day administrative responsibility is in the Clinical Investigations Branch. It is of interest that the Clinical Investigations Branch and the Cancer Therapy Evaluation Program also supervise the treatment contract program of the DCT. The interactions with the Clinical Investigations Branch are primarily those of administration and protocol review. A member of the CIB or the CTEP generally attends all major Cooperative Group meetings to advise the Group membership of research opportunities and administrative changes and also to report on the progress of this Group to the associate director, CTEP.

The second area of intense administrative activity is in the review of protocols. Historically, protocol review was a charge of the Cancer Clinical Investigations Review Committee, a responsibility delegated to it in 1968. At that time, the staff of the Clinical Investigations Branch did preliminary protocol review and circulated the protocol to selected members of the CCIRC. Comments were received and transmitted to the Group chairman. The final disposition of the protocol was negotiated, and the protocol was then registered as approved by the Clinical Investigations Branch and was filed with the IND file for the agents under test. At this time, the Clinical Investigations Branch was in the DCRRC, and this necessitated interaction with the Cancer Therapy Evaluation Program of the DCT. There was thus a dual review. The DCT reviewed the protocol from the point of view of the drug sponsor, and thus the protocol review was a lengthy process which could take up to several months on controversial protocols. After 1975 and the DCT transfer, protocol review was delegated as a responsibility to the Clinical Investigations Branch. The review committee rarely interacted in protocol reviews on a day-to-day basis. The members were used as consultants in selected issues only. The review by the CIB was done by one or more members. The protocol could either be approved, modified, or returned as a result of this review. The Investigational Drug Branch interacted in a major way as the Investigational Drug sponsor. Protocol review has been an important function of the Clinical Investigations Branch. The smoothness of protocol review and the expertise of the CIB staff is vital for a continued flow of meritorious Group studies.

THE FOOD AND DRUG ADMINISTRATION

Prior to 1976, the interactions of the Food and Drug Administration with the Cooperative Group Program were minimal. The sponsor of the new drug holding an IND was usually the Investigational Drug Branch or its predecesor, the Cancer Therapy Evaluation Branch. The IND was duly filed, and the protocols were filed automatically within it. During that period, the FDA maintained a somewhat distant posture in terms of major interaction with the NCI, trusting it to fulfill the requirements of the IND sponsor without constant monitoring. In 1976, this changed. There was a reorganization at the FDA with the Bureau of Drugs. The Section of Oncology became much more active in its IND requirements, especially in the timeliness of submitting annual and periodic reports and the qualifications of investigators. The FDA demanded much more of a role in deciding who was going to study a new drug. This led to a period of upheaval, resulting in the following general resolutions:

a)   Independent investigators who had studied a number of investigational agents over the years were pretty much cut off from the drug supply.

b)   Investigational drugs were reclassified according to their position on the decision network flow and their evidence of efficacy and safety as follows:

> Group A - These are drugs in Phase I and early Phase II. The policy was to make them available to funded and unfunded DCT treatment contractors and to make them available for pilot studies for the Cooperative Groups.

> Group B - This was also called the "new drug studies mechanism". A select group of drugs which had received Phase I and early Phase II are thusly categorized and are available to Cooperative Groups, contractors and cancer centers upon submission and approval of a proper protocol. Some drugs in Group B were offered only to Groups and contractors and not to the centers. A document detailing this mechanism and listing the eligible centers was created. Annual reporting to the DCT is required.

> Group C - These are drugs for which definite activity and indications have been observed by extensive Phase I-III testing. Examples of this class includes daunorubicin, cis-platinum, and hexamethylmelamine. These drugs are in an advanced state of development so that a common protocol prepared by the Investigational Drug Branch staff could be used. The drug could be sent to any qualified medical oncologist who had registered via Form 1573 with the Investigational Drug Branch for treatment of appropriate patients, for the most part as a single agent.

The change has been from the somewhat free-wheeling days of many independent investigators to much intensified regulation. The impact of this on the Cooperative Groups meant the creation of a mechanism to obtain investigational drugs that were currently of interest.

Thus, the pilot study program of the Cooperative Groups evolved. Stated simply, these are pilot studies of new drugs or combinations which are not groupwide studies. They are limited to select institutions having the expertise and the patient resources to carry them out. This allowed the Groups a compromise when a new drug had passed Phase I and an MTD was established. The Cooperative Groups could obtain these drugs for limited use until more expanded Phase I - Phase II testing had been carried out. Only at that point could the drug be moved into the B category where it would be available for groupwide studies. This has been a subject of intense negotiations, and at times considerable conflict between Cooperative Groups, the Investigational Drug Branch, and the Clinical Investigations Branch. Cooperative Groups possess enormous resources, as is also true of the contractors. Cooperative Groups, however, provide a diversity for more adequate field testing trials than research confined to a single institution.

COMMENT

It was the FDA's fear that the information resultant from pilot trials might be inadequate to provide comprehensive documentation of safety and efficacy. The Cooperative Groups created a document in 1976, therefore, which details in a comprehensive fashion the entire organization of the Cooperative Groups, the procedures for obtaining, storing, administration, testing, and monitoring the effects of new drugs, and assurances that all relevant precautions are being taken to insure the safety of human subjects. This detailed document has in effect made the Cooperative Groups responsible to the sponsor for carrying out the intent of the FDA regulations. This process is still evolving. New FDA guidelines are in the wings which will further tighten up regulations regarding who can administer experimental drugs. These will also create additional monitoring requirements and probably on-site monitoring by the FDA. There are suggestions that the Cooperative Groups may have to take over this function themselves and monitor their institutions personally. The negative impact of these regulations on creating imaginative studies by multiple institutions is obvious. The groups may be regulated into a position where their major impact can be almost solely in the area of Phase III trials, fine tuning regimens not of their own creation, whose activity has been suggested in uncontrolled early studies in those institutions favored by DCT as Phase I contractors. Such contracts are limited by the number of new agents requiring testing. Thus, regulations may deter the establishment of a sensible system for going from a new idea to its implementation on trials requiring large numbers of cases. All creativity in clinical cancer research does not reside in the FDA, the NCI staff, or in the few institutions who first encounter a drug. The creativity of the Cooperative Groups must not be lost through regulatory proliferation.

THE ROLE OF THE PEER REVIEW IN COOPERATIVE GROUPS

The peer review committees have had an enormous impact in the shaping of the Cooperative Groups. As in any NIH research program, the government has long considered it a mark of wisdom to separate program administration and peer review. The many chartered committees that perform this function are made of nongovernment experts with the power to review grant applications on their merits and to approve, disapprove, and make budgetary recommendations to the National Cancer Advisory Board which constitutes the final review authority. It is, of course, axiomatic that the Cooperative Group Program has some substantial differences from the traditional grants program. The Cooperative Groups represent a large well-organized program having close administrative ties with the DCT. It is thus apparent that the review process must be responsive to the needs of the program.

The CCIRC (chartered in 1968) attempted to do this and to substitute for a then somewhat small program staff in the following ways. Their charge was to: (a) review grants; (b) conduct national and other conferences, symposia and state-of-the-art presentations to advise the scientific community and the Cooperative Groups of research opportunities; (c) identify gap areas in programs where opportunities existed but were not being investigated; and (d) advise the program staff regarding scientific matters over and above simple grant review. Thus, the history of the CCIRC was intimately entwined with the various divisions in which it resided.

At the time the Cooperative Groups were moved into the DCT, the management concept became a "troika" consisting of: (1) program staff, represented by the Director of the Division of Cancer Treatment, the Associate Director, Cancer Therapy Evaluation Branch, and the Branch Chief, Clinical Investigations Branch; (2) the CCIRC and its executive committee; and (3) the chairmen of the Cooperative Groups and the executive committee of the Group chairmen. The administrative management plan was to have regular meetings of the DCT staff with the executive committee of the Group chairmen followed by a separate meeting between DCT staff and the chief executive of the CCIRC. In this way, information was to be exchanged between program and the Group chairmen and passed back to the CCIRC, so that all three components would be aware of program necessities, of the concerns and issues "out in the field", and conversely the concerns of the review committee. Much valuable advice could be transmitted back to all these components.

Although program and review were separate as far as the actual merit review functions, this interaction of program and review was deemed less than wise by the new Director of the NCI who established a sweeping reorganization of the NCI in July of 1978. The NCI review committees were moved to the DCRRC and a number of the programs residing in the DCRRC such as the Centers Program were moved into other divisions for program administration. Thus, by the separation of review and program, the NCI reaffirmed its original charge. The CCIRC's function will be more sharply limited under the DCRRC. It will no longer conduct symposia and state of the art conferences for the scientific community as a standard function. Rather, it will concentrate strictly on the review process of the scientific merit of grant applications. Only time will tell whether this mechanism will preserve the interest of the overall Cooperative Group Program better than the previous more intense relationship between the parties.

THE IMPACT OF THE COMMISSION FOR PROTECTION OF HUMAN SUBJECTS, THE OFFICE OF PROTECTION FROM RESEARCH RISK, AND THE GENERAL PUBLIC ON COOPERATIVE PROGRAMS

The history of the treatment of human disease has been one of a constant search for improving methods. These methods must be tested on patients who then become human research subjects. There are many well known examples of previous failure to protect the rights of human subjects. Consequently, in the 1960's it became apparent to Congress that there had been numerous flagrant instances of failure to protect the hapless victims of disease. This was affirmed at a worldwide conference in Helsinki. Therefore, Congress instituted a commission to study the impact of research on human subjects, to define the areas where subjects needed the most protection and to make recommendations to DHEW so that appropriate regulations could be created. The upshot of this activity was the establishment of institutional review boards, committees for the protection of human subjects; and it became a requirement that all federally sponsored research must be reviewed at each institution. The institution furnished the Office of Protection from Research Risk with assurances that they were in compliance with the guidelines for the protection of human subjects. This led to the necessity for truly informed consent and the documentation required gradually became more extensive (and burdensome) as the guidelines were expanded and detailed. The protection of minors, pregnant women, fetuses, and prisoners became a matter of intense concern for the Commission and subsequently the institutional review boards.

The current status of this situation is as follows: Each institution participating in federally funded research must have an approved institutional review board and furnish the Office of Protection from Research Risk with a detailed outline of its composition, the names of the persons, and the representation throughout concerned professional and lay segments. Each institution upon doing this can apply for a general assurance which covers all its research programs or special assurances which cover a particular project only. The interest in protection of human subjects has gradually broadened to require ever more full disclosure of physical, emotional, and now financial risks of participating in a research project. Proposed new guidelines include the requirement to disclose the steps that must be taken in case of research related injury and a disclosure of whether compensation is available, the nature of the medical care available (and its reimbursement) or an offer to provide the patient with full information about these matters. If these guidelines are implemented, they will add to what is an already enormous burden for the Cooperative Groups as well as the research community in general.

Further, there are few data to support a conclusion that these processes have improved the protection of patients from risks or have accomplished anything except to drive up the indirect cost rates, reduce direct support for research, and delay the discovery of new knowledge. There is a widespread belief that the ethical are already working hard to comply with federal, institutional and ethical requirements, heavily burdened by additional record keeping, but that the unethical are proceeding unimpeded in their usual behavior.

Frequently, there are prereviews in institutions before a project goes to the institutional review board. Many of these prereview committees have been found necessary because the expertise in highly technical matters may not be extensive enough on an institutional review board. Such boards are supposed to represent a "jury" consisting of the "common denominator" of expertise in the institution. These committees act as consultants to the board, but lengthen the time it takes to activate a protocol. The requirements for ever-increasing disclosure, especially of financial risks, of course, will put all institutions into an awkward position without decreasing risks (from a low level) or increasing patient security (hospitals do not have compensation resources available). The disincentive to participate in research will multiply tremendously, far outstripping any change in the hazards of research. The full impact of this regulatory process is now being investigated under a DCT contract. This will be a very important investigation and hopefully will reassure the scientific community and the DCT that bureaucracy has not obstructed progress in the therapeutic research for cancer. Its chances for doing so seem slim. It remains to be seen whether the study can assess the relative risks to the population of delaying effective cancer therapies, and the impedance which excessive regulation contributes to this delay.

SUMMARY

This brief overview of the "regulatory history" of the Cooperative
Groups suggests a number of conclusions and recommendations:

1. The original impetus for the Cooperative Groups was truly
    investigator-initiated with the National Cancer Institute a
    partner with the scientific community.

2. The administrative responsibilities for the Cooperative
    Groups in the NCI have shifted several times. Subsequent
    shifts, if any, should be made with the full realization that
    these can be and usually are disruptive. The success of the
    Cooperative Group Program is contingent upon continuity of
    administration so that a maximum turnout of energy can be
    expended on research and a minimum on learning new admini-
    strative guidelines.

3. Day-to-day administration of the Cooperative Groups, par-
    ticularly in protocol review, offers the DCT a chance to
    "guide" research, (some believe "control" it). It is certainly
    valid to avoid wasteful duplication and to identify studies
    where a particular treatment is likely to be harmful, unethi-
    cal or unimportant.   The Clinical Investigations Branch
    performs a vital function in this regard. On the other hand,
    zealous application of bureaucratic privilege is not in the
    best interest of any program, especially one involving grants.

4. The proliferation of competing treatment programs in the
    NCI should be viewed with concern. There are currently
    Cooperative Groups, cancer centers, a large contract pro-
    gram, and large cancer control programs as well as organ site
    programs, all competing for the same scarce resources, often
    unnecessarily duplicating each others' efforts and admini-
    strative machinery.

5. The rapid growth of oncology as a specialty has been a major
    force in increasing the size and overall mission of the
    Cooperative Groups. It is desirable to integrate these highly
    trained practitioners into organized programs. Their rela-
    tionship with local cancer centers, with the cancer control
    program, and with the Cooperative Group program should not
    be one of "looking for the best offer". There should be a well
    coordinated plan based upon a coherent NCI philosophy so
    that the resources are used wisely.

6. The involvement of the FDA in the Cooperative Group Program has been quite variable. It is currently militant and promises to be more so. FDA regulations are clear enough. Their mission is to protect the public from drugs and devices, not from disease. Secondarily, it is to promote the flow of effective antitumor agents to the market place, so that they can have general applicability. The problem of a regulatory agency such as the FDA is that it cannot take things on faith, it cannot have a blind trust in the goodness of the investigators, and therefore has to walk the tight rope between excessive monitoring with its inhibition of creativity and adequate protection. It is hoped that there will be wisdom in the FDA so that its conflicting interests can be best served.

7. The rising expectations of the public for full disclosure, informed consent, and protection of human subjects is a major problem. This has been mandated by Congress, and a distinguished commission has been appointed to study this problem. It is, however, apparent that the orderly flow of research ideas may be impeded through excessive review and federal regulations which then protect human subjects to their overall detriment rather than benefit. It is surprising that few, if any, cancer patients are represented on these councils. They consist of persons who are all healthy, and perhaps unprepared to perceive the urgency of therapeutic investigations for cancer.

Cooperative Groups have provided the arena in which creative clinical investigations have influenced one another to better achievements in cancer therapy, which were implemented through the mechanisms of clinical trials, in the premier medical installations of the country. An assault on this clinical investigative resource by ramming amidship or by the excessive barnacles of regulatory bureaucracy will slow the pace and lengthen the voyage.

ATTACHMENT 1

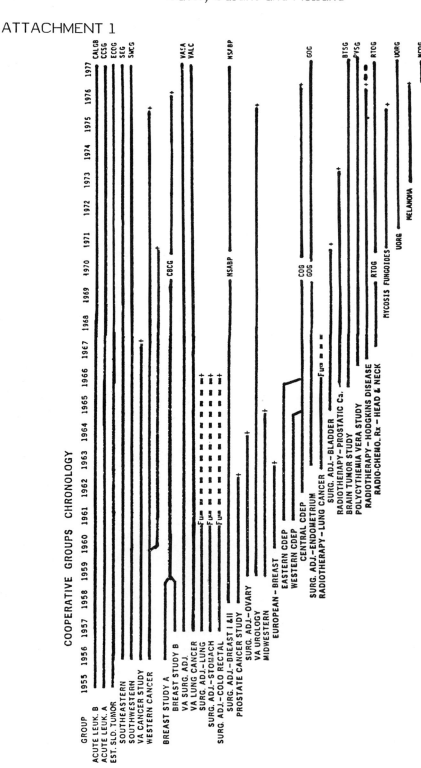

ATTACHMENT 2
Cooperative Group Funding 1970 - 1977*

(DOLLARS IN THOUSANDS)

GROUPS	70	71	72	73	74	75	76	77
CANCER AND LEUKEMIA GROUP B	1,129	1,112	(19)** 1,368	(20) 1,510	(21) 1,969	(20) 2,098	(21) 2,902	(24) 4,279
CENTRAL ONCOLOGY GROUP	594	910	(22) 822	(25) 1,229	(24) 1,524	(25) 1,640	(24) 1,493	(phase out) 255
CHILDREN'S CANCER STUDY GROUP	676	777	(16) 982	(18) 1,281	(18) 1,329	(19) 1,758	(18) 2.630	(20) 2,834
COOPERATIVE BREAST CANCER GROUP	538	424	(10) 477	(9) 443	(9) 525	(9) 781	(phase out) 264	
EASTERN COOPERATIVE ONCOLOGY GROUP	735	686	(11) 1,051	(19) 1,439	(20) 1,680	(24) 2,062	(21) 2,124	(30) 3,725
GYNECOLOGIC ONCOLOGY GROUP	-	334	(12) 421	(19) 891	(20) 1,057	(19) 1,041	(20) 1,947	(18) 1,926
MALIGNANT MELANOMA GROUP	-	-	-	(4) 173	(4) 182	(4) 481	(4) 497	(phase out) 120
NATIONAL SURGICAL ADJUVANT BREAST PROJECT		348	(14) 378	(14) 360	(13) 678	(14) 19	(14) 784	(21) 901
NATIONAL WILMS' TUMOR STUDY GROUP	48	48	(1) 59	(1) 24	(1) 165	(1) 364	(1) 162	(1) 172
NORTHERN CALIFORNIA ONCOLOGY GROUP	-	-	-	-	-	-	-	(1) 550
POLYCYTHEMIA VERA STUDY GROUP	123	92	(1) 91	(1) 85	(1) 219	(1) 333	(1) 445	(2) 491
RADIATION THERAPY ONCOLOGY GROUP	-	-	(16) 597	(17) 523	(11) 719	(12) 887	(19) 1,667	(21) 1,772
RADIO/CHEMOTHERAPY--HEAD AND NECK	145	158	101	(phase out) 45				
RADIOTHERAPY--HODGKIN'S DISEASE	88	114	(3)** 185	(1) 95	(2) 91	(2) 48	(2) 88	(1) 63
RADIOTHERAPY--PROSTATE	23	32	(1) 50	(phase out) 55	8	7	-	-
SOUTHEASTERN CANCER STUDY GROUP	410	422	(14) 678	(15) 771	(17) 905	(17) 1,700	(18) 1,965	(36) 3,333
SOUTHWEST ONCOLOGY GROUP	727	1,007	(22) 1,340	(21) 2,010	(27) 2,459	(31) 3,092	(32) 4,363	(36) 4,693
SURGICAL ADJUVANT RENAL CELL GROUP	123	129	120	135	131------- (phase out)			
URO-ONCOLOGY RESEARCH GROUP	-	-	-	-	(1) 110	(1) 322	(1) 396	(1) 433
VA COOPERATIVE UROLOGICAL RES. GROUP	118	186	281	290	312	334 (phase out)		
WESTERN CANCER STUDY GROUP	356	361	(6) 731	(19) 957	(18) 1,252	(19) 1,268	(phase out-----) 858	41
RELATED RESOURCES								
RADIOLOGIC PHYSICS CENTER	-	116	131	169	219	212	469	320
CANCER CLINICAL COORDINATING CENTER	-	-	195	202	279	458	851	737
LYMPHOMA PATHOLOGY CENTER	49	60	64	88	117	125	172	194
MYCOSIS FUNGOIDES GROUP	-	-	-	38	116	19	64 (phase out)	
(EUROPEAN ORGANIZATION FOR RESEARCH IN THERAPY OF CANCER DATA & COORDINATING CENTER)	12	22	30	25	131	132	216	264

*SCIENTIFIC EVALUATION INCLUDED IN FY 75, 76, 77; EXCLUDES DRUGS
**NUMBER OF GRANTS

REFERENCES

1. Cooperative Group Program Review, November, 1977, prepared by the CTEP.
2. Loeb V: Report of the Education Task Force Cooperative Group Studies, February, 1979.
3. Davis H, Durant JR, Holland JF: Overview of the Cooperative Groups and their interrelationships with the National Cancer Institute and other governmental agencies.
4. Carbone PP, Jacobs EM, Muggia FM: Description of procedures regulating clinical trials within the Cooperative Groups, June, 1976.

23

Impact of cooperative groups

Paul P. Carbone

The Cooperative Groups were initiated in 1955 as multiinstitution study groups to develop concepts and test chemical agents in the therapy of acute leukemias and solid tumors. As a relatively new area of investigation, the initial efforts involved the development of specific methodology, forms, definitions and procedures. Not only were clinicians and pharmacologists involved, but the initial efforts also included statisticians and biometricians. In addition to research, the early mission of Cooperative Groups encompassed the goal of cancer education to attract young people into this new field. The effort also involved the development of standards of optimal cancer care including the application of staging and supportive care. Thus, over the years the groups have had three major purposes: 1) Research, 2) Cancer Care, and 3) Education.

In the intervening 25 years, the Clinical Trials Group concept has become attractive to more individuals at many hospitals, universities and centers. The Groups quickly became involved in a major way in multimodal trials in the late 1960's. More recently, specific specialty groups, such as the Gynecologic Oncology Group and the Lymphoma Pathology Review Panel, are included in Group activities.

The growth of the Cooperative Groups has been evolutionary and modulated by peer review. Over the past 25 years, 36 separate groups have been formed; yet many of these have either gone out of existence and/or been remodeled, so that in 1979 only 14 groups remain active. The molding and reshaping of the Cooperative Groups has been the direct result of peer review. The Cancer Clinical Investigation Review Committee (CCIRC) has approved new Groups and members, as well as

disapproved or denied funding to both prospective and existing individual institutions and Groups.   Not only has the quality review
emphasis been on quantitative estimates of patient numbers entered on
study, but it has consistently involved completeness and promptness of
the data.   More recently the CCIRC has addressed itself to evaluating
the multimodality input into Group activities.   Thus, to participate in
Group funding one must demonstrate not only an ability to provide a
sufficient volume and high-quality data, but also significant contributions from other than medical oncologists.

Not only are the investigator-initiated trial programs of the Cooperative Groups modulated by outside review bodies on a regular basis, but
they also have stringent internal review mechanisms to assure high-
quality performance.   Most Groups have strict membership requirements which usually include a site visit. Each member is also reviewed
at regular intervals for quality and productivity.   Reviews include
patient accession, quality and promptness of records, completeness of
followup, as well as scientific contributions to Group protocol and
manuscript writing. Moreover, each member must have a significant
element of multimodality involvement in its membership as well as
patient accrual.   The Group may approve, warn, put an institution on
probation, or even terminate membership.   This activity is taken
seriously and has resulted in the expulsion of some members and the
voluntary withdrawal of others.   This aspect of review is truly a peer
review system that is unique to Cooperative Group activities.   In other
clinical trials mechanisms no clear-cut ongoing internal review occurs.
The grant or contract review mechanism may, in fact, be NCI staff and
mainly for quantity rather than quality.

IMPACT OF GROUPS

The impact of Cooperative Groups is usually measured in terms of
scientific output, namely through the clinical and/or biological importance of its trial activities.   This chapter will summarize other possible
impacts of the Cooperative Groups.   The data to support these other
accomplishments are, unfortunately, not very quantitative.   However,
based on information and the personal experience of the Group chairmen it is possible to illustrate some of these other impacts.

Of major importance is the fact that a large number of patients
directly participate in the clinical trials programs.   Not all of these
patients have far-advanced, incurable cancers; there are over 130
projects involving surgery and/or surgical adjuvant trials, 200 involving
radiotherapy, and 160 involving immunotherapy.   As we become
involved with more early disease studies and develop more effective

treatments, our active patient base becomes larger.   The Groups are currently following well over 100,000 patients.

There is a larger number being treated at Cooperative Group institutions who were considered for Group studies but were not entered. Likewise, there are equally large numbers of patients whose treatments may have been influenced by Cooperative Group protocols.   Many major institutions, engaged in Cooperative Group clinical trials research, are also doing early or pilot projects as well as secondary protocols that are done prior to Group protocols.   Thus, the total number of patients on whom Group activities impact may be two or three times the actual number of patients put on Group studies.

Another important area is that of the impact on training and utilization of health personnel. Estimates of the number of active participants by specialty are shown on Table 1.   Unfortunately, this estimate is imprecise since there is no uniform way to list members across Groups or to determine the actual involvement of individuals at every institution. In addition to the health professionals we know about, there are countless other students, residents, and fellows, who are exposed to clinical trial activities.   These individuals are involved in rounds, conferences, case discussions about patients and/or studies.   Finally, new specialists, oncology nurses, and data managers have come onto the scene with major responsibilities to collect data and treat patients on protocol studies.   These individuals know the protocols and interact with the patients and other physicians explaining the side effects and

TABLE 1
Health Personnel in Cooperative Groups in 1978

Gynecologists	325
Medical Oncologists	1550
Pathologists	475
Pediatric Oncologists	400
Radiation Oncologists	600
Statisticians	50
Surgeons	850

Residents, Fellows, Students,
Oncology Nurses, Data Managers

practical aspects of the treatments as well as collecting the necessary data.

What kind of impact do the Cooperative Groups have on all these participating health personnel? Firstly, the individuals are exposed to the concepts of clinical trials and the requirements in a first-hand way. In the past the laboratory was considered the prime disciplinary modality to develop rigid scientific approaches in medicine. Currently, clinical trials have become the oncologist's training ground to develop the necessary skills and discipline to do good clinical research. Bringing order to the chaos of the delivery of medical care is a major achievement and attraction of clinical trials. Further evidence for ascribing this aspect as a realistic achievement of clinical trials is the fact that many trainees of oncology programs are keen to continue the association with clinical trials when they relocate to other hospitals. This has led to natural associations for control programs that antedates the centers' program. These young individuals seek and continue their association with the Group. This aspect mushroomed into a large natural resource for cancer control activities in community hospitals.

Another impact of Groups can be estimated by counting the numbers of primary and affiliate member institutions (Table 2). Over 1,000 hospitals are listed as participants in Group efforts. Little is known about the characteristics of these hospitals except that 18 of the 21 comprehensive centers participate. Almost all of the medical schools are associated with one or more of the Cooperative Groups. Likewise, most Veterans Administration hospitals are affiliated with Group activities. An interesting and very informative statistic is that 41 different countries have one or more affiliations with Groups. These individuals are rarely funded to participate, but find it important and necessary to do so.

TABLE 2
Impact: Health Care System

Institutions	650
Affiliates	493
Comprehensive Centers	18
Medical Schools	110
V.A. Hospitals	Most
International	41 countries

In attempting to describe the impact of these institutions' participation in Group studies, there are other indirect attributes that can be sited. With the new Federal regulations requiring institutional review boards for clinical trials, in general, the Group trials proposed and reviewed at these institutional review boards are readily accepted and serve as models for other clinical trial groups at the university. Since many of the other trials are merely interviews or specimen obtaining studies, the cancer clinical trials probably represent most of the therapeutic trials.

Another indirect impact has been the fact that Cooperative Group standards in areas like response, toxicity, and performance status have become the international standards and a reference point for many other clinical trials (Table 3). The design of clinical trials in cancer evolved from efforts to understand the biology of cancer in the human and development of new research methodology. The basic concepts of remission, induction, and maintenance were first defined in the early leukemia protocols. Moreover, important principles of patient selection, multivariate analyses, stratification, and randomization parameters have come from Group trials. In fact, the concept of Phase I, II and III trials in cancer have evolved from the initial studies. The Groups have emphasized pathology review in clinical trials for many years dating back to the origins of the National Surgical Adjuvant Breast Program as well as the Veterans Administration Lung Group. While disappointment exists in the results of the treatment of lung, pancreas, and colorectal neoplasms, much has been learned in a

TABLE 3
Impact: Clinical Trials Methodology

Statistical Design

Protocol Definitions

Response

Toxicity

Stratification

Prognostic Factors

Pathology Review

Natural History

Data Collection

quantitative way about the impact of histology and natural history on survival and response.

Reseach efforts can be easily measured in terms of improved cure rates. This has occurred in certain diseases, particularly lymphomas, childhood cancers, testicular tumors, and more recently in breast cancer. However, little is mentioned about the impact of therapy that occurs when proposed "cures" of uncontrolled observations are subjected to repetition using controlled clinical trials (Table 4). This table illustrates the numerous studies that have disproven the uncontrolled benefits of specific therapies in myeloma, adjuvant therapy of colorectal and lung cancers, certain combinations in colon and lung cancers, as well as immunotherapy in a variety of tumors.

TABLE 4
Research: Cancer Care

Reliability of Uncontrolled Observations

Myeloma	Urethane
Adjuvant Therapy	Colon, Lung
Combinations	Lung, Colon
Immunotherapy	Colon, Melanoma, Breast

Role of Surgery - Radiotherapy

Breast Cancer, Lung, Colon, Wilm's
Head and Neck

Utility of Experimental Therapy

Myeloma, Acute Leukemia, Osteosarcoma

Value of Multimodal Therapy

Breast Cancer, Osteosarcoma, Wilm's

In addition, the Group studies have clarified the relative role of surgery and radiotherapy in several neoplastic diseases. Furthermore, the clinical studies have confirmed and shown the value of experimental therapies in acute leukemia, myeloma, and osteosarcomas, as well as

multimodal efforts in others.   These studies, done as part of Cooperative Group efforts, have eliminated ineffective treatments and
defined more effective nontoxic therapies.   Since these studies are
carried out using the best of statistical design with input from a wide
variety of specialists as well as at multiple institutions, the results are
not easily misinterpreted or biased by investigator selection or enthusiasm.   These results are hard to quantitate but do provide real benefits
to the understanding of cancer as well as the improvement in morbidity
and mortality.

Similar observations can be made relative to the studies of immunotherapy.   In the not too distant past, enthusiasm abounded and results
were highly encouraging (Table 5).   Yet in melanoma no Group study has

TABLE 5
Research - Immunotherapy

Disease	Agent	Group	Result
Melanoma	BCG	SWOG	-
	C. parvum	ECOG	-
		SEG	-
	MER	CALGB	-
Lymphoma - HD	BCG	ECOG	T.E.*
Lymphoma - NHD	BCG	SWOG	T.E.
Ovary	BCG	SWOG	+
AML	BCG	SEG	+
	BCG	SWOG	T.E.
	MER	CALGB	-
	Poly I:C	CALGB	-
	BCG	CCSG	-
	Levamisole	SWOG	-
Myeloma	Levamisole	SWOG	+

*T.E. = Too Early

confirmed the benefit of nonspecific immunostimulation. On the other hand, some preliminary positive results appear to be seen in adult acute leukemia and in ovarian cancer.

In the early 1970's the concept of adjuvant therapy appeared to be a promising way to overcome drug resistance inherent to the treatment

TABLE 6
Research: Surgery

Breast Cancer	NSABP
	SWOG
Childhood Cancer	CCSG
	SWOG
	CALGB
	WTSG
Gastrointestinal Cancer	
Gastric	COG
	ECOG
Colorectal	NSABP
	RTOG
	ECOG
	VASAG
	SWOG
Gynecologic Cancer	GOG
	ECOG
	RTOG
Head and Neck Cancer	RTOG
	ECOG
Lung	VASAG
	ECOG
	SWOG
Urologic Cancer	VAUG
Sarcomas	ECOG
	CALGB
	SWOG
Melanoma	COG
	ECOG
	SWOG

of breast cancer. There were contracts initiated with the feeling that the Cooperative Groups were not able to do these studies. Table 6 shows that, in fact, surgery or surgery plus other modality trials have been in the Groups for years dating back to the 1960's for lung and breast cancer, and the early 1970's for most other tumors. Likewise, radiotherapy trials either alone or in combination have been done since the 1960's in several diseases.

Table 7 shows some of the Group pathology efforts that will undoubtedly provide important answers to cancer biology.

TABLE 7
Clinical Trials: Pathology

Breast	NSABP
	SWOG
Lung	VASAG
	VALG
	SWOG
Lymphoma	SWOG
	ECOG
	SEG
Leukemia	ECOG
	SWOG
	CALGB
	CCSG
Brain Tumors	ECOG
	RTOG
Wilm's	WTSG
Sarcoma	SWOG
Genitourinary	SWOG
Ovary	SWOG

A comment needs to be made at this point relative to the administrative control of Group efforts. Like the evolution of the modern Groups, the administrative responsibility of the National Cancer Institute for the Groups has vacillated under six administrative units dating back to the Cancer Chemotherapy National Service Center. In addition, at least two major reviews of Groups have been held in the past. Currently, the Groups are undergoing another shift with the CCIRC, the major review group located in the Division of Grants and Resources, while the administrative aspects are in the Division of Cancer Treatment and the Clinical Investigation Branch. What changes the next few years will bring cannot be devined. However, the Cooperative Group mechanism has been responsive to changes in the direction of science as well as the administration of NCI. As described, there is an academic tradition among the Group members that creates a "university without walls". Cooperation among university hospitals occurs because each unit retains its identity. Throughout the years, the Group members have developed a way of interacting with each other that is non-threatening.

It has been said that money enforces this type of behavior. In fact, the cooperation exists even when grant monies are not available to all participants. One needs to be cognizant and supportive of this kind of association. The relationships have been built up over many years, and the individual members feel that they lose very little of their autonomy but have the advantages of the larger cooperative effort. To merely shift the monies to create new managers and force new alliances will undoubtedly be disruptive, expensive and artificial. Rarely will the resultant relationships be any better than now - more likely they will not be as good. To set up consortium memberships from geographic areas likewise submerges the individual member behind an organization that could result in difficulties in evaluation and review for the NCI.

It will be necessary to foster a more varied mechanism to do clinical research and not reshuffle the current ones because of administrative pressures. Obviously, more monies need to be found, but at present large amounts of monies are being spent in administrative mechanisms, state of the art demonstrations, NCI-directed studies, as well as Congress-delineated mandates. The result may be to foster easy, quick answers to the various pressure rather than to carefully define priorities and possibilities. The investigator-initiated clinical research effort, like the investigator-initiated basic laboratory program, will provide the most answers at the lowest cost. Investigator-initiated clinical research, whether in the centers or the Cooperative Groups, have provided most of the answers to date. The future is likely to be a repeat of the past. The Cooperative Group mechanism has proven to be flexible and responsive.

24

Cooperative Group
Bibliographies

CANCER AND LEUKEMIA GROUP B

1956 - 1978

1. Holland JF, Frei E, Burchenal JH: Criteria for the evaluation of response to therapy of acute leukemia. VIth International Congress of Hematology, pp.213-214, 1956.

2. Frei E, Holland JF, Schneiderman MA, Pinkel D, Selkirk G, Gold L, Regelson W, Freireich E, Silver R: A comparative study of two regimens of combination chemotherapy in acute leukemia. Blood 13:1126-1148, 1958.

3. Freireich EJ, Frei E, Holland JF, Pinkel D, Selawry O, Rothberg H, Haurani F, Raylor R, Gehan E: Evaluation of a new chemotherapeutic agent in patients with "advanced refractory" acute leukemia. Studies in 6-azauracil. Blood 16:1268-1278, 1960.

4. Hoogstraten B, Schroeder LR, Freireich EJ, Frei E, Holland JF, Pinkel D, Vogel P, Mills SD, Burger EO, Hayes DM, Spurr CL, Kurkcuoglu M, Storrs R, Ebaugh F, Wolman IJ, Haurani F, Gendel B, Gehan E: Cyclophosphamide (cytoxan) in acute leukemia. Preliminary Report. Cancer Chemother Rep 8:116-119, 1960.

5. Selawry OS, Holland JF, Wasserman LR, Hoogstraten B, Stickney JM, Cooper T, James GW, Moon JH, Tocatins L, Haurani F, Ebaugh F, Matthews L, Gendel B, Okel B, Frei E, Freireich EJ, Schroeder ML, Lee SL, Ritz ND, Gehan E: Effect of 2-amino-6-(1-methyl-4-nitro-5 imidazolyl) thio) purine (imidazolylthioguanine; B.W. 57-323) on acute leukemia in man. Cancer Chemother Rep 8:56-60, 1960.

6. Shnider BI, Frei E, Tuohy JH, Gorman J, Freireich EJ, Brindley CO, Clements J: Clinical studies of 6-azauracil. Cancer Res 20:28-33, 1960.

7. Frei E, Franzino A, Shnider B, Costa G, Colsky J, Brindley C, Hosley H, Holland JF, Gold GL, Jonsson U: Clinical studies of vinblastine. Cancer Chemother Rep 12:125-129, 1961.

8. Frei E, Freireich EJ, Gehan E, Pinkel D, Holland JF, Selawry O, Haurani F, Spurr CL, Hayes DM, James GW, Rothberg H, Sodee DB, Rundles RW, Schroeder LR, Hoogstraten B, Wolman IJ, Traggis DG, Cooper T, Gendel BR, Ebaugh F, Taylor R: Studies of sequential and combination antimetabolite therapy of acute leukemia: 6-mercaptopurine and methotrexate. Blood 18:431-454, 1961.

9. Hayes DM, Spurr CL, Schroeder LR, Freireich EJ: A clinical trial of sarcolysin in acute leukemia. Cancer Chemother Rep 12:153-155, 1961.

10. Holland JF, Gehan E, Brindley CO, Dederick MM, Owens AH, Shnider BI, Taylor R, Frei E, Selawry OS, Regelson W, Hall TC: A comparative study of optimal medical care with and without azaserine in multiple myeloma. Clin Pharm & Therap 2:22-28, 1961.

11. Hoogstraten B: Remission maintenance in acute leukemia: A new specific experimental design (Studies by the Acute Leukemia Group B). J Chron Dis, Pergamon Press Ltd. Printed in Great Britain 15:269-272, 1962.

12. Lee SL, Livings D, James WG, Schroeder L, Selawry O, Stickney JM: Morphologic classification of acute leukemias. Cancer Chemother Rep 16:151-153, 1962.

13.   Freireich EJ, Gehan E, Frei E, Schroeder LR, Wolman IF, Anbari R, Burgert EO, Mills SD, Pinkel D, Selawry OS, Moon JH, Gendel BR, Spurr CL, Storrs R, Haurani F, Hoogstraten B, Lee SL: The effect of 6-mercaptopurine on the duration of steroid induced remission in acute leukemia: A model for evaluation of other potentially useful therapy. Blood 21:699-716, 1963.

14.   Holland JF, Regelson W, Selawry OS, Costa G: Methylglyoxal-bis-guanylhydrazone - An active agent against Hodgkin's disease and acute myeloblastic leukemia. Acta Unio Internat Contra Cancrum 20:352-353, 1964.

15.   Frei E, Karon M, Levin RH, Freireich EJ, Taylor RJ, Hananian J, Selawry OS, Holland JF, Hoogstraten B, Wolman IJ, Abir E, Sawitsky A, Lees S, Mills SD, Burgert WO, Spurr CL, Patterson RB, Ebaugh FB, James BW, Moon JH: The effectiveness of combinations of anti-leukemic agents in inducing and maintaining remission in children with acute leukemia. Blood 26:642-656, 1965.

16.   Frei E, Spurr CL, Brindley CO, Selawry O, Holland JF, Rall DP, Wasserman LR, Hoogstraten B, Shnider BI, McIntyre OR, Matthews LB, Miller SP: Clinical studies of dichloromethotrexate. Clin Parmacol and Therapeut 6:160-171, 1965.

17.   Frei E, Carbone PP, Shnider BI, Gold GL, Colsky J, Franzino A, Krant MJ, Brena GP, Owens AH, Holland JF, Costa G, Hall TC, Hosley H, Horton J, Tarr N, Salvin LG: Neoplastic disease, treatment with vinblastine. Arch Intern Med 116:846-852, 1965.

18.   Selawry OS, Hananian J, Wolman IJ, Abir E, Chevalier L, Gourdeau R, Denton R, Gussoff BD, Levy R, Burgert O, Mills SD, Blom J, Jones B, Patterson RB, McIntyre OR, Haurani FI, Moon JH, Hoogstraten B, Kung FH, Sheehe PR, Frei E, Holland JF: New treatment schedule with improved survival in childhood leukemia - intermittent parenteral vs. daily oral administration of methotrexate for maintenance of induced remission. JAMA 194:75-81, 1965.

19.   Gailani SD, Armstrong JG, Carbone PP, Tan C, Holland JF: Clinical trial of vinleurosine sulfate. A new drug derived from vinca rosea linn. Cancer Chemother Rep 50:95-103, 1966.

20.   Holland JF, Hosley H, Scharlau C. Carbone PP, Frei E, Brindley CO, Hall TC, Shnider BI, Gold GL, Lasagna L, Owens AH, Miller SP: A controlled trial of urethane treatment in multiple myeloma. Blood 27:328-342, 1966.

21.   Karon M, Freireich EJ, Frei E, Taylor R, Wolman IJ, Djerassi I, Lee SL, Sawitsky A, Hananian J, Selawry O, James D, George P, Patterson RB, Burgert O, Haurani FI, Oberfield RA, Macy CT, Hoogstraten B, Blom J: The role of vincristine in the treatment of childhood acute leukemia. Clin Pharm & Therap 7:332-339, 1966.

22.   Seibert DJ, Hayes DM, Cooper T, Blom J, Ebaugh FG: Intravenous urethane (ethyl carbamate) therapy of multiple myeloma. Cancer 19:710-712, 1966.

23.   Storrs RC, Wolman IJ,.Gussoff B, Hananian J: Remission maintenance in acute lymphocytic leukemia with hydroxyurea. Cancer Res 26:241-244, 1966.

24.   Burgert EO, Glidewell O: Dactinomycin in Wilms' tumor. JAMA 199:464-468, 1967.

25.   Hayes DM, Costa J, Moon JH, Hoogstraten B, Harley JB: Combination therapy with thioguanine and azaserine for multiple myeloma. Cancer Chemother Rep 51:235-238, 1967.

26.   Hoogstraten B, Sheehe PR, Cuttner J, Cooper I, Kyle RA, Oberfield RA, Townsend SR, Harley JB, Hayes DM, Costa G, Holland JF: Melphalan in multiple myeloma. Blood 30:74-83, 1967.

27.   Jones B, Kung F, Nyhan WL, Hananian J, Blom J, Burgert EO, Mills SD, Treat C, Wolman IJ, Chevalier L, Denton R, Sheehe P, Glidewell O, Holland JF: Chemotherapy of the leukemic transformation of lymphosarcoma. J Pediatr 70:442-448, 1967.

28.   Kyle RA, Carbone PP, Lynch JJ, Owens AH, Costa G, Silver RT, Cuttner J, Harley JB, Leone LA, Shnider BI, Holland JF: Evaluation of tryptophan mustard in patients with plasmacytic myeloma. Cancer Res 27:510-515, 1967.

29.   Regelson W, Holland JF, Gold GL, Lynch J, Olson KB, Horton J, Hall TC, Krant M, Colsky J, Miller SP, Owens A: 6-Mercaptopurine intravenously at weekly intervals to patients with advanced cancer. Cancer Chemother Rep 51:277-282, 1967.

30.   Regelson W, Holland JF, Talley RW: Clinical pharmacologic study of kethoxal bis (thiosemicarbazone) in advanced cancer. Cancer Chemother Rep 5:171-177, 1967.

31.   Salmon SE, Samal BA, Hayes DM, Hosley H, Miller SP, Schilling A: Role of gamma globulin for immunoprophylaxis in multiple myeloma. N Eng J Med 277:1336-1340, 1967.

32.   Carbone P, Spurr C, Schneiderman N, Scotto J, Holland J, Schnider B, Hayes D, Serbert D, Haurani F, Levy R, Moon J, Hoogstraten B, Cuttner J, Silver R, Herovitz H, Leone L, Albala M, Gailani S, MacDonald R, Townsend S, Hood A, Bloom J: Management of patients with malignant lymphoma: A comparative study with cyclophosphamide and vinca alkaloids. Cancer Res 28:811-822, 1968.

33.   Ellison RR, Holland JR, Weil M, Jacquillat C, Boiron M, Bernard J, Sawitsky A, Rosner F, Gussoff B, Silver RT, Karanas F, Cuttner J, Spurr CL, Hayes DM, Blom J, Leone LA, Haurani F, Kyle R, Hutchison JL, Forcier RJ, Moon JH: Arabinosyl cytosine: A useful agent in the treatment of acute leukemia in adults. Blood 32:507-523, 1968.

34.   Selawry OS, Holland JF, Wolman IJ: Effect of vincristine on malignant solid tumors in children. Cancer Chemother Rep 52:497-500, 1968.

35.   Selawry OS, Holland JF, Glidewell O: Relationship of methotrexate dose schedule to stage of disease in children with acute lymphocytic leukemia. Cancer Chemother Separatum 8:127-139, 1968. (Verlag der Wiener Med. Akademie).

36.   Burgert EO, Glidewell O, Mills SD, Nyhan WL, Kung F, Lee SL, Sawitsky A, Patterson RB, Wolman IJ, Moon JH, Jones B, Corner J, Chevalier L, Selawry O, Holland JF: Acute lymphocytic leukemia in children. Maintenance therapy with methotrexate administered intermittently. JAMA 207:923-928, 1969.

37.   Cuttner J, Glidewell OJ: Combination of melphalan and prednisone in poor risk patient with multiple myeloma. Presented at the Amer. Soc. of Clinical Oncology, San Francisco, California, 1969.

38.   Hernandez K, Pinkel D, Lee S, Leone L: Chemotherapy with 6-azauridine for patients with leukemia. Cancer Chemother Rep 53:203-207, 1969.

39.   Hoogstraten B, Costa J, Cuttner J, Forcier JR, Leone LA, Harley JF, Glidewell OJ: Intermittent melphalan therapy in multiple myeloma. JAMA 209:251-253, 1969.

40.   Hoogstraten B, Owens A, Lenhard R, Glidewell O, Leone L, Olson K, Harley J, Townsend S, Miller S, Spurr C: Combination chemotherapy in lymphosarcoma and reticulum cell sarcoma. Blood 33:370-378, 1969.

41.   Ogawa M, Kochwa S, Smith C, Ishizaka K, McIntyre OR: Clinical aspects of IgE myeloma. N Eng J of Med 281:1217-1220, 1969.

42.   Sawitsky A, Desposito F, Treat C, Wolman IJ, Kung FH, Nyhan WL, Sinks LL, Jones B, Edmonson JH, Burgert EO, Rausen AR, Patterson R, Storrs RC, Glidewell O: Vincristine and cyclophosphamide therapy in generalized neuroblastoma. Am J Dis Child 119:308-313, 1970.

43.   Glidewell O, Holland JF: Clinical trials of the ALGB in acute lymphocytic leukemia of childhood. Presented at the Vth International Symposium on Comparative Leukemia Research, Padova, Italy, 1971.

44.   Jones B, Holland JF, Morrison AR, Lee SL, Sinks LF, Cuttner J, Rausen AR, King F, Pluss HJ, Haurani FI, Patterson RJ, Blom J, Burgert EO, Moon JH, Chevalier L, Sawitsky A, Albala MM, Forcier RJ, Falkson G, Glidewell O: Daunorubicin in the treatment of advanced childhood lymphoblastic leukemia. Cancer Res 31:84-90, 1971.

45.   Ohnuma T, Rosner F, Levy R, Cuttner J, Moon J, Silver R, Blom J, Falkson G, Burningham R, Glidewell O, Holland J: Treatment of acute leukemia with L-asparaginase Cancer Chemother Rep 55:269-273, 1971.

46.   Rosner F, Glidewell O, Ellison RR, Lee SL, Cuttner J, Gailani S, Morrison AN, Hoogstraten B, Weil M, Leone L, Levy RN, Cooper I, Brunner KW, Serpick A, Burmingham RA, Holland JF: Failure of hydroxyurea and prednisone in the treatment of acute myelocytic leukemia. Cancer Chemother Rep 55:199-204, 1971.

47.   Ellison RR, Hoogstraten B, Holland JF, Levy RN, Lee SL, Silver RT, Leone LA, Cooper T, Oberfield RA, ten Pas A, Blom J, Jacquillat C, Haurani F: Intermittent therapy with 6-mercaptopurine and methotrexate given intravenously to adults with acute leukemia. Cancer Chemother Rep 56:535-542, 1972.

48.   Gailani S, Holland JF, Falkson G, Leone L, Burningham R, Larsen V: Comparison of treatment of metastatic gastrointestinal cancer with 5-FU to a combination of 5-FU with cytosine arabinoside. Cancer 29:1308-1313, 1972.

49.   Harley JB, Schilling A, Glidewell O: Ineffectiveness of fluoride therapy in multiple myeloma. N Eng J Med 286:1283-1288, 1972.

50. Holland JF, Glidewell O: Chemotherapy of acute lymphocytic leukemia of childhood.   Cancer
     30:1480-1487, 1972.

51. Jones B, Cuttner Y, Levy RN, Patterson RB, Kung F, Pleuss HJ, Falkson G, Treat CL, Haurani F,
     Burgert EO, Rosner F, Carey RW, Lukens J, Blom J, Degnan TJ, Wohl H, Glidewell O, Holland JF:
     Daunorubicin versus daunorubicin plus prednisone versus daunorubicin plus vincristine plus prednisone
     in advanced childhood acute lymphocytic leukemia. Cancer Chemother Rep 56: 729-737, 1972.

52. Spurr C, Hayes DM, McIntyre R, Seibert DJ, Haurani FI, Carey R, Kyle RA, Shapiro L, Townsend SR,
     ten Pas A, Moon JH, Cuttner J, Hoogstraten B, Silver RT, Leone LA, Costa J, Ellison RR, Glidewell O,
     Holland JF, Lee SL, Blom J, Harley JB, Krall JM, Ramanan SV, Shnider B, Krant M, Greenberg M,
     Carbone P, Serpick A, Schilling A, Shadduck R, Feldstein A: Ineffectiveness of fluoride therapy in
     multiple myeloma. N Eng J Med 286:1283-1288, 1972.

53. Band PR, Holland JF, Bernard J, Weil M, Walker M, Rall D: Treatment of central nervous system
     leukemia with intrathecal cytosine arabinoside. Cancer 32:744-748, 1973.

54. Costa G, Engle RL, Schilling A, Carbone P, Kochwa S, Nachman RL, Glidewell O: Melphalan and
     prednisone: An effective combination for the treatment of multiple myeloma. Am J of Med 54:589-
     599, 1973.

55. Ellison RR, Wallace HJ, Hoagland HC, Woolford DC, Glidewell OJ: Prognostic parameters in acute
     myelocytic leukemia as seen in Acute Leukemia Group B. Advances in the Biosciences 14:51-69, 1973.
     Workshop on Prognostic Factors in Human Acute Leukemia, Reisenburg, Germany.

56. Glidewell O, Holland JF: Clinical trials of the ALGB in acute lymphocytic leukemia of childhood. In
     Unifying Concepts of Leukemia, Bibl. Haemt. No 39. RM Dutcher and L Chicho-Branche eds. Basel:
     Karger, pp.1053-1067, 1973.

57. Holland JF, Scharlau C, Gailani S, Krant MJ, Olson KB, Horton J, Shnider BI, Lynch JJ, Owens A,
     Carbone PP, Colsky J, Grob D, Miller SP, Hall TC: Vincristine treatment of advanced cancer: A
     cooperative study of 392 cases. Cancer Res 33:1258-1264, 1973.

58. Hoogstraten B, Holland JF, Kramer S, Glidewell OJ: Combination chemotherapy-radiotherapy for
     Stage III Hodgkin's disease. Arch Int Med 131:425-428, 1973.

59. Kyle AR, Costa G, Cooper MR, Ogawa M, Silver RT, Glidewell O, Holland JF: Evaluation of aniline
     mustard in patients with multiple myeloma. Cancer Res 33:956-960, 1973.

60. Lee SL, Glidewell O: Cytology and survival in acute lymphatic leukemia of children. In Recent
     Results in Cancer Research, Vol. 43. G Mathe, P Pouillart, L Schwarzenberg, Eds. Berlin: Springer-
     Verlag, pp.29-34, 1973.

61. Nissen NI, Stutzman L, Holland JF, Glidewell OJ: Chemotherapy of Hodgkin's disease in studies by
     Acute Leukemia Group B. Arch Int Med 131:396-401, 1973.

62. Stutzman L, Glidewell O: Multiple chemotherapeutic agents for Hodgkin's disease: Comparison of
     three routines: A cooperative study by Acute Leukemia Group B. JAMA 225:1201-1211, 1973.

63. Wallace HJ, Holland JF, Glidewell OF, Ellison RR, Weil M, Carey RW, Schwartz JM, Hoagland HC,
     Henderson ES, Wiernik P, Yates JW: Therapy of acute myelocytic leukemia - Acute Leukemia Group B
     Studies. Proc. of First International Meeting of the Therapy of Acute Leukemia, Rome, Italy, 1973.

64. Weil M, Glidewell OJ, Jacquillat C, Levy R, Serpick AA, Wiernik PH, Cuttner J, Hoogstraten B,
     Wasserman L, Ellison RR, Gailani S, Brunner K, Blom J, Boison M, Bernard J, Holland JF: Daunoru-
     bicin in the therapy of acute granulocytic leukemia. Cancer Res 33:921-928, 1973.

65. Cortes EP, Holland JF, Wang JJ, Sinks LF, Blom J, Senn H, Bank A, Glidewell O: Amputation and
     adriamycin in primary osteosarcoma. N Eng J Med 291:998-1000, 1974.

66. Hayes DM, Ellison RR, Glidewell O, Holland JF, Silver RT: Chemotherapy for the terminal phase of
     chronic myelocytic leukemia. Cancer Chemother Rep 58:233-247, 1974.

67. Jones B, Kung F, Chevalier L, Forman EN, Rausen AR, Koch K, Desposito F, Maurer H, Jacquillat C,
     Degnan TJ, Pluess H, Desforges J, Patterson RB, Glidewell O, Holland JF: Chemotherapy of
     reticuloendotheliosis, comparison of methotrexate plus prednisone versus vincristine plus prednisone.
     Cancer 34:1011-1017, 1974.

68. Kyle RA, Seligman BR, Wallace HJ, Silver RT, Glidewell O, Holland JF: Multiple myeloma resistant
     to melphalan treated with cyclophosphamide, prednisone and chloroquine. Cancer   Chemother Rep
     59:557-562, 1975.

69. McIntyre RO, Kochwa S, Weksler B, Glidewell O, Woolford D, Costa G, Leone L, Cuttner J, Holland J: Correlation of abnormal immunoglobulin with clinical features in myeloma. Arch Int Med 135:46-52, 1975.

70. Moon JH, Gailani S, Cooper MR, Hayes DM, Rege VB, Blom J, Falkson G, Maurice P, Brunner K, Glidewell O, Holland JF: Comparison of the combination of 1:3 bis (2-chlorethyl) 1-nitrosourea (BCNU) and vincristine with two dose schedules of 5-(3,3-dimethyl-1-triazino) imidazole 4-carboxamide (DTIC) in the treatment of disseminated malignant melanoma. Cancer 35:368-371, 1975.

71. Glidewell OJ, Holland JF: Comparative prognosis of the acute leukemias. In Comparative Leukemia Research, J Clemmesen and DS Yohn, eds. New York: S. Karger, 1976.

72. Holland JF, Glidewell O, Ellison RR, Carey RW, Schwartz J, Wallace HJ, Hoagland HC, Wiernick P, Rai K, Bekesi G, Cuttner J: Acute myelocytic leukemia. Arch Intern Med 136:1377-1381, 1976.

73. Lee SL, Kopel S, Glidewell O: Cytomorphological determinations of prognosis in acute lymphoblastic leukemia of children. Sem in Oncol 3:209-217, 1976.

74. Sawitsky A, Rai KR, Aral I, Silver RT, Glicksman AS, Carey RW, Scialla S, Cornell CJ, Seligman B, Shapiro L: Mediastinal irradiaton of chronic lymphocytic leukemia. Am J of Med 61:892-896, 1976.

75. Jones B, Holland JF, Glidewell O, Jacquillat C, Weil M, Pochedly C, Sinks L, Chevallier L, Maurer HM, Koch K, Falkson G, Patterson R, Seligman B, Sartorius J, Kung F, Haurani F, Stuart M, Burgert EO, Ruymann F, Sawitsky A, Forman E, Pluess H, Truman J, Hakami N: Optimal use of L-asparaginase in acute lymphocytic leukemia. Med & Ped Onc 3:387-400, 1977.

76. Maurer HM, Moon T, Donaldson M, Fernandez C, Gehan EA, Hammond D, Hays DM, Lawrence W, Newton W, Ragab A, Raney B, Soule EH, Sutow WW, Tefft M: The intergroup rhabdomyosarcoma study: A preliminary report. Cancer 40:2015-2026, 1977.

77. Maurer H, Moon T, Donaldson M, Fernandez C, Gehan E, Hammond D, Hays D, Lawrence W, Newton W, Ragab A, Raney B, Soule E, Sutow W, Tefft M: Preliminary results of the intergroup rhabdomyosarcoma study (IRS). In Management of Primary Bone and Soft Tissue Tumors, M.D. Anderson Hospital and Tumor Institute, Year Book Medical Publishers, Inc., pp.317-332, 1977.

78. McIntyre OR, Rai K, Glidewell O, Holland JF: Polyriboinosinic: Polyribocytidylic acid as an adjunct to remission maintenance therapy in acute myelogenous leukemia. In Immunotherapy of Cancer: Present Status of Trials in Man, WD Terry and D Windhorst, eds. New York: Raven Press, pp.423-440, 1977.

79. Nissen NI, Pajak T, Glidewell O, Blom H, Flaherty M, Hayes D, McIntyre R, Holland J: Overview of four clinical studies of chemotherapy for Stage III and IV non-Hodgkin's lymphomas by the Cancer and Leukemia Group B. Cancer Treat Rep 61:1097-1107, 1977.

80. Perez C, Razek A, Tefft M, Nesbit M, Burgert O, Kissane J, Vietti T, Gehan E: Analysis of local tumor control in Ewing's sarcoma: Preliminary results of a cooperative intergroup study. Cancer 40:2864-2873, 1977.

81. Sawitsky A, Rai KR, Glidewell O, Silver T: Comparison of daily versus intermittent chlorambucil and prednisone therapy in the treatment of patients with chronic lymphocytic leukemia. Blood 50:1049-1059, 1977.

82. Kung FH, Nyhan WL, Cuttner J, Falkson G, Lanzkowsky P, DelDuca V, Nawabi U, Koch K, Pleuss H, Freeman A, Burgert EO, Leone LA, Ruymann F, Patterson RB, Degman T, Hakami N, Pajak TF, Holland JF: Vincristine, prednisone, and L-asparaginase in the induction of remission in children with acute lymphocytic leukemia following relapse. Cancer 41:460-467, 1978.

83. Maurice P, Glidewell O, Jacquillat C, Silver R, Carey R, TenPas A, Cornell C, Burningham R, Nissen N, Holland JF: Comparison of methyl-CCNU and CCNU in patients with advanced forms of lymphoma. Cancer 41:1658-1663, 1978.

84. Silver R, Sawitsky A, Rai K, Holland JF, Glidewell O: Guidelines for protocol studies in chronic lymphocytic leukemia. Am J Hematol 4:343-358, 1978.

85. Forcier RJ, McIntyre OR, Nissen NI, Pajak TF, Glidewell OJ, Holland JF: Combination chemotherapy of non-Hodgkin's lymphoma. Accepted for publication in Medical and Pediatric Oncology.

86. Hoogstraten B, Glidewell OJ, Holland JF, Blom J, Stutzman L, Nissen NI: Long term follow-up of combination chemotherapy-radiotherapy of Stage III Hodgkin's disease. Accepted for publication in Cancer.

87. Nissen N, Pajak TF, Glidewell OJ, Pedersen-Bjergaard J, Stutzman L, Falkson G, Cuttner J, Blom J, Leone L, Sawitsky A, Coleman M, Haurani F, Spur C, Jones B, Seligman B, Cornell C, Henry P, Seen H, Brunner K, Martz G, Maurice P, Holland JF: A Comparative study of BCNU containing 4-drug program versus MOPP versus 3-drug combinations in advanced Hodgkin's disease. Accepted for publication in Cancer.

88. Wiernik P, et al: Comparative study of daunorubicin, ara-C and thioguanine, and DNR, ara-C and thioguanine in acute myelocytic leukemia. Accepted for publication in Medical and Pediatric Oncology.

89. Wiernik P, Jones B, Weinberg V, Holland JF: Present day results in young patients with acute nonlymphocytic leukemia. Accepted for publication in Proc Second International Symposium on Therapy of Acute Leukemia, Rome, 1978.

90. Stutzman L, Pajak T: A 10-year followup of combination chemotherapy of Hodgkin's disease by Cancer and Acute Leukemia Group B. Accepted for publication in the Proceedings of   International Cancer Conference.

CENTRAL ONCOLOGY GROUP

1971-1977

1.   Ansfield FJ, Ramirez G, Korbitz BC, Davis HL: Five-drug therapy for advanced breast cancer, Phase I study. Cancer Chemother Rep 55:183-187, 1971.

2.   Shingleton WW, Sedransk N, Johnson RO: Systemic chemotherapy of mammary carcinoma. Annals of Surg 173:913-919, 1971. Oncology 26:287-296, 1972.

3.   Johnson RO, Wolberg WH: Cellular kinetics and their implications for chemotherapy of solid tumors, especially cancer of the colon. Cancer 28:208-212, 1971.

4.   Larsen RR, Hill II GJ: Improved systemic chemotherapy for malignant melanoma. Am J of Surg 122:36-41, 1971.

5.   duPriest RW, Massey WH, Fletcher WS: The search for new cancer drugs: Streptozotocin. Am Surg 38:514-520, 1972.

6.   Hill GJ, Grage TB, Wilson WL, Ansfield FJ: 5-Fluorouracil intravenous infusion for 48 hours, repeated every two weeks. J Surg Oncol 4:60-70, 1972.

7.   Troetel WM, Weiss AJ, Stambaugh JE, Laucius JF, Manthei RW: Absorption, distribution, and excretion of 5-azacytidine in man. Cancer Chemother Rep 56:405-411, 1972.

8.   Weiss AJ, Stambaugh JE, Mastrangelo MJ, Laucius JF, Bellet RE: A Phase I study of 5-azacytidine. Cancer Chemother Rep 56:413-419, 1972.

9.   Belej MA, Troetel WM, Weiss AJ, Stambaugh JE, Manthei RW: The absorption and metabolism of dibromodulcitol in patients with advanced cancer. Clin Pharm Ther 13:563-572, 1972.

10.   Lowe DK, Fletcher WS, Horowitz IJ, Hyman MD: Management of chylothorax secondary to lymphoma. Surg, Gyn and Obstet 135: 35-38, 1972.

11.   Huntington MC, duPriest RW, Fletcher WS: Intra-arterial bleomycin therapy in inoperable squamous cell carcinomas. Cancer 31:153-158, 1973.

12.   Mastrangelo MJ, Grage TB, Bellet RE, Weiss AJ: A Phase I study of emetine hydrochloride in solid tumors. Cancer 31:1170-1175, 1973.

13.   Lindell TD, Moseley HS, Fletcher WS: Combination CCNU and bleomycin therapy for squamous cell carcinoma. Am Surg 40:281-289, 1974.

14.   Burg JR, Moseley HS, Lindell TD, Kremkau EL, Fletcher WS: Evaluation of cardiac function during adriamycin therapy. J Surg Oncol 6:519-529, 1974.

15.   Hill GJ, Ruess R, Berris R, Philpott GW, Parkin P: Chemotherapy of malignant melanoma with dimethyl triazeno imidazole carboxamide (DTIC) and nitrosourea derivatives (BCNU, CCNU). Ann of Surg 180:167-174, 1974.

16.   Davis HL, Ramirez G, Ellerby RA, Ansfield FJ: Five-drug therapy in advanced breast cancer. Cancer 34:239-245, 1974.

17.   Brady LW, Antoniades J, Prasasvinichai S, Torpie RJ, Asbell SO, Glassburn JR: Preoperative radiation therapy. Cancer 34:960-964, 1974.

18.   duPriest RW, Huntington MC, Massey WH, Weiss AJ, Wilson WL, Fletcher WS: Streptozotocin therapy in 22 cancer patients. Cancer 35:358-367, 1975.

19.   Altman SJ, Fletcher WS, Andrews NC, Wilson WL, Pischer T: Yoshi 864, a Phase I study. Cancer 35:1145-1147, 1975.

20.   Dowell KE, Armstrong DM, Aust JB, Cruz AB: Systemic chemotherapy of advanced head and neck malignancies. Cancer 35: 1116-1120, 1975.

21.   Sparks FC, Mosher MB, Hallauer WC, Silverstein MJ, Rangel D, Passaro E, Morton DL: Hepatic artery ligation and postoperative chemotherapy for hepatic metastases: Clinical and pathophysiological results. Cancer 35:1074-1082, 1975.

22.   Cortese AJ, Cornell GN: Radical mastectomy in the aged female. J Am Geriatrics Soc 23:337-342, 1975.

23.   Yaeger RA, Eidemiller LR, Fletcher WS: Multimodality therapy in the treatment of regionally inoperable melanomas and sarcomas. Surg, Gyn, and Obstet 141:367-370, 1975.

24.   Hill GJ, Sicard GA, Metter GE, Mantz CA, Nelson PJ: Quimioterapie e immunoterapia del melanoma maligno. Dermatologia 19:167-172, 1975.

25.   Sasaki T, McConnell DB, Moseley HS, Merhoff GC, Fletcher WS: A clinical trial of CCNU in advanced ovarian carcinoma. J Surg Oncol 7:347-350, 1975.

26.   Wilson WL, Van Ryzin J, Weiss AJ, Frelick RW, Moss SE: A Phase III study in lung carcinoma comparing hexamethylmelamine to dibromodulcitol Oncology 31:293-309, 1975.

27.   Hill GJ: Cancer chemotherapy: Practical comments on current techniques. Chapter 3 of textbook Practice of Surgery, Vol 2, Walter Ballinger and Theodore Drapanas, eds. CV Mosby Co, pp. 43-89, 1975.

28.   Ramirez G, Klotz JH, Strawitz JG, Wilson WL, Cornell GN, Madden RE, Minton JP: Combination chemotherapy in breast cancer, a randomized study of 4 vs 5 drugs. Oncology 32:101-108, 1975.

29.   Grage TB: Adjuvant therapy in the management of breast cancer. Chapter in book Cancer Management, JS Najarian and JP Delaney eds, 1975.

30.   Johnson RO, Metter GE, Wilson WL, Hill GJ, Krementz ET: A Phase I evaluation of DTIC and other studes in malignant melanoma in the Central Oncology Group. Cancer Treat Rep 60:183-187, 1976.

31.   Wilson WL, Andrews NC, Frelick RW, Nealon TF, Bick RL, Adams T: Preliminary report on the use of CCNU, adriamycin and hexamethylmelamine in carcinoma of the lung. Cancer Treat Rep 60:269-271, 1976.

32.   Takeuchi O, DiVecchia L, Bronn DG, Pace WG, Minton JP: The role of estrogen receptors in predicting subsequent therapy for recurrent breast cancer. Ohio Med J 72, March 1976.

33.   Sasaki GH, Leung BS, Fletcher WS: Therapeutic value of nafoxidine hydrochloride in the treatment of advanced carcinoma of the human breast. Surg, Gyn and Obstet 142:560-564, 1976.

34.   Sasaki GH, Leung BS, Fletcher WS: Levodopa test and estrogen receptor assay in prognosticating responses of patients with advanced cancer of the breast to endocrine therapy. Ann of Surg 183:392-396, 1976.

35.   Hill GJ, Johnson RO, Metter GE, Wilson WL, Davis HL, Grage TB, Fletcher WS, Golomb FM, Cruz AB: Multimodal surgical adjuvant therapy for a broad spectrum of tumors in humans. Surg, Gyn and Obstet 142:882-892, 1976.

36.   Carter RD, Krementz ET, Hill GJ, Metter GE, Fletcher WS, Golomb FM, Grage TB, Minton JP, Sparks FC: DTIC and combination therapy for melanoma: I. Studies with DTIC, BCNU, CCNU, vincristine and hydroxyurea (COG Protocol 7130). Cancer Treat Rep 60:601-609, 1976.

37.   Klotz JH: Truncated geometric response - Duration of response models for clinical trials. J Am Stat Assoc 71:331-334, 1976.

38.   Weiss AJ, Metter GE, Fletcher WS, Wilson WL, Grage TB, Ramirez G: Studies on adriamycin using a weekly regimen demonstrating its clinical effectiveness and lack of cardiac toxicity. Cancer Treat Rep 60:813-822, 1976.

39.   Kraybill WG, Anderson DD, Lindell TD, Fletcher WS: Islet cell carcinoma of the pancreas: Effective therapy with 5-fluorouracil, streptozotocin, and tuberciden. Am Surg 42:467-470, 1976.

40.   Minton JP, Matthews RH, Wisenbaugh TW: Elevated adenosine 3', 5'-Cyclic monophosphate levels in human and animal tumors in vivo. J Natl Cancer Inst 57:39-41, 1976.

41.   Grage TB: Preoperative radiation in the treatment of rectal cancer. Chapter in book Controversy in Surgery., Philadelphia: WB Saunders Co, 1976.

42.   Cruz AB, Metter GE, Armstrong DM, Aust JB, Fletcher WS, Wilson WL, Richardson JD: Treatment of advanced malignancy with CCNU, a Phase II cooperative study with long-term followup. Cancer 38:1069-1076, 1976.

43. Moseley HS, Sasaki T, McConnell DB, Merhoff GC, Wilson WL, Grage TB, Weiss AJ, Fletcher WS: A randomized pilot study comparing two regimens in the treatment of squamous cell carcinoma. J Surg Onc 8:35-42, 1976.

44. Young VL, Kashmiri R, Hazen ZR, Meeker WR: Usefulness of serial carcinoembryonic antigen (CEA) determinations in monitoring chemotherapy. Southern Med J 69:1274-1276, 1976.

45. Minton JP: Precise selection of breast cancer patients with bone metastasis for endocrine ablation. Surgery 80:513-517, 1976.

46. Ansfield FJ, Klotz JH, Nealon TF, Ramirez G, Minton JP, Hill GJ, Wilson WL, Davis HL, Cornell GN: A Phase III study comparing the clinical utility of four regimens of 5-fluorouracil - A preliminary report. Cancer 39:34-40, 1977.

47. Grage TB, Metter GE, Cornell GN, Strawitz JG, Hill GJ, Frelick RW, Moss SE: Adjuvant chemotherapy with 5-fluorouracil after surgical resection of colorectal carcinoma (COG Protocol 7041). A preliminary report. Am J Surg 133:59-66, 1977.

48. Weiss AJ, Metter GE, Nealon TF, Keenan JP, Ramirez G, Swaminathan A, Fletcher WS, Moss SE, Manthei RW: A Phase II study of 5-azacytidine in solid tumors. Cancer Treat Rep, Vol 61, No 1, 1977.

49. Klotz J, Teng J: One-way layout for counts and the exact enumeration of the Kruskal-Wallis H distribution with ties. J Am Stat Assoc 72:165-169, 1977.

50. Weiss AJ, Cantor RI: Evaluation of daunorubicin in adenocarcinoma of the large intestine. Cancer Treat Rep 60:1667-1670, 1976.

51. Bick RL, Kovacs I, Fekete LF: A new two-stage functional assay for antithrombin-III (heparin cofactor): Clinical and laboratory evaluation. Thrombosis Research 8:745-756, 1976.

52. Grage TB, Metter GE, Cornell GN, Strawitz J, Hill GJ, Frelick RW, Moss SE: The role of 5-fluorouracil as an adjuvant to the surgical treatment of large bowel cancer. Chapter in book Adjuvant Therapy of Cancer, SE Salmon and SE Jones, eds. Amsterdam: Elsevier/North-Holland Biomedical Press, pp.259-263, 1977.

53. Weiss AJ, Manthei RW: Experience with the use of adriamycin in combination with other anticancer agents using a weekly schedule, with particular reference to lack of cardiac toxicity. Cancer 40:2046-2052, 1977.

CHILDREN'S CANCER STUDY GROUP

1955-Present

1. Burchenal J: Therapy of acute leukemia in children. Proc VII Cong Intl Soc Hematol, pp. 322-331, 1958.

2. Burchenal J, Heyn R, Sutow W, Freireich E, Whittington R, Louis J: Investigations in acute leukemia. Conferences on Experimental Clinical Cancer Chemotherapy. National Cancer Institute Monography 3:149-168, 1960.

3. Carter R, Brubaker C, Leikin S, Louis J, Severo N, Wolff J, Murphy M: The frequency of the various morphologic types of childhood leukemia and their response to certain chemotherapeutic agents. Cancer Chemother Rep 16:165-168, 1960.

4. Hartmann J, Erlandson M, Murphy M, Origenes M, Sitarz A: The clinical evaluation of 5-fluoro-2'-deoxyuridine in acute leukemia in children. Cancer Chemother Rep 8:84-96, 1960.

5. Heyn R, Brubaker C, Burchenal J, Cramblett H, Wolff J: The comparison of 6-mercaptopurine with the combination of 6-mercaptopurine and azaserine in the treatment of acute leukemia in children: Results of a cooperative study. Blood 15:350-359, 1960.

6. Krivit W, Bentley H: Use of 5-fluorouracil in the management of advanced malignancies in childhood. Am J Dis Child 100:217-227, 1960.

7. Pierce M, Hall J, Ozon N: The effect of 6-mercaptopurine riboside in 20 cases of childhood leukemia previously treated with purine antimetabolites. Cancer Chemother Rep 14:121-128, 1961.

8. Leikin S: Leukemia: Current concepts in therapy. Pediatr Clinics of N Am 9:753-767, 1962.

9. Sullivan M, Beatty E, Hyman C, Murphy M, Pierce M, Severo N: A comparison of the effectiveness of standard dose 6-mercaptopurine, combination 6-mercaptopurine and DON, and high-loading 6-mercaptopurine therapies in the treatment of acute leukemia in children: Results of a cooperative study. Cancer Chemother Rep 16:161-165, 1962.

10. Sullivan M, Beatty E, Hyman C, Murphy M, Pierce M, Severo N: A comparison of the effectiveness of standard dose 6-mercaptopurine, combination 6-mercaptopurine and DON, and high-loading 6-mercaptopurine therapies in treatment of the acute leukemias of childhood: Results of a cooperative study. Cancer Chemother Rep 18:83-95, 1962.

11. Wolff J, Pratt C, Sitarz A: Chemotherapy of metastatic retinoblastoma. Cancer Chemother Rep 16:435-437, 1962.

12. Heyn R, Newton W, Carter R: Elderfield pyrimidine mustard in acute leukemia in children - a Phase I study. Cancer Chemother Rep 33:51-55, 1963.

13. Hartmann J, Origenes M, Murphy M, Sitarz A, Erlandson M: Effects of 2'-deoxy-5-fluorouridine and 5-fluorouracil on childhood leukemia. Cancer Chemother Rep 34:51-53, 1964.

14. Origenes M, Beatty E, Brubaker C, Hammond D, Hartmann J, Shore N, Williams K: Trial of hydroxyurea in cancer in children. Cancer Chemother Rep 37:41-46, 1964.

15. Origenes M, Beatty E, Brubaker C, Hammond D, Hartmann J, Shore N, Williams K: Oxylone in acute leukemia in children. Cancer Chemother Rep 37:35-40, 1964.

16. Hyman C, Bogle J, Brubaker C, Williams K, Hammond D: Central nervous system involvement by leukemia in children. I. Relationship to systemic leukemia and description of clinical and laboratory manifestations. Blood 25:1-12, 1965.

17. Hyman C, Bogle J, Brubaker C, Williams K, Hammond D: Central nervous system involvement by leukemia in children. II. Therapy with intrathecal methotrexate. Blood 25:13-22, 1965.

18. Sitarz A, Heyn R, Murphy M, Origenes M, Severo N: Triple drug therapy with actinomycin D, chlorambucil, and methotrexate in metastatic solid tumors in children. Cancer Chemother Rep 45:45-51, 1965.

19. Sitarz A, Heyn R, Murphy M, Origenes M, Severo N: Triple drug therapy with actinomycin D, chlorambucil, and methotrexate in metastatic solid tumors in children. In Year Book of Cancer, pp.295-298, 1965.

20. Hartmann J, Beatty E, Hammond D, Murphy M, Origenes M, Severo N: Clinical study of fluorometholone in acute leukemia in children. Cancer Chemother Rep 50:339-345, 1966.

21. Hartmann J: The case for a children's cancer center. CA, A Cancer J for Clinicians 72-74, 1966.

22. Heyn R, Beatty E, Hammond D, Louis J, Pierce M, Murphy M, Severo N: Vincristine in the treatment of acute leukemia in children. Pediatrics 38:82-91, 1966.

23. Jenkin R: Ewing's sarcoma - A study of treatment methods. Clin Radiol 17:97-106, 1966.

24. Krivit W, Brubaker C, Hartmann J, Murphy M, Pierce M, Thatcher G: Induction of remission in acute leukemia of childhood by combination of prednisone and either 6-mercaptopurine or methotrexate. J Pediatr 68:965-968, 1966.

25. Pierce M, Shore N, Sitarz A, Murphy M, Louis J, Severo N: Cyclophosphamide therapy in acute leukemia of childhood. Cancer 19:1551-1560, 1966.

26. Hartmann J: The physician and the children's cancer center. Supplement, Pediatr 40:523-531, 1967.

27. Jenkin R, Peters M, Darte J: Hodgkin's disease in children. Am J of Roentgenology Rad Therapy and Nuc Med 1:222-226, 1967.

28. Sharp H, Nesbit M, White J, Krivit W: Renal and hepatic pathology following initial remission of acute leukmia induced by prednisone. Cancer 20:1395-1402, 1967.

29. Sharp H, Nesbit M, D'Angio G, Krivit W: Addition of local radiation after bone marrow remission in acute leukemia in children. Cancer 20:1403-1404, 1967.

30. Shore N, Hartmann J: Preliminary evaluation of daunomycin in children with acute leukemia. Path Biol 15:939, 1967.

31. Wolff J, Brubaker C, Murphy M, Pierce M, Severo N: Prednisone therapy of acute childhood leukemia: Prognosis and duration of response in 330 treated patients. J Pediatr 70:626-631, 1967.

32. Brubaker C, Gilchrist G, Hammond D, Hyman C, Shore N, Williams K: Induction of remission in acute leukemia with prednisone and intravenous methotrexate. J Pediatr 73:623-625, 1968.

33. Evans A: Vincristine in the treatment of children with acute leukemia. Cancer Chemother Rep 52:469-471, 1968.

34. Evans A: If a child must die... N Eng J Med 278:138-142, 1968.

35. Howard J, Albo V, Newton W: Cytosine arabinoside: Results of a cooperative study in acute childhood leukemia. Cancer 21:341-345, 1968.

36. Krivit W, Brubaker C, Thatcher G, Pierce M, Perrin E, Hartmann J: Maintenance therapy in acute leukemia of childhood, comparison of cyclic vs. sequential methods. Cancer 21:352-356, 1968.

37. Leikin S, Brubaker C, Hartmann J, Murphy M, Wolff J, Perrin E.: Varying prednisone dosage in remission induction of previously untreated childhood leukemia. Cancer 21:346-351, 1968.

38. Newton W, Sayers M, Samuels L: Intrathecal methotrexate therapy for brain tumors in children. Cancer Chemother Rep 52:257-261, 1968.

39. Pierce M, Brubaker C, Wolff J: Thiopurines in the treatment of acute childhood leukemia. Cancer Chemother Rep 52:321-328, 1968.

40. Sitarz A, Brubaker C, Hartmann J, Leikin S, Murphy M, Wolff J, Perrin E: Induction of remission in childhood leukemia with vincristine and 6-mercaptopurine and methotrexate, administration in sequence after prednisone. Cancer 21:920-925, 1968.

41. Wolff J, Krivit W, Newton W, D'Angio G: Single versus multiple dose dactinomycin therapy of Wilm's tumor. N Eng J Med 279: 290-294, 1968.

42. Breslow N: On large sample sequential analysis with applications to survivorship data. J Appl Prob 6:261-274, 1969.

43. Evans A, Heyn R, Newton W, Leikin S: Vincristine sulfate and cyclophosphamide for children with metastatic neuroblastoma. JAMA 207:1325-1327, 1969.

44.   Evans A, Heyn R, Nesbit M, Hartmann J: Evaluation of mitomycin C in the treatment of metastatic osteogenic sarcoma. Cancer Chemother Rep 53:297-298, 1969.

45.   Finklestein J, Hittle R, Hammond D: Evaluation of a high dose cyclophosphamide regimen in childhood tumors. Cancer 23:1239-1242, 1969.

46.   Freedman M, Finklestein J, Gilchrist G, Hammond D, Higgins G, Hyman C, Shore N, Williams K, Karon M: Preliminary evaluation of cyclophosphamide and cytosine arabinoside in acute leukemia of children. Cancer Chemother Rep 53:299-303, 1969.

47.   Grosfeld J, Clatworthy W, Newton W: Combined therapy in childhood rhabdomyosarcoma: An analysis of 42 cases. J of Pediatr Surg 4:637-645, 1969.

48.   Hammond D: Use of cytosine arabinoside in childhood acute leukemia. In Conference on Ara-C (cytosine arabinoside hydrochloride-NSC-63878): Development and application Natl Cancer Inst, Bethesda, 1969.

49.   Jenkin R: Medulloblastoma in childhood: Radiation therapy. Canadian Med Assoc J 100:51-53, 1969.

50.   Leikin S, Brubaker C, Hartmann J, Murphy M, Wolff J: The use of combination therapy in leukemia remission. Cancer 24:427-432, 1969.

51.   Pierce M, Borges W, Heyn R, Wolff J, Gilbert E: Epidemiological factors and survival experience in 1770 children with acute leukemia - Treated by members of Childrens Cancer Study Group A between 1957 and 1964. Cancer 23:1296-1304, 1969.

52.   Sayers M, Newton W, Samuels L: Intrathecal methotrexate therapy of brain tumors of childhood. Ann NY Acad Sci 159:608-613, 1969.

53.   Breslow N, Zandstra R: A note on the relationship between bone marrow lymphocytosis and remission duration in acute leukemia. Blood 36:246-249, 1970.

54.   Breslow N: A generalized Kruskal-Wallis test for comparing K samples subject to unequal patterns of censorship. Biometricka 57:579-594, 1970.

55.   Breslow N: Sequential modification of the UMP test for binomial probabilities. J Am Stat Assoc 63:639-648, 1970.

56.   Evans A, Gilbert E, Zandstra R: The increasing incidence of central nervous system leukemia in children. Cancer 26:404-409, 1970.

57.   Jenkin R, Rider W, Sonley M: Ewing's sarcoma - A trial of adjuvant total-body irradiation. Radiology 96:151-155, 1970.

58.   Krivit W, Gilchrist G, Beatty E: The need for chemotherapy after prolonged complete remission in acute leukemia of childhood. J Pediatr 76:138-141, 1970.

59.   Breslow N, McCann B: Statistical estimation of prognosis for children with neuroblastoma. Cancer Res 31:2098-2103, 1971.

60.   Evans A, D'Angio G, Randolph J: A proposed staging for children with neuroblastoma. Cancer 27:374-378, 1971.

61.   Freedman M, Finklestein J, Hammond D, Karon M: The effect of chemotherapy on acute myelogenous leukemia in children. J Pediatr 78:526-532, 1971.

62.   Koop C, Johnson D: Neuroblastoma: An assessment of therapy in reference to staging. J Pediatr Surg 6:595-599, 1971.

63.   Lahey E: Histiocytosis X. In Practice of Medicine. New York: Harper and Row, 1971.

64.   Samuels L, Newton W, Heyn R: Daunorubicin therapy in advanced neuroblastoma. Cancer 27:831-834, 1971.

65.   Evans A: Treatment of neuroblastoma. Cancer 30:1595-1599, 1972.

66.   Finklestein J, Albo V, Ertel I, Karon M, Hammond D: 5-(3,3-dimethyl-l-triazeno) imidazole-4-carboxamide in the treatment of advanced acute lymphocytic leukemia in children. Cancer Chemother Rep 56:523-526, 1972.

67. Ortega J, Finklestein J, Ertel I, Hammond D, Karon M: Effective combination treatment of advanced acute lymphocytic leukemia with cytosine arabinoside and L-asparaginase. Cancer Chemother Rep 56:363-368, 1972.

68. Karon M, Sieger L, Leimbrock S, Finklestein J, Nesbit M, Swaney J: 5-azacytidine: A new active agent for the treatment of acute leukemia. Blood 42:359-365, 1973.

69. Leikin S, Evans A, Heyn R, Newton W: The impact of chemotherapy on advanced neuroblastoma. Survival of patients diagnosed in 1956, 1962, and 1966-68 in Children's Cancer Study Group A. J Pediatr 84:131-134, 1973.

70. Breslow N: Covariance analysis of censored survival data. Biometrics 30:89-99, 1974.

71. Evans A, Baehner R, Chard R, Leikin S, Pang E, Pierce M: Comparison of daunorubicin with adriamycin in the treatment of late-stage childhood solid tumors. Cancer Chemother Rep 58: 671-676, 1974.

72. Heyn R, Holland R, Newton W, Tefft M, Breslow N, Hartmann J: The role of combined chemotherapy in the treatment of rhabdomyosarcoma in children. Cancer 34:2128-2142, 1974.

73. Heyn R, Nesbit M, Joo P, Karon M, Borges W, Hammond D, Breslow N: Effect of BCG in the duration of the first remission in children with acute lymphoid leukemia. In Neoplasm Immunity: BCG Vaccination. Evanston: Schori Press, 1974.

74. Miller D, Sonley M, Karon M, Breslow N, Hammond D: Additive therapy in the maintenance of remission in acute lymphoblastic leukemia of childhood: The effect of the initial leukocyte count. Cancer 34:508-517, 1974.

75. Wolff J, D'Angio G, Hartmann J, Krivit W, Newton W: Long-term evaluation of single versus multiple courses of actinomycin D therapy of Wilm's tumor. N Eng J Med 290:84-86, 1974.

76. Albo V, Movassaghi N, Sitarz A, Hammond D, Weiner J, Reed A: Cyclophosphamide maintenance therapy after a second remission of childhood acute lymphoblastic leukemia: Comparative clinical trial (standard dose versus intermittent high dose versus cyclophosphamide plus cytosine arabinoside. Cancer Chemother Rep 59:1097-1102, 1975.

77. Finklestein J, Albo V, Ertel I, Hammond D: 5-(3,3-dimethyl-1-triazeno)imidazole-4-carboxamide in the treatment of solid tumors in children. Cancer Chemother Rep 59:351-357, 1975.

78. Heyn R, Joo P, Karon M, Nesbit M, Shore N, Breslow N, Weiner J, Reed A, Hammond D: BCG in the treatment of acute lymphocytic leukemia. Blood 46:431-442, 1975.

79. Heyn R: The role of chemotherapy in the management of soft tissue sarcomas. Cancer 35:921-924, 1975.

80. Lahey E: Histiocytosis X - Comparison of three treatment regimens. J Pediatr 87:179-183, 1975.

81. Lahey E: Histiocytosis X - An analysis of prognostic factors. J Pediatr 87:184-189, 1975.

82. Leikin S, Bernstein I, Evans A, Finklestein J, Hittle R, Klemperer M: Use of combination adriamycin and DTIC in children with advanced stage IV neuroblastoma. Cancer Chemother Rep 59: 1015-1018, 1975.

83. Sitarz A, Albo V, Movassaghi N, Karon M, Hammond D, Weiner J, Reed A: Dibromodulcitol compared with cyclophosphamide as remission maintenance therapy in previously treated children with acute lymphoblastic leukemia or acute undifferentiated leukemia: Possible effectiveness of reducing the incidence of central nervous system leukemia. Cancer Chemother Rep 59:989-994, 1975.

84. Bernstein I, Wright P: Immunology and immunotherapy of childhood neoplasia. Pediatr Clin of N Am 23:93-109, 1976.

85. Chilcote R, Baehner R, Hammond D: Septicemia and meningitis in children splenectomized for Hodgkin's disease. N Eng J Med 295:789-800, 1976.

86. D'Angio GJ, Evans AE, Breslow N, Beckwith B, Bishop H, Feigl P, Goodwin W, Leape LL, Sinks LF, Sutow W, Tefft M, Wolff J: The treatment of Wilm's tumor: Results of the National Wilm's Tumor Study. Cancer 38:633-646, 1976.

87. D'Angio G, Meadows A, Mike V, Harris C, Evans A, Jaffe N, Newton W, Schweisguth O, Sutow W, Morris-Jones P: Decreased risk of radiation associated second malignant neoplasms in actinomycin-D treated patients. Cancer 37:1177-1185, 1976.

88.   Evans A, Albo V, D'Angio G, Finklestein J, Leikin S, Santulli T, Weiner J, Hammond D: Cyclophos-
      phamide treatment of patients with localized and regional neuroblastoma. Cancer 38:655-660, 1976.

89.   Evans A, Albo V, D'Angio G, Finklestein J, Leikin S, Santulli T, Weiner J, Hammond D: Factors
      influencing survival of children with nonmetastatic neuroblastoma. Cancer 38:661-666, 1976.

90.   Evans A, Gerson J, Schnaufer L: Spontaneous regression of neuroblastoma. Natl Cancer Inst Monogr
      44:49-54, 1976.

91.   Nesbit M, Kersey J, Finklestein J, Weiner J, Simmons R: Immunotherapy and chemotherapy in
      children with neuroblastoma. J Natl Cancer Inst 57:717-720, 1976.

92.   Nesbit M, Sonley M, Hammond D: Usefulness of cytosine arabinoside and prednisone in refractory
      childhood lymphoblastic leukemia. Med and Pediatr Oncol 2:61, 1976.

93.   Nesbit M, Krivit W, Heyn R, Sharp H: Acute and chronic effects of methotrexate on hepatic,
      pulmonary, and skeletal systems. Cancer 37:1048-1054, 1976.

94.   Pendergrass TW: Congenital anomalies in children with Wilm's tumor. Cancer 37:403-409, 1976.

95.   Tefft M, D'Angio GJ, Grant W: Postoperative radiation therapy for residual Wilm's tumor. Review of
      Group III patients in the National Wilm's Tumor Study. Cancer 37:2768-2772, 1976.

96.   Wolff J: Chemotherapeutic management of Wilm's tumor. In Wilm's Tumor, Carl Pochedly and Denis
      Miller, Eds., pp. 205-214, 1976.

97.   Evans A, Bernstein I, Finklestein J, Klemperer M, Leikin S, Weiner J, Hammond D: Methyl-CCNU for
      patients with previously treated metastatic neuroblastoma - A Phase II study. Cancer Treat Rep
      61:83-85, 1977.

98.   Hays D, Sutow W, Lawrence W, Moon T, Tefft M: Rhabdomyosarcoma: Surgical therapy in extremity
      lesions in children. Ortho Clinics of N Am 8:883-902, 1977.

99.   Heyn R, Holland R, Joo P, Johnson D, Newton W, Tefft M, Breslow N, Hammond D: Treatment of
      rhabdomyosarcoma in children with surgery, radiotherapy and chemotherapy. Med and Pediatr Oncol
      3:21-32, 1977.

100. Krivit W: Overwhelming postsplenectomy infection. Am J Hematol 2:193-201, 1977.

101. Lawrence W, Hays D, Moon T: Lymphatic metastasis with childhood rhabdomyosarcoma. Cancer
      39:556-559, 1977.

102. Maurer H, Moon T, Donaldson M, Fernandez C, Gehan E, Hammond D, Hays D, Lawrence W, Newton
      W, Ragab A, Raney B, Soule E, Sutow W, Tefft M: Preliminary results of the Intergroup
      Rhabdomyosarcoma Study. In Management of Primary Bone and Soft Tissue Tumors. Chicago: Year
      Book Medical Publishers, Inc., 1977.

103. Maurer H, Moon T, Donaldson M, Fernandez C, Gehan E, Hammond D, Hays D, Lawrence W, Newton
      W, Ragab A, Raney B, Soule E, Sutow W, Tefft M: The Intergroup Rhabdomyosarcoma Study: A
      preliminary report. Cancer 40:2015-2026, 1977.

104. Ortega J, Nesbit M, Donaldson M, Hittle R, Weiner J, Karon M, Hammond D: L-asparaginase,
      vincristine, and prednisone for induction of first remission in acute lymphocytic leukemia. Cancer Res
      37:535-540, 1977.

105. Ramsay N, Coccia P, Krivit W, Bloomfield C, Nesbit M: Vinblastine, procarbazine, and cytosine
      arabinoside in combination for reinduction of childhood acute myelocytic leukemia. Cancer
      Treat Rep 60:1683-1685, 1977.

106. Tefft M, Fernandez C, Moon T: Rhabdomyosarcoma: Response with chemotherapy prior to radiation
      in patients with gross residual disease. Cancer 39:665-670, 1977.

107. Van Dyke J, Jenkin R, Leung P, Cunningham J: Medulloblastoma: Treatment technique and radiation
      dosimetry. J Rad Oncol Biol Phys 2:993-1005, 1977.

108. Ablin A, Bleyer W, Finklestein J, Hartmann J, Leikin S, Hammond D: Failure of moderate - dose
      prolonged - infusion methotrexate and citrovorum factor rescue in patients with previously treated
      metastatic neuroblastoma - a Phase II study. Cancer Treat Rep 62:1097-1099, 1978.

109.   Beckwith J, Palmer N: Histopathology of Wilm's tumor. <u>Cancer</u> 41:1937-1948, 1978.

110.   Bernstein I, Evans A, Finklestein J, Klemperer M, Hittle R, Leikin S, Hammond D: Phase II study of the failure of vincristine and bleomycin for previously treated children with metastatic neuroblastoma. <u>Cancer Treat Rep</u> 62:1201-1202, 1978.

111.   Breslow N, Palmer N, Hill L, Buring J, D'Angio G: Wilm's tumor: Prognostic factors for patients without metastases at diagnosis. <u>Cancer</u> 41:1577-1589, 1978.

112.   Breslow N: Perspectives on the statistician's role in cooperative clinical research. <u>Cancer</u> 41:326-332, 1978.

113.   Bleyer W: The clinical pharmacology of methotrexate - New applications of an old drug. <u>Cancer</u> 41:36-51, 1978.

114.   Chard R, Finklestein J, Sonley M, Nesbit M, McCreadie S, Weiner J, Sather H, Hammond D: Increased survival in childhood acute non-lymphocytic leukemia after treatment with prednisone, cytosine arabinoside, 6-thioguanine, cyclophosphamide and vincristine (PATCO) combination chemotherapy. <u>Med and Pediatr Oncol</u> 4:263-273, 1978.

115.   D'Angio G, Clatworthy H, Evans A, Newton W, Tefft M: Is the risk of morbidity and rare mortality worth the cure? <u>Cancer</u> 41:377-380, 1978.

116.   Hammond D, Bleyer A, Hartmann J, Hays D, Jenkin R: The team approach to the managment of pediatric cancer. <u>Cancer</u> 41:29-35, 1978.

117.   Krivit W, Hammond D: Vindesine: A Phase II study by the Childrens Cancer Study Group. <u>Current Chemother</u> 1331-1334, 1978.

118.   Maurer H (For the IRS Committee): Rhabdomyosarcoma in childhood and adolescense. <u>Curr Prob in Cancer</u> 2:3-36, 1978.

119.   Raney B, Hays D, Lawrence W, Soule E, Tefft M, Donaldson M: Paratesticular rhabdomyosarcoma in childhood. <u>Cancer</u> 42:729-736, 1978.

120.   Ruebesh T, Weinstein R, Baehner R, Wolff D, Bartlett M, Gonzales-Crussi F, Sulzer A, Schultz M: An outbreak of pneumocystis pneumonia in children with acute lymphocytic leukemia. <u>Am J Dis Child</u> 132:143-148, 1978.

CLINICAL DRUG EVALUATION PROGRAM

1963-1975

1. Good, JD, Hickey, RG, Tidrick RT: Oxylone as a palliative agent in advanced mammary cancer. Cancer Chemother Rep 31:49-52, 1963.

2. Johnson RO: Preliminary Phase II trials with 1-aminocyclopentane carboxylic acid.   Cancer Chemother Rep 32: 67-71, 1963.

3. Ansfield FJ: Phase I study of azotomycin. Cancer Chemother Rep 46:37-40, 1965.

4. Wilson WL, de la Garza JG: Phase I study of hexamethylmelamine. Cancer Chemother Rep 48:49-52, 1965.

5. Weeth JB, Segaloff A: Massive estrogen therapy: Phase I study of hexestrol. Cancer Chemother Rep 48:53-56, 1965.

6. Gurland J, Johnson RO: How reliable are tumor measurements? JAMA 194:973-978, 1965.

7. Aust JB, Roux K: A Phase I study of NSC 1026 in cancer patients. Cancer Chemother Rep 49:63-64, 1975.

8. Gurland J, Johnson RO: A case for using only the maximum diameter in measuring tumor lesions. Cancer Chemother Rep 50:119-124, 1966.

9. Johnson RO, Bisel HF, Andrews NC, Wilson WL, Rochlin DB, Segaloff A, Krementz ET, Aust JB, Ansfield FJ: A Phase I study of NSC 17256E. Cancer Chemother Rep 50:671-673, 1966.

10. WIlson WL, Bisel HF, Krementz ET, Lien RC, Prohaska J: Further clinical evaluation of 5-FUDR. Cancer Chemother Rep 51:85-90, 1967.

11. Andrews NC, Wilson WL: Phase II study of methotrexate in solid tumors. Cancer Chemother Rep 51:471-474, 1967.

12. Schroeder JM, Weeth JB: A Phase II evaluation of flurometholone. Cancer Chemother Rep 51:525-534, 1967.

13. Mason JH, Wilson WL, Ansfield FJ, Rochlin DB, Grage TB: Phase I clinical study of acetophenone 2-demethyl-amino-4-dihydroxyhydrochloride. Cancer Chemother Rep 52:297-299, 1968.

14. Weiss AJ, Ramirez G, Grage TB, Strawitz J, Goldman L, Downing V: A Phase II study of azotomycin. Cancer Chemother Rep 52:611-614, 1968.

15. Mrazek RG, Andrews NC, Bisel HF, Wilson WL, Hummel RP: Phase II clinical study of hexestrol. Cancer Chemother Rep 52:751-753, 1968.

16. Wilson WL, Schroeder JM, Bisel HF, Mrazek RG, Hummel RP: Phase II study of hexamethylmelamine. Cancer 23:132-136, 1969.

17. Bisel HF, Ansfield FJ, Mason JH, Wilson WL: Clinical studies with tuberciden administered by direct intravenous injection. Cancer Res 30:76-78, 1970.

18. Grage TB, Rochlin DB, Weiss AJ, Wilson WL: Clinical studies with tuberciden administered after absorption into human erythrocytes. Cancer Res 30:79-81, 1970.

19. Wilson WL, Bisel JF, Cole D, Rochlin DB, Ramirez G, Madden RE: Prolonged low-dosage administration of hexamethylmelamine. Cancer 25:568-570, 1970.

20. Aust JB, Andrews NC, Schroeder JM, Lawton RL: Phase II study of 1-amino-cyclopentanecarboxylic acid in patients with cancer --Clinical note. Cancer Chemother Rep 54:237-239, 1970.

      Addendum: Separate work done by Dr NC Andrews in Leiomyosarcomas only. Cancer Chemother Rep 54:240-241, 1970.

21. Wilson WL, Hurley JD, Mrazek RG: Phase II study of alanine mustard. Cancer Chemother Rep 54:361-363, 1970.

22. Andrews NC, Weiss AJ, Ansfield FJ, Rochlin DB, Mason J: Phase I study of dibromodulcitol. Cancer Chemother Rep 55:61-65, 1971.

23. Ansfield FJ, Ramirez G: Phase I and II studies of 2'-deoxy-5-(trifluoro-methyl)-uridine. Cancer Chemother Rep 55:205-208, 1971.

24. Ramirez G, Weiss AJ, Rochlin DB, Bisel HF: Phase II study of 17256E (6 Alpha-methyl pregn-4-ene-3, 11, 20-trione). Cancer Chemother Rep 55:265-268, 1971.

25. Wagner DE, Ramirez G, Weiss AJ, Hill GJ: Combination Phase I-II study of imidazole carboxamide. Oncology 26:310-316, 1971.

26. Weiss AJ, Wilson WL: Evaluation of the combination of hexamethylmelamine and methotrexate in carcinoma of the lung. Cancer Chemother Rep 55:299-302, 1971.

27. Wilson WL, Weiss AJ, Andrews NC: Photosensitization of pseudourea. Cancer Chemother Rep 55:525, 1971.

28. Hill GJ, Sedransk N, Rochlin DB, Bisel HF, Andrews NC, Fletcher WS, Schroeder JM, Wilson WL: Mithramycin therapy of testicular tumors. Cancer 30:900-908, 1972.

29. Kogler J, Hill GJ, Sedransk N, Cole DR, Weiss AJ, Wilson WL: Phase II study of carbestrol in patients with solid tumors. Cancer Chemother Rep 56:641-647, 1972.

30. Ramirez G, Wilson WL, Grage TB, Hill GJ: Phase II evaluation of 1,3-bis(2-chloroethyl)-1-nitrosourea (BCNU) in patients with solid tumors. Cancer Chemother Rep 56:787-789, 1972.

31. Hill GJ, Larsen RR: Cancer Chemotherapy: I. Methods, agents and overall results in 400 patients. Oncology 26:206-222, 1972.

32. Hill GJ, Larsen RR, Sas EM, Cohen BI, Irish TJ, Kandel E, Kogler J: Cancer chemotherapy: II. Results of 603 courses of therapy in 400 consecutive patients followed for 18-52 months. Oncology 27:137-152, 1973.

33. Andrews NC, Weiss AJ, Wilson WL, Nealon T: Phase II study of dibromodulcitol. Cancer Chemother Rep 58:653-660, 1974.

34. Davis HL, Rochlin DB, Weiss AJ, Wilson WL, Andrews NC, Madden RE, Sedransk N: Cytosine arabinoside toxicity and antitumor activity in human solid tumors. Oncology 29:190-200, 1974.

35. Grage TB, Weiss AJ, Wilson WL, Reynolds V: Phase I studies of porfiromycin in solid tumors. J Surg Oncol 7:415-420, 1975.

36. Wilson WL, Weiss AJ, Ramirez G: Phase I study of L-asparaginase: The use of L-asparaginase in the common human solid tumors. Oncology 32:109-117, 1975.

EASTERN COOPERATIVE ONCOLOGY GROUP

1957 - 1978

1.   Regelson W, Zuckerman P, Holland JF: Coordinate grid mapping technique in medicine. Cancer 10:436-437, 1957.

2.   Wells C, Ajmone-Marsan C, Frei E, Tuohy J, Shnider B: Electroencephalographic and neurological changes induced in man by the administration of 1,2,4-triazine-3,5 (2H,4H) dione (6-azauracil). Electroencephalography, Montreal 9:325-332, 1957.

3.   Zubrod CG: Experimental design in clinical trials of antitumor drugs. Proc Third Nat Cancer Conf, Philadelphia: J.B. Lippincott & Co., pp.443-446, 1957.

4.   Zuckerman P, Regelson W, Holland JF: Coordinate grid mapping technique in medicine. Med and Illus 7:10-12, 1957.

5.   Holland JF, Regelson W: Studies of phenylalanine nitrogen mustard in metastatic malignant melanoma of man. Ann N Y Acad Sci 68:1122-1125, 1958.

6.   Zubrod CG: Clinical investigations in cancer chemotherapy. J Chron Dis 8:183-190, 1958.

7.   Zubrod CG: Neoplastic disease (cancer). Ann Rev Med 9:287-302, 1958.

8.   Zubrod CG: Procedures recommended for the clinical trial of alkylating agents. Ann N Y Acad Sci 68:1246, 1958.

9.   Brindley CO, Markoff E, Schneiderman MA: Direct observation of lesion size and number as a method of following the growth of human tumors. Cancer 12:139-146, 1959.

10. Gold GL, Hall TC, Shnider BI, Selawry O, Colsky J, Owens AH, Dederick MM, Holland JF, Brindley CO, Jones R: A clinical study of 5-fluorouracil. Cancer Res 19:935-939, 1959.

11. Gold GL, Shnider BI: Some unusual syndromes associated with neoplastic disease. Ann Intern Med 51:890-896, 1959.

12. Holland JF: Cancer chemotherapy: Its principles and practice. Westchester Co Med Bull 27:19-28, 1959.

13. Shnider BI, Gold GL: Recent developments in cancer chemotherapy. Med Ann D C 28:637-643, 1959.

14. Brindley CO, Colsky J, Dederick M, Holland JF, Owens AH, Shnider BI, Frei E, Hreschyshyn MM, Nevinny HB, Uzer Y, Jones R: Clinical trials of the cytostatic agent A-139 or 2,5-bis-(1-aziridinyl)-3, 6-bis-(2-methoxyethoxy-p-benzoquinone). Cancer Res 20:1580-1583, 1960.

15. Chalmers TC, Dederick MM: A comparison of x-ray therapy and chemotherapy in the treatment of bronchogenic carcinoma. Natl Cancer Inst Monogr No. 3. Conference on Experimental Cancer Chemotherapy, pp.85-105, 1960.

16. Colsky J, Franzino A, Majima H, Jones R: Human pharmacologic studies with actinomycin D (PA 126-P). Cancer Chemother Rep 8:27-32, 1960.

17. Condit PT, Levy AM, Shnider BI, Oviedo RG: Some effects of S,2-aminoethylisothiouronium bromide hydrobromide (AET) in man. Cancer 13:842-849, 1960.

18. Costa G, Holland JF: Clinical studies with psicofuranine. Cancer Chemother Rep 8:33-35, 1960.

19. Jones R, MD, Chairman. Drs. CG Zubrod D Karnofsky, and B Baker, Members Panel: Use of alkylating agents and the future of these agents. Natl Cancer Inst Monogr No. 3. Conference on Experimental Cancer Chemotherapy, pp.127-147, 1960.

20. Jones R, Jonsson U, Colsky J, Lessner H, Franzino A: Cancer Chemotherapy: Present status and future prospect. Proc Fourth National Cancer Conference, pp.175-182, 1960.

21. Lane M, Lipowska B, Hall TC, Colsky J: Observations on the clinical pharmacology of 5-bis (2'-chlorethyl) aminouracil (uracil mustard). Cancer Chemother Rep 9:31-36, 1960.

22. Lasagna LC: Planning clinical chemotherapy studies. Natl Cancer Inst Monogr No. 3. Conference on Experimental Cancer Chemotherapy, pp.45-49, 1960.

23. Lee LE, Chairman: Curreri A, Shnider B, Colsky J, Jonsson U, Close H, Members. Panel: Investigation of therapy in solid tumors. Natl Cancer Inst Monogr No. 3. Conf on Experimental Cancer Chemotherapy, pp.71-83, 1960.

24. Rundles RW, Chairman: Lukes R, Ackerman L, Holland J, Spear P, Scott JL, Spurr CL, Members. Panel: Investigations in malignant lymphomas. Natl Cancer Inst Monogr No. 3. Conf on Exp Cancer Chemother, pp.193-227, 1960.

25. Segaloff A, Chairman: Bisel HF, Hall TC, Escher GC, Noer RJ, Members. Panel: Investigations in breast carcinoma. Natl Cancer Inst Monogr No. 3. Conf on Exp Cancer Chemother, pp.257-276, 1960.

26. Selawry OS, Holland JF: Tolerance to weekly doses of 2-amino-6- (1-methyl-4-nitro-5-imidazolyl) thio purine (B.W. 57-323) in humans. Cancer Chemother Rep 8:53-55, 1960.

27. Shnider BI, Gold GL, Hall TC, Dederick M, Nevinny HB, Potee KG, Lasagna L, Owens AH, Hreschyshyn M, Selawry O, Holland JF, Jones R, Colsky J, Franzino A, Zubrod CG, Frei E, Brindley C: Preliminary studies with cyclophosphamide. Cancer Chemother Rep 8:106-111, 1960.

28. Shnider BI, Frei E, Tuohy J, Gorman J, Freireich EJ, Brindley CO, Clements J: Clinical studies of 6-azauracil. Cancer Res 20:28-33, 1960.

29. Skipper HE, Chairman: Bernard R Baker, Ralph Jones, Members. Panel: Basis for seeking new types and structures for chemotherapeutic agents. Natl Cancer Inst Monogr No. 3. Conf Exp Cancer Chemother, pp.59-69, 1960.

30. Uzer Y, Shnider BI, Gold GL: A double blind study with iproniazid in patients with far-advanced cancer. Abtibiot Med Clin Ther 7:777-781, 1960.

31. Zubrod CG, MD, Chairman: Drs J Ipsen, E Frei, L Lasagna, M Lipsett, E Gehan, and G Escher, Members. Panel: Newer techniques and some problems in cooperative group studies. Natl Cancer Inst Monogr No. 3. Conf Exp Cancer Chemother, pp.277-292, 1960.

32. Zubrod CG, Schneiderman M, Frei E, Brindley CO, Gold GL, Shnider BI, Oviedo R, Gorman J, Jones R, Jonsson U, Colsky J, Chalmers T, Ferguson B, Dederick M, Holland J, Selawry O, Regelson W, Lasagna L, Owens AH: Appraisal of methods for the study of chemotherapy of cancer in man: Comparative therapeutic trial of nitrogen mustard and triethylene-thiophosphoramide. J Chron Dis 11:7-33, 1960.

33. Frei E, Franzino A, Shnider BI, Costa G, Colsky J, Brindley CO, Hosley H, Holland JF, Gold GL, Jonsson U: Clinical studies of vinblastine. Cancer Chemother Rep 12:125-129, 1961.

34. Holland JF, Gehan EA, Brindley CO, Dederick MM, Owens AH, Shnider BI, Taylor R, Frei E, Selawry O, Regelson W, Hall TC: A comparative study of optimal medical care with and without azaserine in multiple myeloma. Clin Pharmacol Ther 2:22-28, 1961.

35. Krant MJ, Neyman A, Levene MB, Hall TC: Radiation sensitization in mammals with BUDR: Preliminary Report. Radiat Res 14:479-480, 1961.

36. Lasagna L, Owens AH, Shnider BI, Gold GL: Toxicity after large doses of noscapine. Cancer Chemother Rep 15:33-34, 1961.

37. Regelson W, Holland JF: Initial clinical study of parenteral methylglyoxal bis(guanylhydrazone) diacetate. Cancer Chemother Rep 11:81, 1961.

38. Carey RW, Hall TC, Finkel H: A comparison of two dosage regimens for vincristine. Cancer Chemother Rep 27:91-96, 1962.

39. Chalmers TC: Combination of radiotherapy and chemotherapy in the treatment of carcinoma of the lung. Cancer Chemother Rep 16:463-465, 1962.

40. Condit P, Shnider BI, Owens A: Studies on the folic vitamins. VII. The effects of large doses of amethopterin in patients with cancer. Cancer Res 22:706-712, 1962.

41. Costa G, Hreschyshyn M, Holland JF: Initial clinical studies with vincristine. Cancer Chemother Rep 24:39-44, 1962.

42. Gold GL, Salvin LG, Shnider BI: A comparative study with three alkylating agents: mechlorethamine, cyclophosphamide, and uracil mustard. Cancer Chemother Rep 16:417-419, 1962.

43. Gold GL, Shnider BI: Unsuspected hazards of oncolytic drugs. Med Ann D C 31:143-146, 1962.

44. Hall TC: A comparative study of 5-fluorouracil (FU), 5-fluorodeoxyuridine (FUDR), and methotrexate (MTX) - Progress Report. Cancer Chemother Rep 16:391-396, 1962.

45. Hall TC: Medical Progress: Chemotherapy of cancer. N Eng J Med 266:129-134, 178-185, 238-245, 289-296, 1962.

46. Hall TC: Recent advances in chemotherapy of solid tumors. Med Sci 2:31-48, 1962.

47. Hall TC, Krant MJ, Lloyd JG, Patterson WB, Ishihara A, Potee KG, Lovina TO, Mullen JM: Treatment of localized inoperable neoplasms with intraarterial infusions of 8-azaguanine. Cancer 15:1156-1164, 1962.

48. Hreschyshyn MM, Holland JF: Chemotherapy in patients with gynecologic cancer. Am J Obstet Gynecol 83:468-489, 1962.

49. Krant MJ, Iszard DM, Abadi A, Carey RW: Treatment of multiple myeloma with 1-aminocyclopentanecarboxylic acid. Cancer Chemother Rep 22:59-64, 1962.

50. Miller SP, Brenner S: Combination therapy with Cobalt-60 and chlorambucil in the treatment of disseminated ovarian carcinomatosis. Cancer Chemother Rep 16:455-462, 1962.

51. Owens AH, Shnider BI, Gold GL, Brindley CO, Miller SP: Clinical toxicity after graded doses of alanine mustard. Cancer Chemother Rep 21:143-145, 1962.

52. Owens AH: Predicting anticancer drug effects in man from laboratory animal studies. J Chron Dis 15:223-228, 1962.

53. Shnider BI: Early clinical trials with anticancer agents: Phase I and Phase II studies. A. Dosage schedules and routes of administration. Cancer Chemother Rep 16:61-67, 1962.

54. Shnider BI: Early human trials with anticancer agents. J Chron Dis 15:229-236, 1962.

55. Carbone PP, Bono V, Frei E, Brindley CO: Clinical studies with vincristine. Blood 21:640-647, 1963.

56. Colsky J: The clinical investigator and evaluation of new drugs. Am J Hosp Pharm 20:517, 1963.

57. Colsky J, Shnider B, Jones R, Nevinny H, Hall T, Regelson W, Selawry O, Owens AH, Brindley CO, Frei E, Uzer Y: A comparative study of 9-alpha-bromo-11-keto progesterone and prednisolone in the treatment of advanced carcinoma of the female breast. Cancer 16:502, 1963.

58. Costa G, Carbone PP, Gold GL,, Owens AH, Miller SP, Krant MJ, Bono VJ: Clinical trial of vinblastine in multiple myeloma. Cancer Chemother Rep 27:87-89, 1963.

59. Dederick MM, Hall TC, Nevinny HB, Potee KG: Preliminary report on human toxicity study of streptovitacin A. Cancer Chemother Rep 27:81-86, 1963.

60. Hall TC, Dederick MM, Nevinny HB: Prognostic value of response to therapeutic castration of patients with breast cancer. Cancer Chemother Rep 31:47-48, 1963.

61. Krant MJ, Chalmers TC, Dederick MM, Hall TC, Levene MB, Muench H, Shnider BI, Gold GL, Hunter C, Bersack SR, Owens AH, Deleon N, Dickson RJ, Brindley CO, Brace KC, Frei E, Gehan E, Salvin LG: Comparative trial of chemotherapy and radiotherapy in patients with non-resectable cancer of the lung. Am J Med 35:363-373, 1963.

62. Nevinny HB, Hall TC: In situ determination of the antitumor effect of chemotherapeutic coumpounds. Proc 2nd Int Symp Chemother, Naples, 3:219-225, 1963.

63. Regelson W, Holland JF: Clinical experiment with methylglyoxal bis (guanylhydrazone) diacetate. Cancer Chemother Rep 27:15-26, 1963.

64. Brindley CO, Salvin LG, Potee KG, Lipowska B, Shnider BI, Regelson W, Colsky J: Further comparative trial of triethylenethiophosphoramide and mechlorethamine in patients with melanoma and Hodgkin's disease. J Chron Dis 17:19-30, 1964.

65. Carbone PP, Freireich EJ, Frei E, Rall DP, Karon M, Brindley CO: The effectiveness of methylglyoxal bis(guanylhydrazone) in human malignant disease. Acta Union Int Contre Cancer 20:340-343, 1964.

66. Carbone PP, Frei E, Owens AH, Olson KG, Miller SP: 6-Thioguanine therapy in patients with multiple myeloma. Cancer Chemother Rep 36:59-62, 1964.

67. Fishbein WN, Carbone PP, Owens AH, Kelly MG, Rall DP, Tarr NA: Preliminary studies with 5-bis (2-chlorethyl)amino-dl-tryptophan in animals and man. Cancer Chemother Rep 42:19-24, 1964.

68. Regelson W, Holland JF, Frei E, Gold GL, Hall TC, Krant M, Miller SP: Comparative clinical toxicity of 6-MP and 6-mercaptopurine ribonucleoside administered intravenously to patients with advanced cancer. Cancer Chemother Rep 36:41-48, 1964.

69. Carbone PP, Krant MJ, Miller SP, Hall TC, Shnider BI, Colsky J, Horton J, Hosley H, Miller JM, Frei E, Schneiderman MA: The feasibility of using randomization schemes early in the clinical trials of new chemotherapeutic agents: Hydroxyurea. Clin Pharmacol Ther 6:17-24, 1965.

70. DeVita VT, Carbone PP, Owens AH, Gold GL, Krant MJ, Edmonson J: Clinical trials with 1,3 bis (2-chlorethyl)-1-nitrosourea (BCNU). Cancer Res 25:1876-1881, 1965.

71. Ellison RR: Clinical pharmacologic study of hadacidin. Cancer Chemother Rep 46:31-36, 1965.

72. Foley HT, Shnider BI, Gold GL, Matias PI: Phase I studies with thiocarzolamide. Cancer Chemother Rep 47:83-86, 1965.

73. Foley HT, Shnider BI, Gold GL, Uzer Y: Phase I studies with pyrazole. Cancer Chemother Rep 44:45-48, 1965.

74. Frei E, Spurr CL, Brindley CO, Selawry O, Holland JF, Rall DP, Wasserman LR, Hoogstraten B, Shnider BI, McIntyre OR, Matthews LB, Miller SP: Clinical studies of dichloromethotrexate. Clin Pharmacol Ther 6:160-171, 1965.

75. Frei E, Carbone PP, Shnider BI, Gold GL, Colsky J, Franzino A, Krant MJ, Brena G, Owens AH, Holland JF, Costa G, Hall TC, Hosley H, Horton J, Tarr N, Salvin LG: A study of vinblastine in the treatment of patients with neoplastic disease. Arch Intern Med 116:846-852, 1965.

76. Horton J, Olson KB: Combination therapy with 5-fluorouracil, mitomycin C, vincristine, and thioTEPA in advanced cancer. Cancer Chemother Rep 49:59-61, 1965.

77. Nevinny HB, Krant MJ, Moore EW: Metabolic studies of the effects of methotrexate. Metabolism 14:135-140, 1965.

78. Olson KB, Hall TC, Horton J, Hosley HF: Thalidomide (N-phthaloyl glutamimide) in the treatment of advanced cancer. Clin Pharmacol Ther 6:292-297, 1965.

79. Regelson W, Holland JF, Myers WPL, Hall TC: Clinical study of O-phenylenediamine in melanoma. Cancer Chemother Rep 45:41-44, 1965.

80. Colsky J, Shnider BI, Franzino A, Perez J: Observations in patients with metastatic malignancy treated with duazomycin A. Clin Pharmacol Ther 7:352-358, 1966.

81. Costa G, Carbone PP, Engle R, Schilling A: Prednisone and L-phenylalanine mustard (L-PAM): An effective combination in the treatment of multiple myeloma in man. Proc Internat Cancer Cong, Tokyo, 1966.

82. Dawson JJ, Hall TC, Schneiderman MA, Shnider BI, Owens AH, Andrews JR, Baxter DH, Brenner S, Hunter C, Levene MB, Sheehan FR, White B: The objective evaluation of change in tumor size in lung cancer patients with non-measurable disease. Cancer 19:415-420, 1966.

83. Finkel HE, Yount WJ, Salmon SE, Schilling A: Current concepts in the therapy of multiple myeloma. Med Clin North Am 50:1569-1578, 1966.

84. Foley HT, Shnider BI, Gold GL, Rius J: A pilot study of methotrexate, duazomycin A, and radiation therapy in carcinoma of the lung. J New Drugs 6:105-111, 1966.

85. Holland JF, Hosley H, Scharlau C, Carbone PP, Frei E, Brindley CO, Hall TC, Shnider BI, Gold GL, Lasagna L, Owens AH, Miller SP: A controlled trial of urethane treatment in multiple myeloma. Blood 27:328-342, 1966.

86. Khung CL, Hall TC, Piro AJ, Dederick MM: A clinical trial of oral 5-fluorouracil. J Clin Pharmacol Ther 7:527-533, 1966.

87. Nathanson L, Hall TC, Dederick MM, Yount WJ, Miller S: Initial pharmacology studies of three types of combination chemotherapy. Cancer Chemother Rep 50:259-264, 1966.

88. Salmon SE, Yount WJ, Shadduck RK, Hall TC, Schilling A: O-DL-sarcolysin in solid tumors. Cancer Chemother Rep 50:685-692, 1966.

89. Cavins JA, Hall TC, Olson KB, Khung CL, Horton J, Colsky J, Shadduck RK: Initial toxicity study of sangivamycin. Cancer Chemother Rep 51:197-200, 1967.

90. Eastern Cooperative Group in Solid Tumor Chemotherapy: Comparison of antimetabolites in the treatment of breast and colon cancr. JAMA 200:770-778, 1967.

91. Foley HT, Shnider BI, Gold GL, Matias P, Colsky J, Miller SP: Phase I studies of porfiromycin. Cancer Chemother Rep 51:283-293, 1967.

92. Hall TC, Dederick MM, Chalmers TC, Krant MJ, Shnider BI, Lynch JJ, Holland JF, Ross C, Koons CR, Owens AH, Frei E, Brindley C, Miller SP, Brenner S, Hosley HF, Olson KB: A clinical pharmacologic study of chemotherapy and x-ray therapy in lung cancer. Am J Med 43:186-193, 1967.

93. Horton J, Olson KB, Cunningham TJ, Sullivan JM: Epodyl in advanced cancer involving the brain and other organs. Cancer 20:1837-1840, 1967.

94. Kyle RA, Carbone PP, Lynch JJ, Owens AH, Costa G, Silver RT, Cuttner J, Harley JB, Leone LA, Shnider BI, Holland JF: Evaluation of tryptophan mustard in patients with plasmacytic myeloma. Cancer Res 27:510-515, 1967.

95. Nathanson L, Hall TC, Rutenberg A, Shadduck RK: Clinical toxicologic study of cyclohexylamine salt of N,N-bis (2-chlorethyl) phosphorodiamidic acid. Cancer Chemother Rep 51: 35-39, 1967.

96. Olson KB, Hall TC, Horton J, Nathanson L: Combination cancer chemotherapy. Proc Int Cong Chemother, Vienna, Austria, pp. 257-263, 1967.

97. Regelson W, Holland JF, Gold GL, Lynch J, Olson KB, Horton J, Hall TC, Krant M, Colsky J, Miller SP, Owens A: 6-Mercaptopurine given intravenously at weekly intervals to patients with advanced cancer. Cancer Chemother Rep 51:277-282, 1967.

98. Salmon SE, Samal BA, Hayes DM, Hosley H, Miller SP, Schilling A: Role of gamma globulin for immunoprophylaxis in multiple myeloma. N Eng J Med 277:1336-1340, 1967.

99. Yount WJ, Hall TC, Schilling A, Shadduck RK: DL-ortho-sarcolysin in treatment of multiple myeloma. Cancer Chemother Rep 51:517-523, 1967.

100. Carbone PP, Spurr C, Schneiderman M, Scotto J, Holland JF, Shnider B (ECOG & CALGB): Management of patients with malignant lymphoma; A comparative study with cyclophosphamide and vinca alkaloids. Cancer Res 28:811-822, 1968.

101. Ellison RR, Nadler SH, Shnider B, Gold GL, Horton J, Colsky J, Franzino A, Krant MJ, Hall TC: Clinical trial of hadacidin at three fractionated dose levels. Cancer Chemother Rep 52:425-431, 1968.

102. Gailani SD, Holland JF, Nussbaum A, Olson KB: Clinical and biochemical studies of pyridoxine deficiency in patients with neoplastic diseases. Cancer 21:975-988, 1968.

103. Horton J, Olson KB, Cunningham T, Sullivan J: Comparison of a combination of 5-fluorouracil, mitomycin C, triethylenethiophosphoramide, and fluoxymesterone with 5-fluorouracil alone in patients with advanced cancer. Cancer Chemother Rep 52:597-600, 1968.

104. Khung CL, Hall TC, Kelley RM, Grogan RH, Griffiths CT: Preliminary clinical trial of DL-metasarcolysin for advanced carcinoma of the breast. Cancer Chemother Rep 52:413-416, 1968.

105. Dennis L, Baig M, Angeles A, Shnider BI: The effect of pyran co-polymer on the hemostatic mechanism. Proc Am Soc Clin Pharmacol Chemother, 1969.

106. Hoogstraten B, Owens AH, Lenhard RE, Glidewell OJ, Leone LA, Olson KB, Harley JB, Townsend SR, Miller SP, Spurr CL: Combination of chemotherapy in lymphosarcoma and reticulum cell sarcoma. Blood 33:370-378, 1969.

107. Nathanson L, Hall TC, Schilling A, Miller S: Concurrent combination chemotherapy of human solid tumors: Experience with a three-drug regimen and review of the literature. Cancer Res 29:419-425, 1969.

108. Olson KB, Horton J, Pratt KL, Paladine WJ, Cunningham T, Sullivan J, Hosley H, Treble DH: 1-Acetyl-2 picolinoyl-hydrazine in the treatment of advanced cancer. Cancer Chemother Rep 53:291-296, 1969.

109. Stolbach L, Krant MJ, Mitchell ML: The effect of 6-medroxyprogesterone acetate (Provera) on (131 I) tri-iodothyronine resin sponge acetate. J Endocrinol 43:309-319, 1969.

110. Gold G, Shnider BI, Salvin LG, Schneiderman MA, Colsky J, Owens AH, Krant MJ, Miller SP, Frei E, Hall TC, Spurr CL, McIntyre OR, Hoogstraten B, Holland JF: The use of mechlorethamine, cyclophosphamide, and uracil mustard in neoplastic disease: A controlled study. J Clin Pharmacol 10:110-112, 1970.

111. Perlia CP, Gubisch NJ, Wolter J, Edelberg D, Dederick MM, Taylor SG: Mithramycin treatment of hypercalcemia. Cancer 25:389-397, 1970.

112. Burke PJ, Owens AH, Colsky J, Shnider BI, Edmonson JH, Schilling A, Brodovsky HS, Wallace HJ, Hall TC: A clinical evaluation of a prolonged schedule of cytosine arabinoside. Cancer Res 30:1512-1515, 1970.

113. Moon JH, Edmonson JH: Procarbazine and multiple myeloma. Cancer Chemother Rep 54:245-248, 1970.

114. Jehn UW, Nathanson L, Schwartz RS, Skinner M: In vitro lymphocyte stimulation by a soluble antigen from malignant melanoma. N Eng J Med 283:329-333, 1970.

115. Horton J, Olson KB, Sullivan J, Reilly C, Shnider B, FACP, and Eastern Cooperative Oncology Group: 5-FU in cancer: An improved regimen. Ann Intern Med 73:897-900, 1970.

116. Horton J, Baxter DH, Olson KB, and Eastern Cooperative Oncology Group: The management of metastases to the brain by irradiation and corticosteroids. Amer J Roentgenol Rad Ther & Nucl Med CXI, No. 2:334-336, 1971.

117. Cohen JL, Krant MJ, Shnider BI, Matias PI, Horton J, Baxter D: Radiation plus 5-fluorouracil: Clinical demonstration of an additive effect in bronchogenic carcinoma. Cancer Chemother Rep 55:253-258, 1971.

118. Shnider BI, and the Eastern Cooperative Oncology Group: The use of chemotherapy in lung cancer (controlled trials). Med Ann D C 40:489-495, 1971.

119. Slayton RE, Shnider BI, Elias E, Horton J, Perlia CP: New approach to the treatment of hypercalcemia. Clin Pharmacol Ther 12:833-837, 1971.

120. Nathanson L, Wolter J, Horton J, Colsky J, Shnider BI, Schilling A: Characteristics of prognosis and response to an imidazole carboxamide in malignant melanoma. Clin Pharmacol Ther 12: 955-962, 1971.

121. Harley JB, Schilling A, Glidewell O: Ineffectiveness of fluoride in multiple myeloma. N Eng J Med 286:1283-1288, 1972.

122. Costanza M, Nathanson L, Lenhard R, Wolter J, Colsky J, Oberfield R, Schilling A: Therapy of malignant melanoma with imidazole carboxamide and bis-chloroethyl nitrosourea. Cancer 30:1457-1461, 1972.

123. Nathanson L: Regression of intradermal malignant melanoma after intralesional injection of mycobacterium bovis strain BCG. Cancer Chemother Rep 56:659-665, 1972.

124. Rossof AH, Slayton RE, Perlia CP: Preliminary clinical experience with cis-diamminedichloro-platinum (II), CACP. Cancer 30:1451-1456, 1972.

125. Wampler GL, Mellette SJ, Kuperminc M, Regelson W: Hexamethylmelamine in the treatment of advanced cancer. Cancer Chemother Rep 56:505-514, 1972.

126. Costa G, Engle RL, Schilling A, Carbone P, Kochwa S, Nachman RL, Glidewell O: Melphalan and prednisone: An effective combination for the treatment of multiple myeloma. Am J Med 54:589-599, 1973.

127. Lenhard R: Eastern Cooperative Oncology Group Studies. Arch Intern Med 131:418-420, 1973.

128. Holland JR, Scharlau C, Gailani S, Krant MJ, Olson KB, Horton J, Shnider BI, Lynch JJ, Owens A, Carbone P, Colsky J, Miller SP, Hall TC: Vincristine treatment of advanced cancer. Cancer Res 33:1258-1264, 1973.

129. Rege VB, Owens AH: BCNU in the treatment of advanced Hodgkin's disease, lymphosarcoma, and reticulum cell sarcoma. Cancer Chemother Rep 58:383-392, 1974.

130. Shnider BI, Colsky J, Jones R, Carbone PP: Effectiveness of methyl-GAG administered intra-muscularly. Cancer Chemother Rep 58:689-695, 1974.

131. Shnider BI, Baig M, Serpick A, Kayhoe DE: Combination therapy with 5-fluorouracil, cyclophos-phamide, vincristine and methotrexate. J Clin Pharmacol 15:69-72, 1975.

132. Fisher B, Carbone P, Economou SG, Frelick R, Glass A, Lerner H, Redmond C, Zelen M, Band P, Katrych D, Wolmark N, Fisher ER: L-phenylalanine mustard (L-PAM) in the management of primary breast cancer. A report of early findings. New Eng J Med 292:117-122, 1975.

133. Horton J, Mittelman A, Taylor SG, Jurkowitz L, Bennett JM, Ezdinli E, Colsky J, Hanley JA: Phase II trials with procarbazine, streptozotocin, 6-thioguanine, and CCNU in patients with metastatic cancer of the large bowel. Cancer Chemother Rep 59:333-340, 1975.

134. Miller SP, Brenner S, Horton J, Stolbach L, Shnider BI, Pocock S: Comparative evaluation of combined radiation-chlorambucil treatment of ovarian carcinomatosis. Cancer 36:79-84, 1975.

135. Taylor SG, Pocock SJ, Shnider BI, Colsky J, Hall TC: Clinical studies of 5-fluorouracil + premarin in the treatment of breast cancer. Med & Pediatric Oncology 1:113-121, 1975.

136. Carbone P, Costello W: Eastern Cooperative Oncology Group Studies with DTIC. Cancer Treatment Rep 60:193-198, 1976.

137. Shnider BI, Baig M, Colsky J: A Phase I study of 5-azacytidine. J Clin Pharmacol 16:205-212, 1976.

138. Costanza ME, Nathanson L, Costello WG, Wolter J, Brunk JF, Colsky J, Hall T, Oberfield RA, Regelson W: Results of a randomized study comparing DTIC with TIC mustard in malignant melanoma. Cancer 37:1654-1659, April 1976.

139. Edmonson JH, Lagakos S, Stolbach L, Perlia CP, Bennett JM, Mansour EG, Horton J, Regelson W, Cumings FJ, Israel L, Brodsky I, Shnider BI, Creech R, Carbone PP: Mechlorethamine plus CCNU in the treatment of inoperable squamous and large cell carcinoma of the lung. Cancer Treatment Rep 60:625-627, 1976.

140. Bennett JM, Bakemeier RF, Carbone PP, Ezdinli E, Lenhard RE: Clinical trials with BCNU in malignant lymphomas by the Eastern Cooperative Oncology Group. Cancer Treat Rep 60:739-745, 1976.

141. Knight EW, Lagakos S, Stolbach L, Colsky J, Horton J, Israel L, Bennett J, Perlia C, Regelson W, Carbone PP: Adriamycin in the treatment of far-advanced lung cancer. Cancer Treat Rep 60:939-941, 1976.

142. Edmonson JH, Lagakos SW, Selawry OS, Perlia CP, Bennett JM, Muggia FM, Wampler G, Brodovsky HS, Horton J, Colsky J, Mansour EG, Creech R, Stolbach L, Greenspan EM, Levitt M, Israel L, Ezdinli EZ, Carbone PP: Cyclophosphamide and CCNU in the treatment of inoperable small cell carcinoma and adenocarcinoma of the lung. Cancer Treat Rep 60:925-932, 1976.

143. Moertel CG, Hanley JA: The effect of measuring error on the results of therapeutic trials in advanced cancer. Cancer 38:388-394, 1976.

144. Moertel CG, Mittelman JA, Bakemeier RF, Engstrom P, Hanley J: Sequential and combination chemotherapy of advanced gastric cancer. Cancer 38:678-682, 1976.

145. Cannellos GP, Pocock SJ, Taylor SG, Sears ME, Klaassen DJ, Band PR: Combination chemotherapy for metastatic breast carcinoma. Cancer 38:1882-1886, 1976.

146. Lerner HJ, Band PR, Israel L, Leung BS: Phase II study of tamoxifen: Report of 74 patients with Stage IV breast cancer. Cancer Treat Rep 60:1431-1435, 1976.

147. Lenhard RE, Prentice RL, Owens AH, Bakemeier R, Horton J, Shnider BI, Stolbach L, Berard CW, Carbone PP: Combination chemotherapy of the malignant lymphomas. Cancer 38:1052-1059, 1976.

148. Ezdinli E, Pocock S, Berard CW, Aungst CW, Silverstein M, Horton J, Bennett J, Bakemeier R, Stolbach L, Perlia C, Brunk SF, Lenhard RE, Klaassen DJ, Richter P, Carbone P: Comparison of intensive versus moderate chemotherapy of lymphocytic lymphomas. Cancer 38:1060-1068, 1976.

149. Douglass HO, Lavin PT, Moertel CG: Nitrosoureas: Useful agents for the treatment of advanced gastrointestinal cancer. Cancer Treat Rep 60:769-780, 1976.

150. Moertel CG, Douglass HO, Hanley J, Carbone PP: Phase II study of methyl-CCNU in the treatment of advanced pancreatic carcinoma. Cancer Treat Rep 60:1659-1661, 1976.

151. Selawry O, Krant M, Scotto J, Kazam E, Schneiderman M, Olson K, Shnider B, Edmonson J, Holland J, Taylor S: Methotrexate compared with placebo in lung cancer. Cancer 40:4-8, 1977.

152. Carbone PP, Bauer M, Band P, Tormey D: Chemotherapy of disseminated breast cancer. Cancer 39:2916-2922, 1977.

153. Fisher B, Glass A, Redmond C, Fisher ER, Barton B, Such E, Carbone P, Economou S, Foster R, Frelick R, Lerner H, Levitt M, Margolese R, Mac Farlane J, Plotkin D, Shibata H, Volk H: L-phenylalanine mustard (L-PAM) in the management of primary breast cancer. Cancer 39:2883-2903, 1977.

154. O'Connell MJ, Silverstein MN, Kiely JM, White WL: Pilot study of two adriamycin-based regimens in patients with advanced malignant lymphomas. Cancer Treat Rep 61:65-68, 1977.

155. DeWys WD: Comparison of adriamycin and 5-Fluorouracil in advanced prostatic cancer. Cancer Chemother Rep 59:215-217, 1975.

156. Bennett JM, Lenhard RE, Ezdinli E, Johnson GJ, Carbone PP, Pocock SJ: Chemotherapy of non-Hodgkin's lymphomas: Eastern Cooperative Oncology Group Experience. Cancer Treat Rep 61:1079-1083, 1977.

157. Band PR, Canellos GP, Sears M, Israel L, Pocock SJ: Phase II trial with bleomycin, CCNU and streptozotocin in patients with metastatic cancer of the breast. Cancer Treat Rep 61:1365-1367, 1977.

158. DeWys WD, Bauer M, Colsky J, Cooper RA, Creech R, Carbone PP: Comparative trial of adriamycin and 5-Fluorouracil in advanced prostatic cancer-Progress Report. Cancer Treat Rep 61:325-328, 1977.

159. Elias EG, Band PR, Mittelman A, Colsky J, Regelson W, Shnider BI, Hanley JA: Clinical evaluation of two weekly dose schedules of 'IC-140'. Oncology 31:273-279, 1975.

160. Moertel CG, Douglass HO, Hanley J, Carbone PP: Treatment of advanced adenocarcinoma of the pancreas with combinations of streptozotocin plus 5-Fluorouracil and streptozotocin plus cyclophosphamide. Cancer 40:605-608, 1977.

161. Costanza ME, Nathanson L, Schoenfeld D, Wolter J, Colsky J, Regelson W, Cunningham T, Sedransk N: Results with methyl-CCNU and DTIC in metastatic melanoma. Cancer 40:1010-1015, 1977.

162. Carbone PP: Tumor biology and clinical trials: The Richard and Hinda Rosenthal Foundation Award Lecture. Cancer Res 37:4239-4245, 1977.

163. Horton J, Begg CG, Arseneault J, Bruckner H, Creech R, Hahn RG: Comparison of adriamycin with cyclophosphamide in patients with advanced endometrial cancer. Cancer Treat Rep 62:159-161, January, 1978.

164. Cunningham, TJ, Schoenfeld D, Nathanson L, Wolter J, Patterson WB, Cohen MH: A controlled study of adjuvant therapy in patients with Stage I and II malignant melanoma. In Immunotherapy of Cancer: Present Status of Trials in Man, edited by WD Terry & D Windhorst. New York: Raven Press, pp.19-26, 1978.

165. Cohen MH, Pocock SJ, Savlov ED, Lerner HJ, Colsky J, Regelson W, Carbone PP: Phase I-II trial of intramuscularly administered bleomycin. Europ J Cancer 13:49-53. Pergamon Press, 1977. Printed in Great Britain.

166. Ezdinli EZ, Costello W, Lenhard RE, Bakemeier R, Bennett JM, Berard CW, Carbone PP: Survival of nodular versus diffuse pattern lymphocytic poorly differentiated lymphoma. Cancer 41:1990-1996, 1978.

GYNECOLOGIC ONCOLOGY GROUP

1975-1978

1. Hreschyshyn MM, for the Gynecologic Oncology Group: Description of the GOG, its structure and functions. Treatment of women with cervical cancer, Stage IIIB and IV confined to the pelvis with hydroxyurea or placebo both in combination with radiation therapy. Gynecol Oncol 3:251-257, 1975.

2. McGowan L, Bunnag B: The evaluation of therapy for ovarian cancer. Gynecol Oncol 4:375-383, 1976.

3. Creasman WT, Boronow R, Marrow CP, DeSaia PJ, Blessing J, for Gynecologic Oncology Group: Adenocarcinoma of the endometrium: Its metastatic lymph node potential. A preliminary report. Gynecol Oncol 4:239-243, 1976.

4. Morrow CP, DiSaia PJ, Mangan C, Lagasse L: Continuous pelvic arterial infusion with bleomycin for squamous carcinoma of the cervix recurrent after irradiation therapy. Cancer Treat Rep 61:1403-1405, 1977.

5. Omura G, DiSaia PJ, Blessing J, Boronow R, Hreshchyshyn M, Park R: Chemotherapy of mustard-resistant ovarian adenocarcinoma: A randomized trial of CCNU and methyl-CCNU. Cancer Treat Rep 61:1533-1535, 1977.

6. Gall SA, Creasman WT, Schmidt HJ, DiSaia PJ, Mittelstaedt L, for the Gynecologic Oncology Group: Toxic manifestations following IV corynebacterium administration to patients with ovarian and cervical carcinoma. In press, Am J of Obstet and Gynecol.

NATIONAL SURGICAL ADJUVANT PROJECT FOR BREAST CANCER

1970 - 1978

1. Noer RJ: Breast adjuvant chemotherapy: Effectiveness of thio-TEPA (triethylenethiophosphoramide) as adjuvant to radical mastectomy for breast cancer. Ann of Surg 154:629-647, 1961.

2. Noer RJ: Thio-TEPA with radical mastectomy in the treatment of breast cancer. Am J of Surg 106:405-412, 1963.

3. Cohn I, Slack NH, Fisher B: Complications and toxic manifestations of surgical adjuvant chemotherapy for breast cancer. Surg, Gynecol and Obstet 127:1201-1209, 1968.

4. Fisher B, Ravdin RG, Ausman RK, Slack NH, Moore GE, Noer RJ, and cooperating investigators: Surgical adjuvant chemotherapy in cancer of the breast: Results of a decade of cooperative investigation. Ann of Surg 168:337-356, 1968.

5. Fisher B, Slack NH, Ausman RK, Bross IDJ: Location of breast carcinoma and prognosis. Surg, Gynecol and Obstet 129:705-716, 1969.

6. Fisher B, Slack NH, Bross IDJ and cooperating investigators: Cancer of the Breast: Size of neoplasm and prognosis. Cancer 24:1071-1080, 1969.

7. Fisher B: Prospects for control of metastases. Cancer 24:1286-1289, 1969.

8. Fisher B: Systemic chemotherapy as an adjuvant to surgery in the treatment of breast cancer. Cancer 24:1286-1289, 1969.

9. Fisher B, Ravdin RG, Ausman RK, Slack NH, Moore GE, Noer RJ: Present status of surgical adjuvant chemotherapy in the treatment of breast cancer. In Chemotherapy of Cancer. WH Cole ed. Philadelphia, Pennsylvania: Lea & Febiger, Chapter 9, Section IV, pp. 300-311, 1970.

10. Fisher B, Moore GE, Ravdin RG, Ausman RK, Slack NH, Noer RJ: Surgical adjuvant chemotherapy in the treatment of breast cancer. In Breast Cancer: Early and Late, A Collection of Papers Presented at the Thirteenth Annual Clinical Conference on Cancer, held at the University of Texas M.D. Anderson Hospital and Tumor Institute, Houston, Texas, 1968, Chicago, Illinois: Year Book Medical Publishers, Inc., pp.135-153, 1970.

11. Fisher B, Slack NH: Number of lymph nodes examined and the prognosis of breast carcinoma. Surg, Gynecol and Obstet 131:79-88, 1970.

12. Fisher B, Slack NH, Cavanaugh PJ, Gardner B, Ravdin RG, and cooperating investigators: Post-operative radiotherapy in the treatment of breast cancer: Results of the NSABP Clinical Trial. Ann of Surg 172:711-732, 1970.

13. Ravdin RG, Lewison EF, Slack NH, Dao TL, Gardner B, State D, Fisher B: Results of a clinical trial concerning the worth of prophylactic oophorectomy for breast carcinoma. Surg, Gynecol and Obstet 131:1055-1064, 1970.

14. Fisher B: Present status of the management of regional lymph nodes and planned clinical trials. Am J of Roentgenology, Radium Therapy and Nuclear Med 111:123-129, 1971.

15. Fisher B: Status of adjuvant therapy: Results of the National Surgical Adjuvant Breast Project Studies on oophorectomy, postoperative radiation therapy, and chemotherapy - other comments concerning clinical trials. Cancer 28:1654-1658, 1971.

16. Fisher B: Surgical adjuvant therapy for breast cancer. Cancer 30:1556-1564, 1972.

17. Slack NH, Bross IDJ, Nemoto T, Fisher B: Experiences with bilateral primary carcinoma of the breast. Surg, Gynecol and Obstet 136:433-440, 1973.

18. Fisher ER, Gregorio R, Redmond C, Vellios F, Sommers SC, Fisher B: Pathological findings from the National Surgical Adjuvant Breast Project (Protocol #4) I. Observations concerning the multicentricity of mammary cancer. Cancer 35:247-254, 1975.

19. Fisher B, Carbone P, Economou SG, Frelick R, Glass A, Lerner H, Redmond C, Zelen M, Band P, Katrych DL, Wolmark N, Fisher ER, and other cooperating investigators: L-phenylalanine mustard (L-PAM) in the management of primary breast cancer: A report of early findings. N Eng J Med 292:117-122, 1975.

20. Fisher B, Slack N, Katrych D, Wolmark N: Ten-year follow-up results of patients with carcinoma of the breast in a cooperative clinical trial evaluating surgical adjuvant chemotherapy. Surg, Gynecol and Obstet 140:528-534, 1975.

21. Fisher B, Wolmark N: New concepts in the management of primary breast cancer. Cancer 36:627-632, 1975.

22. Fisher ER, Gregorio RM, Fisher B, with the assistance of Redmond RC, Vellios F, Sommers SC and cooperating investigators: The pathology of invasive breast cancer: A syllabus derived from findings of the National Surgical Adjuvant Breast Project (Protocol #4). Cancer 36:1-85, 1975.

23. Fisher ER, Gregorio R, Fisher B: Prognostic significance of histopathology. In New Aspects of Breast Cancer - Risk Factors in Breast Cancer, Volume 2, BA Stoll ed. London,England: Heinemann Medical Books Ltd., pp.83-109, 1976.

24. Fisher ER, Gregorio R, Redmond C, Dekker A, Fisher B: Pathologic findings from the National Surgical Adjuvant Breast Project (protocol #4) II. The significance of regional node histology other than sinus histiocytosis in invasive mammary cancer. Am J of Clin Pathology 65:21-30, 1976.

25. Fisher B, Rubin H, Sartiano G, Ennis L, Wolmark N: Observations following corynebacterium parvum administration to patients with advanced malignancy: A Phase I study. Cancer 38:119-130, 1976.

26. Fisher ER, Gregorio RM, Redmond C, Kim WS, Fisher B: Pathologic findings from the National Surgical Adjuvant Breast Project (Protocol #4) III. The significance of extranodal extension of axillary metastases. Am J of Clin Pathology 65:439-444, 1976.

27. Fisher B: Some thoughts concerning the primary therapy of breast cancer. In Recent Results In Cancer Research, Vol. 57, G. St.-Arneault, P Band, L Israel eds. Berlin Heidelberg, Germany: Springer-Verlag, pp.150-163, 1976.

28. Fisher B: Results of the prospective study on treatment of breast cancer. In Advances in Cancer Surgery, JS Najarian, JP Delancy eds. New York, New York: Stratton Intercontinental Medical Book Corp., pp.483-488, 1976.

29. Fisher ER, Fisher B: Role of regional lymph nodes. In Secondary Spread in Breast Cancer, BA Stoll, ed. London, England: Heinemann Medical Books Ltd., pp.45-59, 1977.

30. Fisher B: Attempts at combined modality therapy. In Breast Cancer   Management - Early and Late, BA Stoll, ed. London, England: Heinemann Medical Books Ltd., pp.53-56, 1977.

31. Fisher B: Surgery of primary breast cancer. In Breast Cancer: Advances In Research and Treatment - Volume 1: Current Approaches to Therapy, W McGuire, ed. New York, New York: Plenum Publishing Corp., pp.1-42, 1977.

32. Fisher B, Wolmark N: Systemic adjuvant (combined modality) therapy in the treatment of primary breast cancer. In Breast Cancer: Advances in Research and Treatment -Volume 1: Current Approaches to Therapy, WL McGuire, ed. New York, New York: Plenum Publishing Corp., pp.125-163, 1977.

33. Fisher B: Biological and clinical considerations regarding the use of surgery and chemotherapy in the treatment of primary breast cancer. Cancer 40:574-587, 1977.

34. Fisher ER, Fisher B: Relationship of pathologic and some clinical discriminants to the spread of breast cancer. Internat J of Radiat Oncol, Biol and Phys 2:747-750, 1977.

35. Fisher B, Montague E, Redmond C, Barton B, Borland D, Fisher ER, Deutsch M, Schwarz G, Margolese R, Donegan W, Volk H, Konvolinka C, Gardner B, Cohn I, Lesnick G, Cruz A, Lawrence W, Nealon T, Butcher H, Lawton R, and other NSABP investigators: Comparison of radical mastectomy with alternative treatments for primary breast cancer: A first report of results from a prospective randomized clinical trial. Cancer 39:2827-2839, 1977.

36. Fisher B, Glass A, Redmond C, Fisher ER, Barton B, Such E, Carbone P, Economou S, Foster R, Frelick R, Lerner H, Levitt M, Margolese R, Mac Farlane J, Plotkin D, Shibata H, Volk H, and other cooperative investigators: L-Phenylalanine mustard (L-PAM) in the management of primary breast cancer: An update of earlier findings and a comparison with those utilizing L-PAM plus 5-Fluorouracil (5-FU). Cancer 39:3883-3903, 1977.

37. Fisher ER, Redmond C, Fisher B: A perspective concerning the relationship of duration of symptoms to treatment failure in patients with breast cancer. Cancer 40:3160-3167, 1977.

38. Fisher B: Adjuvant chemotherapy in the primary management of breast cancer. Med Clin of North America 61:953-965, 1977.

39. Fisher B: The operative management of primary breast cancer. Internat J of Radiat Oncol, Biol and Phys 2:989-992, 1977.

40. Fisher B, Redmond C, and participating NSABP Investigators: Studies of the National Surgical Adjuvant Breast Project (NSABP). In Adjuvant Therapy of Cancer, SE Salmon, SE Jones, eds. Amsterdam, Netherlands: Elsevier/North-Holland Biomedical Press, pp.67-81, 1977.

41. Fisher B: Combination of loco-regional and systemic therapy in the treatment of primary breast cancer. In Breast Cancer: Progress in Clinical and Biological Research, Volume 12, Proceedings of the International Breast Cancer Conference, held in Lucerne, Switzerland, 1976, ACW Montague, GL Stonesifer, EF Lewison, eds. New York, New York: Alan R. Liss, Inc., pp.387-390, 1977.

42. Fisher B: Results of adjuvant chemotherapy with L-PAM in operable mammary cancer. In Proceedings of the XVII Postgraduate Course on the Cancer of the Breast, Milano, Italy, 1976, U Veronesi, A Perussia, H Emmanuelli, M De Lena, eds. Milano: Casa Editrice Ambrosiana, pp.309-313, 1977.

43. Fisher ER, Gregorio RM, Redmond C, Fisher B: Tubulolobular invasive breast cancer: A variant of lobular invasive cancer. Human Pathology 8:679-683, 1977.

44. Fisher B: Cooperative clinical trials in primary breast cancer: A critical appraisal. Cancer 31:1271-1286, 1977.

45. Fisher B: Adjuvant chemotherapy in breast cancer. Internat J of Radiat Oncol, Biol, and Phys 4:295-298, 1978.

46. Fisher ER, Palekar AS, Gregorio RM, Redmond C, Fisher B: Pathological findings from the National Surgical Adjuvant Breast Project (Protocol #4) IV. Significance of tumor necrosis. Cancer in press.

47. Fisher ER, Palekar A, Rockette H, Redmond C, Fisher B: Pathologic findings from the National Adjuvant Breast Project (Protocol #4) V. Significance of axillary nodal micro and macrometastases. Cancer in press.

48. Fisher ER, Swamidoss S, Lee CH, Rockette H, Redmond C, Fisher B: Detection and significance of occult axillary node metastases in patients with invasive breast cancer. Cancer in press.

POLYCYTHEMIA VERA STUDY GROUP

1968 - 1978

1. Dameshek W: The case for phlebotomy in polycythemia vera. Blood 32:488-491, 1968.

2. Gilbert HS: Problems relating to control of polycythemia vera: The use of alkylating agents. Blood 32:500-505, 1968.

3. Laszlo J: Effective treatment of polycythemia vera with phenylalanine mustard. Blood 32:506, 1968.

4. Osgood EE: The case for 32P treatment in polycythemia vera. Blood 32:492-499, 1968.

5. Wasserman LR: The treatment of polycythemia vera. Blood 32:483-487, 1968.

6. Gilbert HS, Krauss S, Pasternack B, Herbert V, Wasserman LR: Serum vitamin B12 content and unsaturated vitamin B12 binding capacity (UB BC) in myeloproliferative disease. Value in differential diagnosis and as parameters of disease activity. Ann of Intern Med 71:719-729, 1969.

7. Binder RA, Gilbert HS: Muramidase in polycythemia vera. Blood 36:228-232, 1970.

8. Gilbert HS: A reappraisal of the "myeloproliferative disease" concept. Mount Sinai J of Med 4:426-435, 1970.

9. Lau P, Cornwell CG, Williams WJ: Mucopolysaccharide synthesis by human bone marrow in short-term suspension cultures. J Lab Clin Med 76:739, 1970.

10. Brown SM, Gilbert HS, Krauss S, Wasserman LR: Spurious (relative) polycythemia: A nonexistent disease. Amer J of Med 50:200-207, 1971.

11. Pasternack B, Gilbert HS: Planning the duration of long-term survival time studies designed for accrual by cohorts. J Chron Dis 24:681-700, 1971.

12. Silver RT: Polycythemia, in Diagnostic Approaches in Presenting Syndromes. J Barondness, ed. Baltimore: Williams & Wilkins, 1971.

13. Wasserman LR: The management of polycythemia vera. Brit J of Haem 21:371, 1971.

14. Cooper MR, DeChatelet LR, McCall CE, Spurr CL: The activated phagocyte of polycythemia vera. Blood 40:366-374, 1972.

15. Lau P, Gottlieb AJ, Williams W: Mucopolysaccharide sulfation in normal and leukemic leucocytes. Blood 40:725, 1972.

16. Berger, S, Aledort LM, Gilbert HS, Hanson JP, Wasserman LR: Abnormalities of platelet function in patients with polycythemia vera (PV). Cancer Res 33:2683, 1973.

17. Najean Y, et al (Paris): Choice of treatment in polycythemia vera. 1. Efficacy of chemotherapy. La Nouvelle Presse Medicale, 1973.

18. Smith JR, Kay NE: Polycythemia-1973. Laboratory and clinical evaluation. Postgraduate Medicine 54:141-147, 1973.

19. Wasserman LR: Cigarette smoking and secondary polycythemia. JAMA 224:12, 1973.

20. Laszlo J: Recent advances in the management of polycythemia vera and related diseases. Postgraduate Medicine, 1974.

21. Wasserman LR: Polycythemia Vera. Method of Louis R. Wasserman, M.D. In Current Therapy. HF Conn, ed. Philadelphia: WB Saunders Co., 1974.

22. Wasserman LR: Myeloproliferative disorders: A new international study. JAMA. Letter to the Editor, 1974.

23. Berlin NI: Polycythemia vera. Method of Nathaniel I. Berlin. In Current Therapy. HF Conn, ed. Philadelphia: WB Saunders Co, pp.292-294, 1975.

24. Loeb V: Treatment of polycythemia vera. Clinics in Hemat 4:2, 1975.

25. Weinfeld A, et al (Sweden): Megakaryocyte quantifications in relation to thrombokinetics in primary thrombocythaemia and allied diseases. Scand J Haematol, pp.75-81, 1975.

26. Yu T, Weinreb NJ, Wittman R, Wasserman LR: Secondary gout associated with myeloproliferative disorders. Seminars in Arthritis and Rheumatism 5:247, 1975.

27. Seminars in Hematology, Vol. XII No. 4, (October) 1975.

    Berlin NI: Introduction, pp. 335-337.
    Berlin NI: Diagnosis and classification of the polycythemias, pp. 339-351.
    Balcerzak SP, Bromberg PA: Secondary polycythemia, pp. 353-381.
    Weinreb NJ, Shih CF: Spurious polycythemia, pp. 397-407.
    Laszlo J: Myeloproliferative disorders (MPD): Myelofibrosis, myelosclerosis, extramedullary hemato-
        poiesis, undifferentiated MPD and hemorrhagic thrombocythemia, pp. 409-432.
    Ellis JT, Silver RT, Coleman M, Geller SA: The bone marrow in polycythemia vera, pp. 433-444.

28. Seminars in Hematology, Vol. XIII, No. 1 (January) 1976.

    Zanjani ED: Hematopoietic factors in polycythemia vera, pp. 1-12.
    Wurster-Hill D, Whang-Peng J, McIntyre OR, Hsu LY, Hirschhorn K, Modan B, Pisciotta AV, Pierre R,
        Balcerzak SP, Weinfeld A, Murphy S: Cytogenetic studies in polycythemia vera, pp. 13-32.
    Landaw SA: Acute leukemia in polycythemia vera, pp. 33-48.
    Wasserman LR: The treatment of polycythemia vera, pp. 57-77.
    Silverstein MN: The evolution into and the treatment of late stage polycythemia vera, pp. 79-84.

29. Adamson J, Fialkow P, Murphy S, Prchal JF, Steinmann L: Polycythemia vera: Stem cell and probable clonal origin of the disease. N Eng J Med 295:913, 1976.

30. Berlin NI, Wasserman LR: Association between systemically administered radioisotopes and subsequent malignant disease. Cancer 37:1097, 1976.

31. Hoffman R, Zanjani ED, Vila J, Zalusky R, Lutton JD, Wasserman LR: Diamond-blackfan syndrome: Lymphocyte-mediated suppression of erythopoiesis. Science 193:899, 1976.

32. McIntyre RO, Wurster-Hill DH: Mechanisms responsible for the cytogenetic abnormalities encountered in patients with untreated polycythemia vera. Study from the Polycythemia Vera Study Group. Proc 16th Internat Cong Hematol, Kyoto, 5-11, 1976.

33. Hoffman R, Zanjani ED, Lutton JD, Zalusky R, Wasserman LR: Suppression of erythroid colony formation by lymphocytes from patients with aplastic anemia. N Eng J Med 296:10-13, 1977.

34. Pettit RM, Silverstein MN: Polycythemia vera. In Current Therapy. HF Conn, ed. Philadelphia: WB Saunders Co, pp.323-326, 1976.

35. Prchal JD, Adamson JW, Murphy S, Steinman L, Fialkow PJ: Polycythemia vera: Demonstration of normal and abnormal stem cells and characterization of the in vitro response to erythropoietin (ESF). Clin Res 24:442a, 1976.

36. Laszlo J, Huang AT: Diagnosis and management of myeloproliferative disorders. Current Problems in Cancer Vol. II., No. 1, 1977.

37. Silverstein MN: Myeloproliferative diseases. Postgraduate Med 61:206-210, 1977.

38. Weinreb NJ, Wasserman LR: Polycythemia vera: Method of Neal J. Weinreb, M.D. and Louis R. Wasserman, M.D. In Current Therapy. HF Conn, ed. Philadelphia: WB Saunders Co, pp.332, 1977.

39. Weinfeld A: Polycythemia vera terminating in acute leukemia. Scand J Haematol 19:255-272, 1977.

40. Zanjani ED, Poster J, Burlington, Mann LI, Wasserman LR: Liver as the primary site of erythropoietin formation in the fetus. J Lab and Clin Med 89:640, 1977.

41. Zanjani ED, Lutton JD, Hoffman R, Wasserman LR: Erythroid colony formation by polycythemia vera bone marrow in vitro: Dependence on erythropoietin. J of Clin Invest 59:841, 1977.

42. Smith RJ, Landaw SA: Smokers' polycythemia. N Eng J Med, pp.6-10, 1978.

43. Ellis JT, Peterson P: The bone marrow in polycythemia vera. Pathology Annual. Appleton-Century-Croft. (In Press).

44. Hsu LYF, Pinchiarolo D, Gilbert HS, Wittman R, Hirschhorn K: Partial trisomy of the long term arm of chromosome 1 in myelofibrosis and polycythemia vera. Am J of Hematol. In Press.

RADIOTHERAPY ONCOLOGY GROUP

1974-1978

1.   Zelen M: The randomization and stratification of patients to clinical trials. <u>J of Chron Dis</u> 27:365-375, 1974.

2.   Hendrickson F: Radiaton therapy for metastatic tumors. <u>Seminar In Oncology</u>, Vol 2:1, 1975.

3.   Kramer S: Methotrexate and radiation therapy in the treatment of advanced squamous cell carcinoma of the oral cavity, oropharynx, supraglottic larynx and hypopharynx: A preliminary report of a controlled clinical trial of the Radiation Therapy Oncology Group. <u>Can J of Otolaryngology</u> 4:213-218, 1975.

4.   Johnson R, Gomer C, Ambrus J, Pearce J, Boyle D: An investigation of the pharmacological and radiosentizing effects of the 2-nitroimidazole Ro-07-0582 in primates. <u>Br J Radiol</u> 49:294-295, 1976.

5.   Johnson R, Gomer C, Pearce J: An investigation of the radiosensitizing effects of Ro-07-0582 on hypoxic skin in primates. <u>Internat J of Radiat Oncol, Biol and Phys</u> 1:593-599, 1976.

6.   Hendrickson F: The optimum schedule for palliative radiotherapy of metastasis brain cancer. <u>Internat J of Radiat Oncol, Biol and Phys</u> 2:165-168, 1977.

7.   Rubin P, Salazar O, Scarantino C: Systemic radiation of micrometastases in non-oat cell lung cancer: Occult metastases. <u>Internat J of Radiat Oncol, Biol and Phys</u> 2:63-64, 1977.

8.   Rotman M, Moon S, John M, Choi K, Sall S: Extended field para-aortic radiation in cervical carcinoma: The case for prophylactic treatment. <u>Internat J of Radiat Oncol, Biol and Phys</u> 2:88, 1977.

9.   Rotman M, John M, Moon S, Choi K, Moroson H, Sall S: Management of stage IIB carcinoma of the cervix: A study refuting the combining approach. <u>Internat J of Radiat Oncol, Biol and Phys</u> 2:88, 1977.

10.   Johnson R: Gastrointestinal cancer-colon. (Surgery-Radiotherapy). The role of radiation therapy in the management of rectosigmoid cancer. <u>Cancer</u> 40:595-603, 1977.

11.   Berry H: Hepatic metastases revisited. <u>Internat J of Radiat Oncol, Biol and Phys</u> 2:219-220, 1977.

12.   Johnson R, Hetzel F, Sandhu T, Kowal H: The use of either regional or whole-body hyperthermia as an adjunctive treatment with radiotherapy. To be published in the <u>Proceedings of the Conference on the Clinical Prospects for Hypoxic Cell Sensitizers and Hyperthermia</u>, Madison, Wisconsin, September 29-October 1, 1977.

13.   Kowal H, Sandhu T, Johnson R: Applicator design and microwave frequency selection for local hyperthermia/whole-body hyperthermia equipment suitable for clinical treatment. To be published in the <u>Proceedings of the Conference on the Clinical Prospects for Hypoxic Cell Sensitizers and Hyperthermia</u>, Madison, Wisconsin, September 20-October 1, 1977.

14.   Perez CA: Role of radiation therapy and dose optimization in carcinoma of the lung. <u>Internat Assoc for the Studies of Lung Cancer</u>, May, 1978. (In Preparation).

15.   Perez CA: Report on preliminary randomized dose-fractionation study in carcinoma of the lung. ASTR, October, 1978. (In Preparation)

16.   Fazekas J, Davis L, Kramer S: Intravenous methotrexate as an adjuvant to radiotherapy in the treatment of squamous cell carcinoma of the oral cavity, oropharynx, hypopharynx and supraglottic larynx (The first concluding report of a controlled clinical trial of the RTOG). Submitted to <u>Internat J of Radiat Oncol, Biol and Phys</u>.

17.   Rubin P, Marcial V, Hanley J, Mann S, Brady L: The national study on adjunctive oxygen breathing in the radiation treatment of head and neck. Submitted to <u>J of Radiat Oncol, Biol and Phys</u>.

18.   Kramer S: Therapeutic trials in the management of metastatic brain tumors by different time/dose fraction schemes of radiation therapy. To be published as <u>NCI Monograph No. 46</u>.

19.   Snow J, Gelber R, Kramer S, Davis L,, Marcial V, Lawry L: Evaluation of randomized preoperative and postoperative radiation therapy for supraglottic carcinoma: Preliminary report, presented at the American Laryngological Association, 1978. Submitted to <u>Annals of Otology, Rhinology, Laryngology</u>.

20. Kramer S: Postoperative treatment of malignant gliomas by: 1) Standard radiation therapy, 2) High dose radiation therapy, 3) Standard radiation therapy plus BCNU, 4) Standard radiation therapy plus MeCCNU and DTIC. National Cancer Institute Monograph No. 46.

21. Seydel H, Creech R, Mietlowski W, Perez C: Current clinical trials and future prospects in the management of localized small cell undifferentiated carcinoma of the lung. To be published in Seminars in Oncology.

22. Brown G: Primary irradiation of stage I & II adenocarcinoma of the breast. To be published in the Internat J of Radiat Oncol, Biol and Phys.

23. Gomer C, Johnson R, Hetzel F, Lawrence G: The demonstration of In-vivo misonidazole tumor toxicity using post-radiation hypoxia. To be published in the Br J of Cancer, 1978.

24. Marques R, Stafford B, Flynn N, Sadee W: Determination of metronidazole and misonidazole and their metabolites in plasma and urine by high performance liquid chromatography. Submitted to Journal of Chromatography.

25. Johnson R, Wasserman T, Lawrence G, Gomer C, Jain P, Bhaskaran A, Levine M, Sadee W, Phillips T: Initial clinical and pharmacologic evaluation of misonidazole (Ro-07-0582) in the United States, ASTR work-in-progress. October Supplement Internat J of Radiat Oncol, Biol and Phys.

26. Sandu T, Kowal JR: Microwave applicator design for clinical radiotherapy. Accepted for publication in the Internat J of Radiat Oncol, Biol and Phys.

27. Luk KH, Baker DG, Purser P, Castro JR, Manual F: The use of 2450 Megahertz microwave in cancer therapy. Submitted to J of Am Phys Therapy Assoc.

28. Luk KH, Baker DG, Purser P, et al: Potentiation of radiation with hyperthermia: Preliminary report of clinical experience using 2450 megahertz microwave. Works in Progress Session of the 63rd Scientific Assembly. Presented at Radiologic Society of North American, Chicago, Illinois, December, 1977. Submitted to Radiology.

29. Johnson R, Bicher H, Sandhu T, Kowal H, Kishel S: A whole-body hyperthermia unit designed for simultaneous radiotherapy under conditions of oxygen breathing. ASTR Work-in-Progress. October Supplement to the Internat J of Radiat Oncol, Biol and Phys.

30. Hanley J: Language for the computer generation of medical data forms. Biometrics, in press.

31. Lagakos S, Sommer C, Zelen M: Semi-Markov models for partially censored data. Biometrika, in press.

32. Keller B, Mathewson C: Dosimetry guidelines in treatment planning for the oropharynx. University of Rochester Medical Center, Rochester, New York.

33. Keller B, Mathewson C: Dosimetry guidelines in treatment planning for the urinary bladder. University of Rochester Medical Center, Rochester, New York.

34. Rubin P, Keller B: The range of required tumor lethal doses (RTDL) in the treatment of different human tumors. University of Rochester Medical Center, Rochester, New York.

35. Keller B, Grant W, Oliver G, Suntharalingam N, Hooydonk N: Dosimetry guidelines for treatment planning for the RTOG lung cancer protocols. University of Rochester Medical Center, Rochester, New York.

36. Keller B, Grant W: Dosimetry guidelines in treatment planning for rectal cancer. University of Rochester Medical Center, Rochester, New York.

37. Keller B, Grant W: Dosimetry guidelines in treatment planning for abdominal lymphoma. University of Rochester Medical Center, Rochester, New York.

38. Keller B, Grant W, Suntharalingam N: Dosimetry guidelines in treatment planning for brain tumors. University of Rochester Medical Center, Rochester, New York.

39. Keller B, Grant W, Suntharalingam N, Rubin P, Kramer S: Dosimetry guidelines in treatment planning for cancer of the esophagus, stomach and pancreas. University of Rochester Medical Center, Rochester, New York.

40. Keller B, Grant W, Suntharalingham N: Dosimetry guidelines in treatment planning for cancer of the head and neck. University of Rochester Medical Center, Rochester, New York.

41.   Keller B, Suntharalingam N: <u>Dosimetry guidelines</u> in the treatment for breast cancer. University of Rochester Medical Center, Rochester, New York.

42.   Keller B, Suntharalingam N: <u>Dosimetry guidelines</u> in treatment planning for cancer of the ovary. University of Rochester Medical Center, Rochester, New York.

43.   Keller B, Suntharalingam N: <u>Dosimetry guidelines</u> in treatment planning for cancer of the cervix and endometrium. University of Rochester Medical Center, Rochester, New York.

44.   Keller B, Grant W, Suntharalingam N, Rubin P, Kramer S: <u>Standard Treatment Planning Atlas</u>, June 1975.

SOUTHEASTERN CANCER STUDY GROUP

1956-1978

1.   Greenberg BG: Conduct of cooperative field and clinical trials. The American Statistician June, 1959.

2.   Rundles RW, Grizzle J, Bell WN, Corley CC, Frommeyer WB, Greenberg BG, Luguley J, James GW, Jones R, Larsen WE, Loeb V, Leone LA, Palmer JG, Riser WH, Wilson SJ: Comparison of chlorambucil and myleran in chronic lymphocytic and granulocytic leukemia. Am J Med 27:424-432, 1959.

3.   Huguley CM: Long-term study of chronic lymphocytic leukemia: Interim report after 45 months. Cancer Chemother Rep 16:241-244, 1962.

4.   Johnson CB, Frommeyer WB, Hammack WJ, Butterworth CE: 9-ethyl-6-mercaptopurine: Preliminary clinical observations. Cancer Chemother Rep 20:137-141, 1962.

5.   Liebling ME, Grizzle J, Hammack W, Rundles RW: Comparison of chlorambucil and prednisone with urethan and prednisone regimens in the treatment of multiple myeloma. Cancer Chemother Rep 16:253-255, 1962.

6.   Rundles W, Grizzle J, Bono VH, Jonsson U, Huguley CM, Corley CC: Comparison of CB-1348 (chlorambucil, leukeran) and CB-1364. Cancer Chemother Rep 16:223-230, 1962.

7.   Grizzle JE: Tests of linear hypotheses when the data are proportions. Am J Public Health 19:970-976, 1963. New York: American Public Health Association, Inc., 1963.

8.   Hammack WJ, Frommeyer WB: The clinical use of epoxypropidine (eponate) in multiple myeloma. Cancer Chemother Rep, 28:11-12, 1963.

9.   Huguley CM, Grizzle JR, Rundles W, Bell WN, Corley CC, Frommeyer WB, Greenberg BG, Hammack W, Herion JC, James GW, Larsen WE, Loeb V, Leone LA, Palmer JG, Wilson SJ: Comparison of 6-mercaptopurine and busulfan in chronic granulocytic leukemia. Blood 21:89-101, 1968.

10. Lessner H, Jonsson U, Loeb V, Larsen W: Preliminary clinical experience with trimethylcolchininic acid methyl ether d-tartrate (TMCA) in various malignancies. Cancer Chemother Rep 27:33-38, 1963.

11. Grizzle JE: Multivariate comparison of results of treatment in chronic lymphocytic and chronic granulocytic leukemia. J Chron Dis 17:127-152, 1964. Great Britain: Pergamon Press Ltd.

12. Huguley CM, Vogler WR, Lea JW, Corley CC, Lowrey ME: Acute leukemia treated with divided doses of methotrexate. Arch Intern Med 115:23-28, 1965.

13. Vogler WR, Huguley CM, Kerr W: Toxicity and antitumor effect of divided doses of methotrexate. Arch Intern Med 115:285-293, 1965.

14. Corley CC, Lessner HE, Larsen WE, (Writing Committee for the Southeastern Group): Azathioprine therapy for 'autoimmune' diseases. Am J Med 41:404, 1966.

15. Vogler WR, Bain JA, Huguley CM, Palmer HG, Lowrey MD: Metabolic and therapeutic effects of allopurinol in patients with leukemia and gout. Am J Med 40:548-559, 1966.

16. Vogler WR, Huguley CM, Rundles RW, (Writing Committee for the Southeastern Group): Comparison of methotrexate with 6-mercaptopurine-prednisone in the treatment of acute leukemia in adults. Cancer 20:1221, 1967.

17. Lessner HE, (Writing Committee for Southeastern Group): BCNU (1,3,Bis-(B-chloroethyl)-1-nitrosourea) effects on advanced Hodgkin's disease and other neoplasia. Cancer 22:451, 1968.

18. Huguley CM: Survey of current therapy and of problems in chronic leukemia. In Leukemia-Lymphoma. Chicago: Yearbook Medical Publisher, pp.317, 1969.

19. Laszlo J, Durant JR, Loeb V, (Writing Committee for Southeastern Group): Clinical pharmacologic study of 1-acetyl-2-picolinoyl hydrazine. Cancer Chemother Rep 53:131, 1969.

20. Vogler WR, Jacobs J: Toxic and therapeutic effects of methotrexate-folinic acid (leucovorin) in advanced cancer and leukemia. Cancer 28:894, 1971.

21. Vogler WR, (Writing Committee): Clinical trials of 1-B-D-arabinofuranosyl cytosine and 1,3-bis-(2-chloroethyl)-1-nitrosourea combination in metastatic cancer and acute leukemia. Cancer 27:1081, 1971.

22. Huguley CM: The chronic leukemias. In: Current Therapy, HF Conn, ed. Philadelphia: W.B. Saunders Company, pp.286-288, 1972.

23. Huguley CM: Chronic myelocytic and chronic lymphocytic leukemia. Cancer 30:1583, 1972.

24. Vogler WR: Reticulum cell sarcoma and lymphosarcoma. In Current Therapy, HF Conn, ed. Philadelphia: W.B. Saunders Company, pp.288-290, 1972.

25. Durant JR, Lessner HE, (Writing Committee): Development of four-drug BCNU combination chemotherapy regimens. Cancer 32:277, 1973.

26. Durant JR, Lessner HE, Loeb V, Velez-Garcia E: BCNU-cyclophosphamide, therapy for mixed (MLHL) and histiocytic (HL) lymphomas and Hodgkin's disease (HD). Cancer Chemother Rep 57:103-104, 1973.

27. Knospe WH, Loeb V, Huguley CM: Intermittent chlorambucil (CLB) in the therapy of chronic lymphocytic leukemia (CLL). Cancer Chemother Rep 57:100, 1973.

28. Gams RA, Carpenter JT: Central nervous system complications after combination treatment with adriamycin, & 5-(3,3-Dimethyl-1-Triazeno) Imidazone-4-Carboxamide. Cancer Chemother Rep 58:753, 1974.

29. Knospe WH, Loeb V, Huguley CM, (Writing Committee for Southeastern Group): Biweekly chlorambucil treatment of chronic lymphocytic leukemia. Cancer 33:555, 1974.

30. Lessner HE, Vogler WR, (Writing Committee for Southeastern Group): Toxicity study of BCNU given orally. Cancer Chemother Rep 58:407, 1974.

31. Vogler WR, Arkun S, Velez-Garcia E: A Phase I study of twice-weekly 5-azacytidine. Cancer Chemother Rep 58:895-899, 1974.

32. Vogler WR, Chan YK, (Writing Committee for Southeastern Group): Prolonging remission in myeloblastic leukemia by Tice strain Bacillus-Calmette-Guerin (BCG). Lancet 2:128, 1974.

33. Bartolucci AA: A Bayesian plotting solution to the problem of analyzing survival data modeled by the Weibull distribution. Biometrie Praximetrie, 15:137-144, 1975.

34. Durant JR, Loeb V, Doftman RF, Chan YK: BCNU, cyclophosphamide, vincristine, and prednisone (BCOP): A new regimen for diffuse histiocytic lymphoma. Cancer 36:1936-1944, 1975.

35. Grillo-Lopez AJ, Velez-Garcia E, Corcino JJ, Suau LJ: Fluorouracil mitomicina y metil-CCNU en la terapia de cancer gastrointestinal. Boletin Asociacion Medica de Puerto Rico 67:310-311, 1975.

36. Hammack WJ, Huguley CM, Chan YK: Treatment of myeloma: Comparison of melphalan, chlorambucil and azathioprine. Arch Intern Med 135:157, 1975.

37. Hiramoto RN, Ghanta V, Durant JR: Evaluation of a cooperative group human myeloma protocol using the MOPC-104E myeloma model. Cancer Res 35:1309-1313, 1975.

38. Huguley CM, Durant JR, Moores RR, Chan YK, Dorfman R, Johnson LR: A comparison of nitrogen mustard, vincristine, procarbazine, and prednisone (MOPP) vs. nitrogen mustard in advanced Hodgkin's disease. Cancer 36:1227-1240, 1975.

39. Velez-Garcia E, Suau LJ, Lozada J, Grillo-Lopez AJ, Corcino JJ: Treatment of disseminated Hodgkin's disease with a new five-drug chemotherapy regimen. Boletin Asociacion Medica de Puerto Rico 67:318, 1975.

40. Vogler WR, Groth DP, Garwood FA: Cell kinetics in leukemia: Correlation with clinical features and response to chemotherapy. Arch Intern Med 135:950-954, 1975.

41. Durant JR, Omura GA: Cooperative groups and the study of Hodgkin's disease. Hodgkin's Disease, M Lacher, ed. New York: John Wiley and Sons, 1976.

42. Durant JR, Bartolucci AA, Gams RA, Dorfman RF, Velez-Garcia E: Southeastern Cancer Study Group trials with nitrosoureas in Hodgkin's disease. Cancer Treat Rep 60:781-787, 1976.

43. Hocking RR, Speed FM, Lynn MJ: A class of biased estimators in linear regression. Technometrics 18:425-437, 1976.

44. Israeli ZH, Vogler WR, Mingioli ES, Pirkle JL, Smithwick RW, Goldstein JH: The disposition and pharmacokinetics in humans of 5-azacytidine administered intravenously as a bolus or by continuous infusion. Cancer Res 36:1453, 1976.

45. Kansal V, Omura GA, Soong SJ: Prognosis in adult acute myelogenous leukemia related to performance status and other factors. Cancer 38:329, 1976.

46. Kremer WB, Vogler WR, Chan YK: An attempt at synchronization of marrow cells in acute leukemia: Relationship to therapeutic response. Cancer 37:390-402, 1976.

47. Mesel E, Wirtschafter DD, Carpenter JT, Durant JR, Henke C, Gray EA: Clinical algorithms for cancer chemotherapy--systems for community-based consultant-extenders and oncology centers. Meth of Info in Med 15:168-173, 1976.

48. Omura GA: Sequencing of cytosine arabinoside and daunorubicin in acute myelogenous leukemia. Cancer Treat Rep 60:629-663, 1976.

49. Presant CA, Klahr C, Olander J, Gatewood D: Amphotericin-B plus BCNU in advanced cancer -- Phase I and preliminary Phase II results. Cancer 38:1917-1921, 1976.

50. Presant CA, Kolhouse JF, Klahr C: Adriamycin, BCNU, and cyclophosphamide in refractory adenocarcinoma of the breast and other tumors. Cancer 37:620-628, 1976.

51. Smalley RV, murphy S, Huguley CM, Bartolucci AA: Combination versus sequential five-drug chemotherapy in metastatic carcinoma of the breast. Cancer Res 36:3911-3916, 1976.

52. Vogler WR, Kremer WB, Knospe WH, Omura GA, Tornyos K: Synchronization with phase-specific agents in leukemia and correlation with clinical response to chemotherapy. Cancer Treat Rep 60 No. 12, 1976.

53. Vogler WR, Miller DS, Keller JW: 5-azacytidine: A new drug for treatment of myeloblastic leukemia. Blood 48:331-337, 1976.

54. Bartolucci AA, Dickey JJ: Comparative Bayesian and traditional inference for gamma-modeled survival data. Biometrics 33:343-354, 1977.

55. Bartolucci AA, Fraser MD: Comparative step up and composite tests for selecting prognostic indicators associated with survival. Biometrische Zeitschrift, Biometrical Journal 19:437-448, 1977.

56. Durant JR, Gams RA, Bartolucci AA, Dorfman RF: BCNU with and without COP and cycle-active therapy in non-Hodgkin's lymphoma. Cancer Treat Rep 61:1085-1096, 1977.

57. Ghanta VK, Jones MJ, Woodward DA, Durant JR, Hiramoto RN: Cis-dichlorodiamminino platinum (II) in experimental murine myeloma MOPC 104E. Cancer Res 37:771-774, 1977.

58. Huguley CM: Treatment of chronic lymphocytic leukemia. Cancer Treat Rev 4:261-273, 1977.

59. Knospe WH, Gregory SA, Trobauch FE, Stedronsky JA, Schrek R: Chronic lymphocytic leukemia: Correlation of clinical course and therapeutic response with in vitro testing and morphology of lymphocytes. Am J of Hematol 2:73-101, 1977.

60. Lowenbraun S, Bartolucci AA, Krauss S, Smalley RV: Randomized study of cyclophosphamide (CTX) vs. CTX, adriamycin (ADM) and dimethyl triazeno imidazole carboxamide (DTIC) in small cell lung carcinoma (SCLC). Presented at the American College of Physicians meeting, Dallas, Texas, 1977.

61. Moffitt S: Discriminant analysis for directional data. Proceedings of the American Statistical Association 169, 1977.

62. Rassiga AL, Schwartz HJ, Forman WB, Crum ED: Cytosine arabinoside (ara-C) induced anaphylaxis: Demonstration of antibody and successful desensitization. Blood 50:206, 1977.

63. Omura GA, Vogler WR, Smalley RV, Maldonodo N, Broun GO, Knospe WH, Ahn YS, Faguet GB: Phase II study of β-deoxythioguanisone in adult acute leukemia. Cancer Treat Rep, 1977.

64. Ortbals VW, Leibhaver H, Presant CA, VanAmburg AL, Lee J: Influenza immunization of adult patients with malignant diseases. Ann of Intern Med 87:552, 1977.

65. Smalley RV, Vogel J, Huguley CM, Miller DS: Chronic granulocytic leukemia: Cytogenetic conversion of the bone marrow with cycle-specific chemotherapy. Blood 50:107-114, 1977.

66. Smalley RV, Carpenter JT, Bartolucci AA, Vogel CL, Krauss S: A comparison of cyclophosphamide, adriamycin, 5-Fluorouracil (CAF) vs. cyclophosphamide, methotrexate, 5-Fluorouracil, vincristine, prednisone (CMFVP) in patients with metastatic breast cancer. Cancer 40:625-632, 1977.

67. Tabor E, Geretry RJ, Vogel CL, Bayley A, Anthony P, Baker LF: Hepatitis B virus infection and primary hepatocellular carcinoma. J Natl Cancer Inst 50:1197-1200, 1977.

68. Tornyos K, Silberman H, Solomon A: Phase II study of oral methyl-CCNU and prednisone in previously treated alkylating agent-resistant multiple myeloma. Cancer Treat Rep 61:785-787, 1977.

69. Velez-Garcia E: Twice weekly 5-azacytidine infusion in disseminated metastatic cancer-A Phase II study. Cancer Treat Rep 61: No. 9, 1977.

70. Vogel CL, Bayley AC, Brooker RJ, Anthony PP, Zeigler JL: A Phase II study of adriamycin in patients with hepatocellular carcinoma from Zambia and the United States. Cancer 39:1923, 1977.

71. Vogler WR, Gordon DS, Smalley RV, Trulock P: Serial immunologic assessment during a randomized trial of chemo-immunotherapy in acute myeloblastic leukemia (AML). Int Soc of Exp Hematology, 1977.

72. Bartolucci AA, Dickey JM: Coherent inference methods for exponentially modeled survival data with censoring and unknown guarantee time. An invited paper presentation at the Session on Applications of Bayes Methods in the Health Sciences at the Eastern North American Region Biometric Society Meeting in Lexington, Kentucky March 23, 1978.

73. Presant CA, Bartolucci AA, Smalley RV, Vogler WR, and the SECSG: The effect of C-parvum on combination chemotherapy of disseminated malignant melanoma. In Immunotherapy of Cancer, Present Status of Trials in Man, WD Terry and D Windhorst, eds. New York: Raven Press, pp.113, 1978.

74. Balch CM, Murad TM, Soong SJ, Griffin AL, Halpern NB, Maddox WA: A multifactorial analysis of melanoma. I. Prognostic histopathological features comparing Clark's & Breslow's staging methods. Ann of Surg, In Press.

75. Durant JR, Gams RA, Velez-Garcia E, Bartolucci AA, Wirtschafter D, Dorfman RF: BCNU, velban, cyclophosphamide, procarbazine, and prednisone (BCVPP) in advanced Hodgkin's disease. Cancer, In Press.

76. Fradera J, Velez-Garcia E, Maldonado N, de Leon E: Morphologic tumor markers in human lymphomas. Bol Asoc Med de P R, In Press.

77. Lapes M, Rosenzweig M, Barieri B, Joseph R, Smalley RV: Cellular and humor immunity in NHL: Correlation of immunodeficiencies with clinicopathological factors. Am J Clin Pathol, accepted for publication.

78. Vogel CL, Winton EF, Moore MR, Sohner S: Phase I trial of 1, 2:5, 5-dianhydrogalactitol administered intravenously in a weekly schedule. Cancer Treat Rep, In Press.

79. Vogler WR, Kremer WB: Cell kinetics and RNA synthesis in human leukemia. Proc of the Second International Symposium on Pulse Cytophotometry, In Press.

80. Presant CA, Klahr C: Severe myelosuppression from piperazinedione, cyclophosphamide plus DTIC. Cancer.

81. Vogler WR, Bartolucci AA, Omura GA, Miller DS, Smalley RV, Knospe WH, Goldsmith AS, Chan YK, Murphy S: A randomized clinical trial of remission induction, consolidation and chemoimmunotherapy maintenance in adult acute myeloblastic leukemia. Cancer, Immunology and Immunology 3:163, 1978.

SOUTHWEST ONCOLOGY GROUP

ADULT DIVISION

1960-1978

1. Bergsagel DE, Levin WC: A preclusive clinical trial of cyclophosphamide. Cancer Chemother Rep 8:120-134, 1960.

2. Shullenberger CC: Evaluation of the comparative effectiveness of myleran and 6-MP in the management of patients with chronic myelocytic leukemia. Cancer Chemother Rep 16:203-207, 1962.

3. Skinner W, Bergsagel DE, Truax W: Evaluation of new chemotherapeutic agents in treatment of multiple myeloma. VII. M & B 938. Cancer Chemother Rep 28:13-15, 1963.

4. Thurman WG, Bloedow C, Howe CD, Levin WC, Davis P, Lane M, Sullivan MP, Griffith KM: A Phase I study of hydroxyurea. Cancer Chemother Rep 29:103-107, 1963.

5. Alfrey CP, Karjala RJ, Dale SC, Frenkel EP, Lane M: Erythrokinetic abnormalities with administration of hydroxyurea. Cancer Chemother Rep 40:27-30, 1964.

6. Bergsagel DE, Frenkel EP, Alfrey CP, Thurman WG: Megaloblastic erythropoiesis induced by hydroxyurea. Cancer Chemother Rep 40:15-17, 1964.

7. Bickers JN: Phase II studies of hydroxyurea in adults: Carcinoma of the lung. Cancer Chemother Rep 40:45-46, 1964.

8. Bloedow CE: Phase II studies of hydroxyurea in adults: Miscellaneous tumors. Cancer Chemother Rep 40:39-41, 1964.

9. Davis P: Phase II studies of hydroxyurea in adults: Multiple myeloma and lymphoma. Cancer Chemother Rep 40:51-52, 1964.

10. Frenkel EP, Skinner WN, Smiley JD: Studies on a metabolic defect induced by hydroxyurea. Cancer Chemother Rep 40:19-22, 1964.

11. Griffith KM: Hydroxyurea: Results of a Phase I study. Cancer Chemother Rep 40:33-36, 1964.

12. Sears ME: Erythema in areas of previous irradiation in patients treated with hydroxyurea. Cancer Chemother Rep 40:31-32, 1964.

13. Sears ME, Haut A, Eckles N: Melphalan in advanced breast cancer. Cancer Chemother Rep 50:271-279, 1966.

14. Luce JK, Frenkel EP, Vietti TJ, Isassi AA, Hernandez KW, Howard JP: Clinical studies of 6-methyl mercaptopurine riboside in acute leukemia. Cancer Chemother Rep 51:535-546, 1967.

15. Alexanian R, Haut A, Khan AU, Lane M, McKelvey EM, Migliore PU, Stuckey WJ, Wilson HE: Treatment for multiple myeloma, combination chemotherapy with different melphalan dose regimens. JAMA 208:1680-1685, 1969.

16. Bodey GP, Freireich EJ, Monto RW, Hewlett JS: Cytosine arabinoside therapy for acute leukemia in adults. Cancer Chemother Rep Part I 53:59-66, 1969.

17. Costanzi JJ, Coltman CA: Combination chemotherapy using cyclophosphamide, vincristine, methotrexate and 5-Fluorouracil in solid tumors. Cancer 23:589-596, 1969.

18. Frei E, Bickers JN, Hewlett JS, Lane M, Leary WV, Talley RW: Dose schedule and antitumor studies of arabinosyl cytosine. Cancer Res 29:1325-1332, 1969.

19. Monto RW, Talley RW, Caldwell MJ, Levin WC, Guest MM: Observations on the mechanism of hemorrhagic toxicity in mithramycin therapy. Cancer Res 29:697-704, 1969.

20. Luce JK: Chemotherapy for lymphomas: Current status. Leukemia-Lymphoma, A Collection of Papers Presented at the Fourteenth Annual Clinical Conference on Cancer, 1969, M.D. Anderson Hospital and Tumor Institute, Houston. Chicago: Year Book Medical Publishers, pp.295-304, 1970.

21. Luce JK, Thurman WG, Isaacs BL, Talley RW: Clinical trials with the antitumor agent 5-(3,3-dimethyl-1-triazeno)imidazole-4-carboxamide. Cancer Chemother Rep Part I 54:119-123, 1970.

22.   Talley RW: Investigational and practical chemotherapy of solid tumors. Geriatrics pp.113-125, 1970.

23.   Coltman CA, Dudley GM, Lane M, Costanzi JJ, Haut A, Gehan EA: Further clinical studies of combination chemotherapy using cyclophosphamide, vincristine, methotrexate and 5-Fluorouracil in solid tumors. Am J Med Sci 261:73-78, 1971.

24.   Frei E, Luce JK, Loo TL: Phase I and phototoxicity studies of pseudourea. Cancer Chemother Rep Part I 55:91-97, 1971.

25.   Gottlieb JA, Frei E, Luce JK: Dose-schedule studies with hydroxyurea in malignant melanoma. Cancer Chemother Rep Part I 55:277-280, 1971.

26.   Luce JD, Gamble JF, Wilson HE, Monto RW, Isaacs, BL, Palmer RL, Coltman CA, Hewlett JS, Gehan EA, Frei E: Combined cyclophosphamide, vincristine, and prednisone therapy of malignant lymphoma. Cancer 23:306-317, 1971.

27.   Panettiere F, Coltman CA: Phase I experience with emetine hydrochloride as an antitumor agent. Cancer 27:835-841, 1971.

28.   Alexanian R, Bonnet J, Gehan E, Haut A, Hewlett J, Lane M, Monto R, Wilson H: Combination chemotherapy for multiple myeloma. Cancer 30:382-389, 1972.

29.   Frei E, Luce JK, Talley RW, Vaitkevicius VK, Wilson HE: 5-(3,3-dimethyl-1-triazeno)imidazole-4-carboxamide in the treatment of lymphoma. Cancer Chemother Rep Part I 56:667-670, 1972.

30.   Gottlieb JA, Baker I H, Quagliano JM, Luce JK, Whitecar JP, Sinkovics JG, Rivkin SE, Brownlee R, Frei E: Chemotherapy of sarcomas with a combination of adriamycin and dimethyl triazeno imidazole carboxamide. Cancer 30:1632-1638, 1972.

31.   Gottlieb JA, Frei E, Luce JK: An evaluation of the management of patients with cerebral metastases from malignant melanoma. Cancer 29:701-705, 1972.

32.   Rodriguez LH, Finklestein JB, Shullenberger CC, Alexanian R: Bone healing in multiple myeloma with melphalan chemotherapy. Ann Intern Med 76:551-556, 1972.

33.   Whitecar JP, Bodey GP, Freireich EJ, McCredie KB, Hart JS: Cyclophosphamide, vincristine, cytosine arabinoside, and prednisone (COAP) combination chemotherapy for acute leukemia in adults. Cancer Chemother Rep Part I 56:543-550, 1972.

34.   Bonnet JD, Brownlee RW, Vaitkevicius VK, Talley RW: Response of advanced breast cancer to two dosage regimens of 1,3-bis(2-chloroethyl)-1-nitrosourea BCNU. Cancer Chemother Rep Part I 57:231-234, 1973.

35.   Einhorn LH, McBride CM, Luce JK, Caoili E, Gottlieb JA: Intra-arterial infusion therapy with 5-(3,3-dimethyl-1-triazeno) imidazole-4-carboxamide for malignant melanoma. Cancer 32: 749-755, 1973.

36.   Hewlett JS, Bodey GP, Coltman CA, Freireich EJ, Haut A, McCredie KB: Intermittent guanazole therapy in adult acute leukemia. Clin Pharmacol and Ther 14:271-276, 1973.

37.   Luce JK, Frei E, Gehan EA, Coltman CA, Talley R, Monto RW: Chemotherapy of Hodgkin's disease. Arch Intern Med 131:391-395, 1973.

38.   O'Bryan RM, Luce JK, Talley RW, Gottlieb JA, Baker LH, Bonadonna G: Phase II evaluation of adriamycin in human neoplasia. Cancer 32:1-8, 1973.

39.   Panettiere F, Coltman CA: Splenectomy effects on chemotherapy in Hodgkin's disease. Arch Intern Med 131:362-366, 1973.

40.   Rodriguez V, Hart JS, Freireich EJ, Bodey G, McCredie KB, Whitecar JP, Coltman CA: POMP combination chemotherapy of adult acute leukemia. Cancer 32:69-75, 1973.

41.   Spigel SC, Coltman CA, Costanzi JJ: Disseminated breast carcinoma. Arch Intern Med 132:575-577, 1973.

42.   Talley RW, O'Bryan RM, Gutterman JU, Brownlee RW, McCredie KB: Clinical evaluation of toxic effects of cis-diamminedichloroplatinum -- Phase I clinical study. Cancer Chemother Rep Part I 57:465-471, 1973.

43.   Bodey GP, Coltman CA, Freireich EJ, Bonnet JD, Gehan EA, Haut A, Hewlett JS, McCredie KB, Saiki JH, Wilson HE: Chemotherapy of acute leukemia. Arch Intern Med 133:260-266, 1974.

44. Bodey GP, Hewlett JS, Coltman CA, Rodriguez V, Freireich EJ: Therapy of adult acute leukemia with daunorubicin and L-asparaginase. Cancer 33:626-650, 1974.

45. Gottlieb JA: Combination chemotherapy for metastatic sarcoma. Cancer Chemother Rep Part I 58:265-270, 1974.

46. Gottlieb JA, Baker LH, O'Bryan RM, Luce JK, Sinkovics JG, Quagliana JM: Chemotherapy of metastatic sarcomas using combinations with adriamycin. Biochem Pharmacol, pp.183-192, 1974.

47. Gottlieb JA, Rivkin SE, Spigel SC, Hoogstraten B, O'Bryan RM, Delaney FC, Singhakowinta A: Superiority of adriamycin over oral nitrosoureas in patients with advanced breast carcinoma. Cancer 33:519-526, 1974.

48. Levin WC, Mims CH, Haut A: Dibromomannitol: A clinical study of previously treated patients with refractory chronic myelocytic leukemia and blastic transformation. Cancer Chemother Rep Part I 58:223-227, 1974.

49. Southwest Oncology Group: Cytarabine for acute leukemia in adults. Arch Intern Med 133:251-259, 1974.

50. Caoili EM, Talley RW, Smith F, Salem P, Vaitkivicius VK: Guanazole -- a Phase I clinical study. Cancer Chemother Rep Part I 59:1117-1121, 1975.

51. Costanzi JJ, Vaitkevicius VK, Quagliana JM, Hoogstraten B, Coltman CA, Delaney FC: Combination chemotherapy for disseminated malignant melanoma. Cancer 35:342-346, 1975.

52. Gottlieb JA, Baker LH, O'Bryan RM, Sinkovics JG, Hoogstraten B, Quagliana JM, Rivkin SE, Bodey GP, Rodriguez VT, Blumenschein GR, Saiki JH, Coltman CA, Burgess MA, Sullivan P, Thigpen T, Bottomley R, Balcerzak S, Moon TE: Adriamycin used alone and in combination for soft tissue and bony sarcomas. Cancer Chemother Rep Part III 6:271-282, 1975.

53. Hoogstraten B: Adriamycin in the treatment of advanced breast cancer: studies by the Southwest Oncology Group. Cancer Chemother Rep Part III 6:329-334, 1975.

54. Hoogstraten B, Haas CD, Haut A, Talley RW, Rivkin S, Isaacs BL: CCNU and bleomycin in the treatment of cancer: A Southwest Oncology Group study. Med and Pediatr Oncol 1:95-106, 1975.

55. Southwest Oncology Group Study: Remission maintenance therapy for multiple myeloma. Arch Intern Med 135:147-152, 1975.

56. Tranum BL, Haut A, Rivkin S, Weber E, Quagliana JM, Shaw M, Tucker WG, Smith FE, Samson M, Gottlieb J: A Phase II study of methyl CCNU in the treatment of solid tumors and lymphomas: a Southwest Oncology Group Study. Cancer 35:1148-1153, 1975.

57. Tranum BL, Stephens RL, Lehane DE, Hoogstraten B, Lane M, Haut A: Adriamycin plus 5-Fluorouracil: a Phase I study. Cancer Chemother Rep Part I 59:1163-1165, 1975.

58. Tucker WG, Talley RW, Lane M, Bonnett JD: Treatment of adenocarcinoma with combinations of cyclophosphamide, vincristine, and 5-Fluorouracil. Cancer Chemother Rep Part I 59: 425-427, 1975.

59. Baker LH, Talley RW, Matter R, Lehane DE, Ruffner BW, Jones SE, Morrison FS, Stephens RL, Gehan EA, Vaitkevicius VK: Phase III comparison of the treatment of advanced gastrointestinal cancer with bolus weekly 5-FU vs. methyl CCNU plus bolus weekly 5-FU. Cancer 38:1-7, 1976.

60. Baker LH, Vaitkevicius VK, Gehan E: Randomized prospective trial comparing 5-Fluorouracil to 5-Fluorouracil and methyl CCNU in advanced gastrointestinal cancer. Cancer Treat Rep 60:733-737, 1976.

61. Haas CD, Coltman CA, Gottlieb JA, Haut A, Luce JK, Talley RW, Samal B, Wilson HE, Hoogstraten B: Phase II evaluation of bleomycin. Cancer 38:8-12, 1976.

62. Hoogstraten B, George SL, Samal B, Rivkin SE, Costanzi JJ, Bonnet JD, Thigpen T, Braine H: Combination chemotherapy and adriamycin in patients with advanced breast cancer. Cancer 38:13-20, 1976.

63. McKelvey EM, Gottlieb JA, Wilson HE, Haut A, Talley RW, Stephens R, Lane M, Gamble JF, Jones SE, Grozea PN, Gutterman J, Coltman C, Moon TE: Hydroxyldaunomycin (adriamycin) combination chemotherapy in malignant lymphoma. Cancer 38:1484-1493, 1976.

64. Panettiere FJ, Talley RW, Torres J, Lane M: Porfiromycin in the management of epidermoid and transitional cell cancer: A Phase II study. Cancer Treat Rep 60:907-911, 1976.

65. Shaw MT: The cytochemistry of acute leukemia: A diagnostic and prognostic evaluation. Semin in Oncol 3:219-228, 1976.

66. Alexanian R, Salmon S, Bonnet J, Gehan E, Haut A, Weick J: Combination therapy for multiple myeloma. Cancer 40:2765-2771, 1977.

67. Baker LH, Saiki JH, Jones SE, Hewlett JS, Brownlee RW, Stephens RL, Vaitkevicius VK: Adriamycin and 5-Fluorouracil in the treatment of advanced hepatoma: A Southwest Oncology Group study. Cancer Treat Rep 61:1595-97, 1977.

68. Bearden JD, Coltman CA, Moon TE, Costanzi JJ, Saiki JH, Balcerzak SP, Rivkin SE, Morrison FS, Lane M, Spigel SC: Combination chemotherapy using cyclophosphamide, vincristine, methotrexate, 5-Fluorouracil, and prednisone in solid tumors. Cancer 39:21-26, 1977.

69. Herman TS, Jones SE: Systematic restaging in the management of non-Hodgkin's lymphomas. Cancer Treat Rep 61:1009-1015, 1977.

70. Jones SE, Tucker WG, Haut A, Tranum BL, Vaughn C, Chase EM, Durie BGM: Phase II trial of piperazinedione in Hodgkin's disease, non-Hodgkin's lymphoma, and multiple myeloma: A Southwest Oncology Group study. Cancer Treat Rep 61:1617-1621, 1977.

71. Lehane DE, Lane M, Tranum B, Costanzi J, Padilla F: Phase I trial of combination methotrexate and methyl CCNU in patients with advanced neoplastic diseases. Cancer Treat Rep 61:889-891, 1977.

72. Livingston RB, Heilbrun L, Lehane D, Costanzi JJ, Bottomley R, Palmer RL, Stuckey WJ, Hoogstraten B: Comparative trial of combination chemotherapy in extensive squamous carcinoma of the lung: A Southwest Oncology Group study. Cancer Treat Rep 61:1623-1629, 1977.

73. McKelvey EM, Luce JK, Talley RW, Hersh EM, Hewlett JS, Moon TE: Combination chemotherapy with bis chloroethyl nitrosourea (BCNU), vincristine and dimethyl triazeno imidazole carboxamide (DTIC) in disseminated malignant melanoma. Cancer 39:1-4, 1977.

74. McKelvey EM, Luce JK, Vaitkevicius VK, Talley RW, Bodey GP, Lane M, Moon TE: Bis chloroethyl nitrosourea, vincristine, dimethyl triazeno imidazole carboxamide and chlorpromazine combination chemotherapy in disseminated malignant melanoma. Cancer 39:5-10, 1977.

75. McKelvey EM, Moon TE: Curability of non-Hodgkin's lymphomas. Cancer Treat Rep 61:1185-1190, 1977.

76. O'Bryan RM, Baker LH, Gottlieb JE, Rivkin SE, Balcerzak SP, Grumet GN, Salmon SE, Moon TE, Hoogstraten B: Dose response evaluation of adriamycin in human neoplasia. Cancer 39:1940-1948, 1977.

77. Palmer RL, Samal BA, Vaughn CB, Tranum BL: Phase II evaluation of piperazinedione in metastatic breast carcinoma. Cancer Treat Rep 61:1711-1712, 1977.

78. Panettiere FJ, Coltman CA, Delaney FC: Splenectomy, chemotherapy, and survival in Hodgkin's disease. Arch Intern Med 137:341-343, 1977.

79. Quagliana JM, O'Bryan RM, Baker L, Gottlieb J, Morrison FS, Eyre HJ, Tucker WG, Costanzi J: Phase II study of 5-azacytidine in solid tumors. Cancer Treat Rep 61:51-54, 1977.

80. Shaw MT, Raab SO: Adriamycin in combination chemotherapy of adult acute lymphoblastic leukemia: A Southwest Oncology Group study. Med and Ped Oncol 3:261-266, 1977.

81. Thigpen JT, O'Bryan RM, Benjamin RS, Coltman CA: Phase II trial of Baker's antifol in metastatic sarcoma. Cancer Treat Rep 61:1485-1487, 1977.

82. Wilson HE, Bodey GP, Moon TE, Amare M, Bottomley R, Haut A, Hewlett JS, Morrison F, Saiki JH: Adriamycin therapy in previously treated adult acute leukemia. Cancer Treat Rep 61:905-907, 1977.

83. Cecil JW, Quagliana JM, Coltman CA, Al-Sarraf M, Thigpen T, Groppe CW: Evaluation of VP-16-213 in malignant lymphoma and melanoma. Cancer Treat Rep 62:801-803, 1978.

84. George SL, Hoogstraten B: Prognostic factors in the initial response to therapy by patients with advanced breast cancer. J Nat Cancer Inst 60:731-736, 1978.

85. Hoogstraten B, O'Bryan R, Jones S: 1,2:5,6-Dianhydrogalactitol in advanced breast cancer. Cancer Treat Rep 62:841-842, 1978.

86. Livingston RB, Moore TN, Heilbrun L, Bottomley R, Lehane D, Rivkin SE, Thigpen T: Small-cell carcinoma of the lung: Combined chemotherapy and radiation. Ann Intern Med 88:194-199, 1978.

87. McKelvey EM, Hewlett JS, Thigpen T, Whitecar J: Cyclocytidine chemotherapy for malignant melanoma. Cancer Treat Rep 62: 469-471, 1978.

88. O'Bryan RM, Baker L, Whitecar J, Salmon S, Vaughn C, Hoogstraten B: Cyclocytidine in breast cancer. Cancer Treat Rep 62:455-456, 1978.

89. Samal B, Jones S, Brownlee RW, Morrison F, Hoogstraten B, Caoili E, Baker L: Chromomycin A_3 for advanced breast cancer: A Southwest Oncology Group study. Cancer Treat Rep 62:19-22, 1978.

90. Spigel SC, Stephens RL, Haas CD, Jones SE, Lehane D, Moon TE, Coltman CA: Chemotherapy of disseminated germinal tumors of the testis: Comparison of vinblastine and bleomycin with vincristine, bleomycin, and actinomycin-D. Cancer Treat Rep 62: 129-130, 1978.

91. Watt RW, Saiki JH, Tranum BL, Hoogstraten B: Adriamycin and CCNU in advanced breast cancer. A Southwest Oncology Group study. Cancer Clin Trials pp.9-11, 1978.

92. Baker L, Opipari M, Wilson H, Bottomley R, Coltman CA: Mitomycin C, vincristine and bleomycin study of advanced cervical cancer: Phase II. Accepted by Am J of Obstet and Gynecol, 1977.

93. Buroker T, Kim PN, Groppe C, McCracken J, O'Bryan R, Panettiere F, Coltman CA, Bottomley R, Wilson H, Bonnet J, Thigpen T, Vaitkevicius VK, Hoogstraten B, Heilbrun L: 5-FU infusion with mitomycin-C vs. 5-FU infusion with methyl CCNU in the treatment of advanced colon cancer. Cancer 42:1228-1233, 1978.

94. Coltman CA, Bodey GP, Hewlett JS, Haut AB, Bickers JN, Balcerzak SP, Costanzi JJ, Freireich EJ, McCredie KB, Groppe C, Smith TL, Gehan EA: Chemotherapy of acute leukemia: Comparison of vincristine, cytarabine, and prednisone (OAP) alone and in combination with cyclophosphamide (COAP) or daunorubicin (DOAP). Arch Intern Med 138:1342-1348, 1978.

95. Gottlieb JA, Benjamin RS, Baker LH, O'Bryan RM, Sinkovics JG, Hoogstraten B, Quagliana JM, Rivkin SE, Bodey GP Sr, Rodriguez V, Blumenschein GR, Saiki JH, Coltman CA, Burgess MA, Sullivan P, Thigpen T, Bottomley R, Balcerzak S, Moon TE: The role of DIC (dimethyl triazeno imidazole carboxamide, dacarbazine,) in the chemotherapy of sarcomas. Accepted by Cancer Chemother Rep, November 1975.

96. Moore TN, Livingston R, Heilbrun L, Eltringham J, Skinner O, White J, Tesh D: The effectiveness of prophylactic brain irradiation in small cell carcinoma of the lung. Cancer 41:2149-2153, 1978.

97. Tranum B, Hoogstraten B, Kennedy A, Vaughn, CB, Samal B, Thigpen T, Rivkin S, Smith F, Palmer RL, Costanzi J, Tucker WG, Wilson H, Maloney TR: Adriamycin in combination for the treatment of breast cancer. Cancer 41:2078-2083, 1978.

98. Costanzi JJ: Chemotherapy and BCG in the treatment of disseminated malignant melanoma. In Immunotherapy of Cancer: Present Status of Trials in Man pp.87-93, 1978.

99. Haut A, Talley RW: 5-Fluorouracil and azapicyl (1-acetyl-2-picolinoylhydrazine,) in the treatment of adenocarcinoma of the stomach, colon, and rectum. Submitted to Cancer Treat Rep, December, 1976.

100. Hewlett JS, Bodey GP, Wilson HE, Stuckey WJ: 6-Mercaptopurine and 6-methylmercaptopurine riboside combination in the treatment of adult acute leukemia. Cancer Treat Rep 63:1, 1979.

101. Hynes HE, Vaitkevicius VK, O'Bryan RM, Vaughn CB: Phase II trial of dianhydrogalactitol in patients with advanced gastrointestinal cancer. Submitted to Cancer Treat Rep, December, 1977.

102. Padilla F, Vietti T, Lehane D, Whitecar J, Coltman CA: Phase I trial of intravenous thioguanine. Submitted to Cancer Treat Rep, January, 1976.

103. Baker L, Opipari M, Wilson H, Bottomley R, Coltman CA: Mitomycin-C, vincristine and bleomycin therapy for advanced cervical cancer: Phase II. Am J Obstet Gynecol 52:146-150, 1978.

104. Benjamin RS, Baker LH, O'Bryan RM, Moon TE, Gottlieb JA: Chemotherapy for metastatic osteosarcoma: Studies by the M.D. Anderson Hospital and the Southwest Oncology Group. Cancer Treat Rep 62:237-238, 1978.

SOUTHWEST ONCOLOGY GROUP

PEDIATRIC DIVISION

1960-1978

1.   Fernbach DJ, Sutow WW, Thurman WG, Vietti TJ: Preliminary report clinical trials with cyclophos-
     phamide in children with acute leukemia. Cancer Chemother Rep 8:102-105, 1960.

2.   Thurman WG, Fernbach DJ, Holcomb TM, Sutow WW: A "sensitivity spectrum" protocol for evaluating
     multiple agents against solid tumors. Cancer Chemother Rep 12:131-141, 1961.

3.   Thurman WG, Fernbach DJ, Holcomb TM, Sutow WW, Whitaker JA: Clinical trials with AB-100 in
     children with acute leukemia: Preliminary report. Cancer Chemother Rep 12:105-107, 1961.

4.   Fernbach DJ, Sutow WW, Thurman WG, Vietti TJ: Clinical evaluation of cyclophosphamide. A new
     agent for the treatment of children with acute leukemia. JAMA 182:140-147, 1962.

5.   Fernbach DJ, Sutow WW, Thurman WG, Vietti TJ: Clinical trials with cyclophosphamide in the
     treatment of acute leukemia in children. Cancer Chemother Rep 16:173-176, 1962.

6.   Haddy TB, Whitaker JA, Vietti TJ, Riley HD: Clinical trials with cyclophosphamide (cytoxan) in
     children with Wilms' tumor: preliminary report. Cancer Chemother Rep 25:81-85, 1962.

7.   Porter FS, Holowach J, Thurman WG: Uracil mustard therapy in acute leukemia in children. Cancer
     Chemother Rep 18:79-82, 1962.

8.   Porter FS, Thurman WG, Holcomb TM: Actinomycin P_2 therapy for acute leukemia in children.
     Cancer Chemother Rep 25:97-99, 1962.

9.   Sutow WW: Comparative evaluation of ACTH and hydrocortisone used alone and in sequence with 6-
     mercaptopurine in the treatment of acute leukemia in children: preliminary report of a cooperative
     study. Cancer Chemother Rep 16:157-159, 1962.

10. Sutow WW, Haggard ME, Blattner RJ, Porter FS, Bergsagel DE, Griffith KM: Studies of ACTH,
     hydrocortisone, and 6-mercaptopurine in the treatment of children with acute leukemia. J Pediatr
     61:693-701, 1962.

11. Sutow WW, Sullivan MP: Cyclophosphamide therapy in children with Ewing's sarcoma. Cancer
     Chemother Rep 23:55-60, 1962.

12. Thurman WG: Clinical screening of new agents in children with malignant disease. Cancer Chemother
     Rep 16:431-434, 1962.

13. Sullivan MP, Sutow WW, Taylor G: L-Phenylalanine mustard as a treatment for metastatic osteogenic
     sarcoma in children. J Pediatr 63:227-237, 1963.

14. Sutow WW, Thurman WG, Windmiller J: Vincristine (leurocristine) sulfate in the treatment of children
     with metastatic Wilms' tumor. Pediatrics 32:880-887, 1963.

15. Steinberg J, Haddy TB, Porter FS, Thurman WG: Clinical trials with cyclophosphamide in children
     with soft tissue sarcoma. Cancer Chemother Rep 28:39-41, 1963.

16. Thurman WG, Jones B, Sullivan MP, Sutow WW, Whitaker J, Windmiller J: Actinomycin P_2 in
     malignancies in children. Cancer Chemother Rep 28:43-46, 1963.

17. Fernbach DJ: Pediatric clinical trials with hydroxyurea. Cancer Chemother Rep 40:37-38, 1964.

18. Griffith KM: Hydroxyurea: Results of a Phase I study. Cancer Chemother Rep 40:33-36, 1964.

19. Haddy TB, Fernbach DJ, Watkins WL, Sullivan MP, Windmiller J: Vincristine in uncommon malignant
     disease in children. Cancer Chemother Rep 41:41-45, 1964.

20. Holcomb TM, Haggard ME, Windmiller J: Cyclophosphamide in uncommon malignant neoplasms in
     children. Cancer Chemother Rep 36:73-75, 1964.

21. Thurman WG, Fernbach DJ, Sullivan MP: Cyclophosphamide therapy in childhood neuroblastoma. N
     Eng J Med 270:1336-1340, 1964.

22. Thurman WG, Watkins WL: Study of serum B_{12} and folate in patients treated with hydroxyurea. Cancer Chemother Rep 40:23-25, 1964.

23. Vietti TJ, Berry DH, Fernbach DJ, Lusher J, Sutow WW: Uracil mustard therapy in metastatic Wilms' tumor. Am J Dis Child 108:530-532, 1964.

24. Holcomb TM, Berry DH, Haggard ME, Sullivan MP, Watkins WL, Windmiller J: L-Sarcolysin therapy for acute leukemia in children. Cancer Chemother Rep 48:45-48, 1965.

25. Sullivan MP, Fernbach DJ, Haggard ME, Holcomb TM, Lusher J: L-Phenylalanine mustard in uncommon malignant disease in children. Cancer Chemother Rep 45:63-67, 1965.

26. Vietti TJ, Sullivan MP, Berry DH, Haddy TB, Haggard ME, Blattner RJ: The response of acute childhood leukemia to an initial and a second course of prednisone. J Pediatr 66:18-26, 1965.

27. Fernbach DJ, Griffith KM, Haggard ME, Holcomb TM, Sutow WW, Vietti TJ, Windmiller J: Chemotherapy of acute leukemia in childhood. N Eng J Med 275:451-456, 1966.

28. Sutow WW, Berry DH, Haddy TB, Sullivan MP, Watkins WL, Windmiller J: Vincristine sulfate therapy in children with metastatic soft tissue sarcoma. Pediatrics 38:465-472, 1966.

29. Windmiller J, Berry DH, Haddy TB, Vietti TJ, Sutow WW: Vincristine sulfate in the treatment of neuroblastoma in children. Am J Dis Child 111:75-78, 1966.

30. Fernbach DJ: Chemotherapy for acute leukemia in children: Comparison of cyclophosphamide and 6-mercaptopurine. Cancer Chemother Rep 51:381-387, 1967.

31. Haddy TB, Nora AH, Sutow WW, Vietti TJ: Cyclophosphamide treatment for metastatic soft tissue sarcoma. Am J Dis Child 114:301-308, 1967.

32. Haggard ME: Cyclophosphamide in the treatment of children with malignant neoplasms. Cancer Chemother Rep 51:403-405, 1967.

33. Holcomb TM: Cyclophosphamide in the treatment of acute leukemia in children. Cancer Chemother Rep 51:389-392, 1967.

34. Luce JK, Frenkel EP, Vietti TJ, Isassi AA, Hernandez KW, Howard JP: Clinical studies of 6-methylmercaptopurine riboside in acute leukemia. Cancer Chemother Rep 51:535-546, 1967.

35. Milner AN, Sullivan MP: Urinary excretion of cyclophosphamide and its metabolites: Evidence for the existence of an "active" cyclic metabolite. Cancer Chemother Rep 51:343-345, 1967.

36. Sullivan MP: Cyclophosphamide therapy for children with generalized lymphoma and Hodgkin's disease. Cancer Chemother Rep 51:393-396, 1967.

37. Sutow WW: Cyclophosphamide in Wilms' tumor and rhabdomyosarcoma. Cancer Chemother Rep 51:407-409, 1967.

38. Thurman WG, Donaldson MH: Cyclophosphamide therapy for children with neuroblastoma. Cancer Chemother Rep 51:399-401, 1967.

39. Berry DH, Fernbach DJ, Sutow WW, Vietti TJ: Uracil mustard therapy in uncommon malignant neoplasms in children. Cancer Chemother Rep 52:441-443, 1968.

40. Fernbach DJ, Haddy TB, Holcomb TM, Lusher J, Sutow WW, Vietti TJ: Uracil mustard therapy for children with metastatic neuroblastoma. Cancer Chemother Rep 52:287-291, 1968.

41. Fernbach DJ, Haddy TB, Holcomb TM, Stuckey WJ, Sullivan MP, Watkins WL: L-sarcolysin therapy for children with metastatic neuroblastoma. Cancer Chemother Rep 52:293-296, 1968.

42. Haggard ME: Vincristine therapy for acute leukemia in children. Cancer Chemother Rep 52:477-479, 1968.

43. Haggard ME, Fernbach DJ, Holcomb TM, Sutow WW, Vietti TJ, Windmiller J: Vincristine in acute leukemia of childhood. Cancer 22:438-444, 1968.

44. Holton CP, Lonsdale D, Nora AH, Thurman WG, Vietti TJ: Clinical study of daunomycin in children with acute leukemia. Cancer 22:1014-1017, 1968.

45. Lonsdale D, Berry DH, Holcomb TM, Nora AH, Sullivan MP, Thurman WG, Vietti TJ: Chemotherapeutic trials in patients with metastatic retinoblastoma. Cancer Chemother Rep 52:631-634, 1968.

46.   Sullivan MP: Vincristine therapy for Wilms' tumor. Cancer Chemother Rep 52:481-484, 1968.

47.   Sutow WW: Vincristine therapy for malignant solid tumors in children (except Wilms' tumor). Cancer Chemother Rep 52:485-487, 1968.

48.   Sutow WW, Vietti TJ, Fernbach DJ, Lane DM, Donaldson MH, Berry DH: Combination of vincristine and prednisone in therapy of acute leukemia in children. J Pediatr 73:426-430, 1968.

49.   Holton CP, Vietti TJ, Nora AH, Donaldson MH, Stuckey WJ, Watkins WL, Lane DM: Clinical study of daunomycin and prednisone for induction of remission in children with advanced leukemia. N Eng J Med 280:171-174, 1969.

50.   Sullivan MP, Nora AH, Kulapongs P, Lane DM, Windmiller J, Thurman WG: Evaluation of vincristine sulfate and cyclophosphamide chemotherapy for metastatic neuroblastoma. J of Pediatr 44:685-694, 1969.

51.   Sullivan MP, Vietti TJ, Fernbach DJ, Griffith KM, Haddy TB, Watkins WL: Clinical investigations in the treatment of meningeal leukemia: Radiation therapy regimens vs. conventional intrathecal methotrexate. Blood 34:301-319, 1969.

52.   Lane DM, Haggard ME, Lonsdale D, Starling K, Sullivan MP: Remission induction in childhood leukemia with second course vincristine and prednisone therapy. Cancer Chemother Rep Part I 54:113-118, 1970.

53.   Sutow WW, Fernbach DJ, Thurman WG, Holton CP, Watkins WL: Daunomycin in the treatment of metastatic neuroblastoma. Cancer Chemother Rep Part I 54:283-289, 1970.

54.   Vietti TJ, Sullivan MP, Haggard ME, Holcomb TM, Berry DH: Vincristine sulfate and radiation therapy in metastatic Wilms' tumor. Cancer 25:12-20, 1970.

55.   Wang JJ, Selawry OS, Vietti TJ, Body GP: Prolonged infusion of arabinosyl cytosine in childhood leukemia. Cancer 25:1-6, 1970.

56.   Sullivan MP, Vietti TJ, Haggard ME, Donaldson MH, Krall JM, Gehan EA: Remission maintenance therapy for meningeal leukemia: Intrathecal methotrexate vs. intravenous bis-nitrosourea. Blood 38:680-688, 1971.

57.   Sutow WW, Garcia F, Starling KA, Williams TE, Lane DM, Gehan EA: L-asparaginase therapy in children with advanced leukemia. Cancer 28:819-824, 1971.

58.   Sutow WW, Sullivan MP, Wilbur JR, Vietti TJ, Kaizer H, Nagamoto A: L-phenylalanine mustard administration in osteogenic sarcoma: An evaluation of dosage schedules. Cancer Chemother Rep Part I 55:151-157, 1971.

59.   Sutow WW, Wilbur JR, Vietti TJ, Vuthibhagdee P, Fujimoto T, Watanabe A: Evaluation of dosage schedules of mitomycin-C in children. Cancer Chemother Rep Part I 55:285-289, 1971.

60.   Sutow WW, Vietti TJ, Fernbach DJ, Lane DM, Donaldson MH, Lonsdale D: Evaluation of chemotherapy in children with metastatic Ewing's sarcoma and osteogenic sarcoma. Cancer Chemother Rep Part I 55:67-68, 1971.

61.   Vietti TJ, Starling K, Wilbur JR, Lonsdale D, Lane DM: Vincristine, prednisone and daunomycin in acute leukemia of childhood. Cancer 27:602-607, 1971.

62.   Land VJ, Sutow WW, Fernbach DJ, Lane DM, Williams TE: Toxicity of L-asparaginase in children with advanced leukemia. Cancer 30:339-347, 1972.

63.   Sutow WW, Vietti TJ, Lonsdale D, Talley RW: Daunomycin in the treatment of metastatic soft tissue sarcoma in children. Cancer 29:1293-1297, 1972.

64.   Starling KA, Donaldson MH, Haggard ME, Vietti TJ, Sutow WW: Therapy of histiocytosis X with vincristine, vinblastine, and cyclophosphamide. Am J Dis Child 123:105-110, 1972.

65.   Berry DH, Sutow WW, Vietti TJ, Fernbach DJ, Sullivan MP, Haggard ME, Lane DM: Evaluation of uracil mustard in children with Hodgkin's disease, lymphosarcoma, and soft tissue sarcoma. J Clin Pharmacol 12:169-173, 1973.

66.   Dyment PG, Fernbach DJ, Sutow WW: Hexamethylmelamine for acute leukemia and solid tumors in children. J of Clin Pharmacol 13:111-113, 1973.

67. George SL, Fernbach DJ, Vietti TJ, Sullivan MP, Lane DM, Haggard ME, Berry DH, Lonsdale D, Komp D: Factors influencing survival in pediatric acute leukemia. Cancer 32:1542-1553, 1973.

68. Hoogstraten B, Gottlieb JA, Caolili E, Tucker WG, Talley RW, Haut A: CCNU (1-[2-choroethyl]-3-cyclohexyl-l-nitrosourea) in the treatment of cancer. Phase II study. Cancer 32:38-43, 1973.

69. Land VJ, Dyment PG, Komp D, Humphrey GB, Sullivan MP, Starling KA: 5-Fluorouracil and actinomycin D in the treatment of acute leukemia in children. Cancer Chemother Rep Part I 57:335-339, 1973.

70. Komp DM, Britton HA, Vietti TJ, Humphrey GB: Response of childhood histiocytosis X to procarbazine. Cancer Chemother Rep Part I 58:719-722, 1974.

71. Land VJ, Falletta JM, McMillan CW, Williams TE: Guanazole in the treatment of childhood leukemia. Cancer Chemother Rep Part I 58:715-717, 1974.

72. Starling KA, Sutow WW, Donaldson MH, Land VJ, Lane DM: Drug trials in neuroblastoma: Cyclophosphamide alone; vincristine plus cyclophosphamide; 6-mercaptopurine plus 6-methylmercaptopurine riboside; and cytosine arabinoside alone. Cancer Chemother Rep Part I 58:683-688, 1974.

73. Berry DH, Pullen J, George S, Vietti TJ, Sullivan MP, Fernbach D: Comparison of prednisone, vincristine, methotrexate, and 6-mercaptopurine vs. vincristine and prednisone induction therapy in childhood acute leukemia. Cancer 36:98-102, 1975.

74. Fernbach DJ, George SL, Sutow WW, Ragab AH, Lane DM, Haggard ME, Lonsdale D: Long-term results of reinforcement therapy in children with acute leukemia. Cancer 36:1552-1559, 1975.

75. Humphrey GB, Fernbach DJ, Razek AA, Stuckey WJ, Komp D, George S: Evaluation of daunorubicin and methotrexate in combination as a remission maintenance regimen in the treatment of acute leukemia. Cancer Chemother Rep Part I 59:395-399, 1975.

76. Komp DM, Land VJ, Nitschke R, Cangir A, Dyment P: 5-[3,3-Bis(2-chloroethyl)-1-triazeno]imidazole-4-carboxamide in the treatment of childhood malignancy. Cancer Chemother Rep Part I 59:371-376, 1975.

77. Lonsdale D, Gehan EA, Fernbach DJ, Sullivan MP, Lane DM, Ragab AH: Interrupted vs. continued maintenance therapy in childhood acute leukemia. Cancer 36:341-352, 1975.

78. Pullen DJ, Dyment PG, Humphrey GB, Lane DM, Ragab AH: Combined chemotherapy in childhood rhabdomyosarcoma. Cancer Chemother Rep Part I 59:359-365, 1975.

79. Ragab AH, Sutow WW, Komp DM, Starling KA, Lyon GM, George S: Adriamycin in the treatment of childhood solid tumors. Cancer 36:1561-1571, 1975.

80. Starling KA, Berry DH, Britton HA, Humphrey GB, Vats T, Ragab AH: Three dose regimens of adriamycin for induction of remission in acute leukemia in children: A Southwest Oncology Group Study. Med Pediatr Oncol 1:271-276, 1975.

81. Sullivan MP, Humphrey GB, Vietti TJ, Haggard ME, Lee E: Superiority of conventional intrathecal methotrexate therapy with maintenance over intensive intrathecal methotrexate therapy, unmaintained, or radiotherapy (2000-2500 rads tumor dose) in treatment for meningeal leukemia. Cancer 35:1066-1073, 1975.

82. Sutow WW, Komp D, Vietti TJ, Pinkerton D: Clinical trials with 1-acetyl-2-picolinoylhydrazine in children. Cancer Chemother Rep Part I 59:341-344, 1975.

83. Sutow WW, Sullivan MP, Fernbach DJ, Cangir A, George SL: Adjuvant chemotherapy in primary treatment of osteogenic sarcoma. Cancer 36:1598-1602, 1975.

84. Cangir A, Morgan SK, Land VJ, Pullen J, Starling KA, Nitschke R: Combination chemotherapy with adriamycin and dimethyl triazeno imidazole carboxamide (DTIC) in children with metastatic solid tumors. Med Pediatr Oncol 2:183-190, 1976.

85. D'Angio GJ, Evans AE, Breslow N, Beckwith B, Bishop H, Feigl P, Goodwin W, Leape LL, Sinks LF, Sutow W, Tefft M, Wolff J: The treatment of Wilm's tumor. Cancer 38:633-646, 1976.

86. Komp DM, George SL, Falletta J, Land VJ, Starling KA, Humphrey GB, Lowman J: Cyclophosphamide-asparaginase-vincristine-prednisone induction therapy in childhood acute lymphocytic and nonlymphocytic leukemia. Cancer 37:1243-1247, 1976.

87. Sutow WW, Gehan EA, Vietti TJ, Frias AE, Dyment PG: Multidrug chemotherapy in primary treatment of osteosarcoma. J Bone Joint Surg 58:629-633, 1976.

88. Sutow WW, George S, Lowman JT, Starling KA, Humphrey GB, Haggard ME, Vietti TJ: Evaluation of dose and schedule of L-asparaginase in multidrug therapy of childhood leukemia. Med Pediatr Oncol 2:387-395, 1976.

89. Sutow WW, Thomas D, Steuber CP, Pullen J, Vats T, Bryan JH, Morgan SK: Study of cytosine arabinoside synchronization plus vincristine, prednisone, and L-asparaginase for remission induction in advanced acute leukemia in children. Cancer Treat Rep 60:591-594, 1976.

90. Haggard ME, Cangir A, Ragab AH, Komp D, Falletta J, Humphrey GB: 5-Fluorouracil in childhood solid tumors. Cancer Treat Rep 61:69-71, 1977.

91. Komp DM, Silva-Sosa M, Miale T, Sexauer C, Herson J: Evaluation of a MOPP-type regimen in histiocytosis X: A Southwest Oncology Group study. Cancer Treat Rep 61:855-859, 1977.

92. Komp DM, Vietti TJ, Berry DH, Starling KA, Haggard ME, George SL: Combination chemotherapy in histiocytosis X. A Southwest Oncology Group study. Med Pediatr Oncol 3:267-273, 1977.

93. Lane DM, George SL, Komp D, Lonsdale D, Pullen J, Ragab A, Starling KA: Effects of continuous or discontinuous maintenance therapy on subsequent remission maintenance in childhood leukemia. Cancer 40:2005-2009, 1977.

94. Sexauer CL, Morgan S, van Eys J, Komp DM: Phase II trial of asaley in children with late-stage acute lymphocytic leukemia. Cancer Treat Rep 61:1373-1374, 1977.

95. Shaw MT, Humphrey GB, Lawrence R, Fischer DB: Lack of prognostic value of the periodic acid-schiff reaction and blast cell size in childhood acute lymphocytic leukemia. Am J Hematol 2:237-243, 1977.

96. Sullivan MP, Moon TE, Trueworthy R, Vietti TJ, Humphrey GB, Komp D: Combination intrathecal therapy for meningeal leukemia: Two versus three drugs. Blood 50:471-479, 1977.

97. Nitschke R, Komp DM, Morgan SK, Starling KA, Vietti TJ: Toxicity study of cytosine arabinoside and methotrexate in the maintenance therapy of childhood leukemia. A Southwest Oncology Group study. J Clin Pharmacol 18:131-135, 1978.

98. Nitschke R, Starling KA, Vats T, Bryan H: Cis-diamminedichloroplatinum in childhood malignancies. A Southwest Oncology Group study. Med Pediatr Oncol 4:127-132, 1978.

99. Sutow WW, Gehan EA, Dyment PG, Vietti T, Miale T: Multidrug adjuvant chemotherapy for osteosarcoma: Interim report of the Southwest Oncology Group studies. Cancer Treat Rep 62:265-269, 1978.

100. Cangir A, van Eys J, Berry DH, Hvizdala E, Morgan SK: Combination chemotherapy with MOPP in children with recurrent brain tumors. Accepted by Med Pediatr Oncol, December, 1977.

101. Steuber CP, Humphrey GB, McMillan CW, Vietti TJ: Remission induction in acute myelogenous leukemia using cytosine arabinoside synchronization. Med Pediatr Oncol, 4:337-342, 1978.

102. Trueworthy RC, Sutow WW, Pullen J, Komp DM, Berry DH: Repeated use of L-asparaginase in multidrug therapy of childhood leukemia. Accepted by Med Pediatr Oncol, September, 1978.

103. Padilla F, Vietti T, Lehane D, Whitecar J, Coltman CA: Phase I trial of intravenous thioguanine. Submitted to Cancer Treat Rep, January, 1976.

104. Tefft M: Radiation related toxicities in National Wilm's Tumor Study #1. Int J Radiat Oncol Biol Phys 2:455-468, 1977.

105. Bishop HC, Tefft M, Evans AE, D'Angio GJ: Bilateral Wilm's tumor: Review of 30 National Wilm's Tumor Study Cases. Pediatr Surg 12:631-638, 1977.

106. O'Bryan RM, Baker LH, Gottlieb JE, Rivkin SE, Balcerzak SP, Grumet GN, Salmon SE, Moon TE, Hoogstraten B: Dose response evaluation of adriamycin in human neoplasia. Cancer 39:1940-1948, 1977.

107. Baum E, Land VJ, Joo P, Starling KA, Leikin S, Miale T, Krivit W, Miller D, Chard R, Nesbit ME, Sather H, Hammond D: Cessation of chemotherapy (CH) during complete remission (CR) of childhood acute lymphocytic leukemia (ALL). ASCO 18:290, 1977.

108. Smith SD, Trueworthy RC, Lowman JT: Evaluation of compliance in children with malignancies. AACR 18:243, 1977.

109. Quagliana JM, O'Bryan RM, Baker L, Gottlieb JE, Morrison FS, Eyre HJ, Tucker WG, Costanzi J: Phase II study of 5-azacytidine in solid tumors. Cancer Treat Rep 61:51-54, 1977.

110. Tefft M, Fernandez C, Moon TE (For the IRS Committee): Rhabdomyosarcoma: Response with chemotherapy prior to radiation in patients with gross residual disease. Cancer 39:665-670, 1977.

111. Lawrence W, Hays DM, Moon TE (For the IRS Committee): Lymphatic metastasis with childhood rhabdomyosarcoma. Cancer 556-559, 1977.

112. Maurer HM, Moon TE, Donaldson M, Fernandez C, Gehan EA, Hammond D, Hays DM, Lawrence W, Newton W, Ragab A, Raney B, Soule EH, Sutow WW, Tefft M: The Intergroup Rhabdomyosarcoma Study: A preliminary report. Cancer 40:2015-2026, 1977.

113. Hays DM, Sutow WW, Lawrence W, Moon TE, Tefft M (For the IRS Committee): Rhabdomyosarcoma: Surgical therapy for the extremity lesions of children. Ortho Clin N Amer 8:883-902, 1977.

114. Razek A, Perez CA, Tefft M, Burgert O, Griffin P, Gehan EA, Kissane J, Vietti TJ, Nesbit ME: The role of radiotherapy in the Intergroups Ewing's Sarcoma Study. Inter J Radiat Oncol Biol Phys 2:110, 1977.

115. Perez CA, Razek A, Tefft M, Nesbit NE, Burgert EO, Kissane J, Vietti TJ, Gehan EA: Analysis of local tumor control in Ewing's sarcoma. Preliminary results of a cooperative intergroup study. Cancer 40:2864-2873, 1977.

116. Komp DM, Silva-Sosa M, Miale T, Sexauer C, Herson J: Evaluation of a MOPP-Type regimen in histiocytosis X: A Southwest Oncology Group Study. Cancer Treat Rep 61:855-859, 1977.

117. Breslow N, Palmer N, Hill L, Buring M, D'Angio GJ: Wilm's tumor: Prognostic factors for patients without metastases at diagnosis. Cancer 41:1577-1589, 1978.

118. Leape LL, Breslow N, Bishop HC: The surgical treatment of Wilm's tumor: Results of the National Wilm's Tumor Study. Ann Surg 187:351, 1978.

119. Beckwith JB, Palmer N: Histopathology and prognosis of Wilm's tumor. Results of the National Wilm's Tumor Study. Cancer 41:1937-1948, 1978.

120. The National Wilm's Tumor Study: A report fom Cancer Cooperative Study Group. National Wilm's Tumor Study Committee. Cancer Clin Trials 1:61-65, 1978.

121. D'Angio GJ, Tefft M, Breslow N, Meyer J: Radiation therapy of Wilm's tumor: Results according to dose, field, post-operative timing and histology. Int J Oncol Biol Phys 4:769-780, 1978.

122. Saiki JH, McCredie KB, Vietti TJ, Hewlett JS, Morrison FS, Costanzi JJ, Stuckey WJ, Whitecar J, Hoogstraten B: 5-Azacytidine in acute leukemias: A Southwest Oncology Group Study: Cancer 42:2111-2114, 1978.

123. Soule EH, Newton W, Moon TE, Tefft M (for the IRS Committee): Extra-skeletal Ewing's sarcoma: A preliminary review of 26 cases encountered in the Intergroup Rhabdomyosarcoma study. Cancer 42:259-264, 1978.

124. Tefft M, Fernandez C, Donaldson M, Newton W, Moon TE: Incidence of meningeal involvement by rhabdomyosarcoma of the head and neck in children: A report of the Intergroup Rhabdomyosarcoma Study (IRS). Cancer 242:253-258, 1978.

125. Maurer HM, Donaldson M, Gehan EA, Hammond D, Hays DM, Lawrence W, Lindberg R, Moon TE, Newton W, Ragab A, Raney B, Ruymann F, Soule EH, Sutow W, Tefft M: Rhabdomyosarcoma in Childhood and Adolescence. Curr Prob Cancer 11:March, 1978.

126. Hays D: Intergroup Rhabdomyosarcoma Study (IRS): Am Pediatr Surg Assoc, Newsletter, Aug. 1978.

127. Raney RB, Hays DM, Lawrence W, Moon T, Tefft M (For the IRS Committee): Paratesticular rhabdomyosarcoma in childhood. Cancer 42:729-736, 1978.

128. Tefft M, Razek A, Perez C, Burgert EO, Gehan EA, Griffin P, Kissane J, Vietti TJ, Nesbit ME: Local control and survival related to radiation dose and volume and to chemotherapy in non-metastatic Ewing's sarcoma of pelvic bones. Int J Radiat Oncol Biol Phys 4:367-372, 1978.

129. Lane VJ, Askin FB, Ragab AH, Frankel L: "Late" occult leukemic infiltration of the testes. Blood 52:258, 1978.

VETERAN'S ADMINISTRATION

LUNG CANCER STUDY GROUP

1958 - 1978

1. Kaung D, Walsh S, Sbar S, Patno ME: Hydroxyurea in bronchogenic carcinoma. Cancer Chemother Rep 52: 271-274, 1958.

2. Ferguson DJ, Humphrey EW: 5-Fluorouracil. Cancer Chemother Rep 8: 153, 1960.

3. Ferguson DJ, Humphrey E: Mitomycin C. Cancer Chemother Rep 8: 154, 1960.

4. McCracken S, Wolf J: Preliminary clinical investigation of AB-100. Cancer Chemother Rep 6:52, 1960.

5. Wolf J, Spear PW, Yesner R, Patno ME: Nitrogen mustard and the steroid hormones in the treatment of inoperable bronchogenic carcinoma. Am J Med 29: 1008, 1960.

6. Humphrey EW, Blank N: Clinical experience with streptonigrin. Cancer Chemother Rep 12: 99, 1961.

7. Humphrey EW, Dietrich FS: Clinical experience with the methyl ester of streptonigrin. Cancer Chemother Rep 33: 21, 1963.

8. Spear PW: Clinical trials with mithramycin. Cancer Chemother Rep 29: 109, 1963.

9. Yesner R, Amatruda TT, Rich BL, Gallagher W, Goodman A: Histological type and endocrine manifestations of lung cancer. Clin Res 11: 213, 1963.

10. Bolton BH, Kaung DT, Lawton RL, Woods LA: Hydroxyurea A Phase I study. Cancer Chemother Rep 39:47, 1964.

11. Hyde L, Yee J, Wilson R, Patno ME: Cell type and the natural history of lung cancer. JAMA 193: 52-54, 1965.

12. McCracken S, Aboody A: Continuous intravenous infusion of steptonigrin in patients with bronchogenic carcinoma. Cancer Chemother Rep 46: 23, 1965.

13. Wolf J: Controlled studies of the therapy of nonresectable cancer of the lung: I Methodology. Ann Thorac Surg 1:25, 1965.

14. Yesner R, Gerstle B, Auerbach O: Application of the World Health Organization classification of lung carcinoma to biopsy material. Ann Thorac Surg 1:33, 1965.

15. Wolf J, Higgins G: Chemotherapy in lung cancer. Present status. J Thorac Cardiov Surg 51:449, 1966.

16. Wolf J, Patno ME, Roswit B, D'Esopo N: Controlled study of survival of patients with clinically inoperable lung cancer treated with radiation therapy. Am J Med 40:360, 1966.

17. Auerbach O, Stout AP, Hammond EC, Garfinkel L: Multiple primary bronchial carcinomas. Cancer 20:699-705, 1967.

18. Wolf J: Management of the patient with inoperable bronchogenic cancer. Med Clin N Am 51:563, 1967.

19. Green R, Humphrey E, Close H, Patno ME: Alkylating agents in bronchogenic carcinoma. Am J Med 45:516, 1969.

20. Fink A, Finegold S, Patno ME, Close H, Whittington R: Vinblastine sulfate in the treatment of bronchogenic carcinoma. Cancer Chemother Rep Part I, Vol. 54, No. 6, December 1970.

21. Yesner R, Gelfman NA, Feinstein AR: Correlation of histopathology with manifestations and outcome of lung cancer. JAMA, 211:2081-2086, 1970.

22. Kaung D, Sbar S, Patno ME: Treatment of nonresectable cancer of the lung with hydroxyurea given intermittently. Cancer Chemother Rep 55, Part I, No. 1, February 1971.

23. Mizgerd J, Amick R, Hilal H, Patno ME: Imidazole carboxamide in carcinoma of the lung. Cancer Chemother Rep 55, Part 1, No 1, February 1971.

24. Whittington R, Fairly J, Majima H, Patno ME, Prentice R: BCNU in the treatment of bronchogenic carcinoma. Cancer Chemother Rep 56, Part I, , No 6, December 1972.

25. Kaung D, Wolf J, Hyde L, Zelen M: Preliminary report on the treatment of nonresectable cancer of the lung. Cancer Chemother Rep 38:359-364, 1974.

26. Edlis H, Goudsmit A, Brindley C, Niemetz J: A trial of heparin and cyclophosphamide in lung cancer. Cancer Treat Rep Vol. 60, No. 5, May 1976.

27. Gerstl B, Wong S, Yesner R: Quantitative microscopy of epidermoid lung carcinoma: Correlation with survival time. J of Natl Cancer Inst 56:463-469, 1976.

28. Hyde L, Wolf J, Phillips RW: Combination therapy in lung cancer. JAMA 236: 2480, 1976.

29. Morris JF, Haas H: Sequential chemotherapy for bronchogenic carcinoma. Am Rev Resp Disease 115:142, 1977.

30. Petrovich Z, Mietlowski W, Ohanian M, Cox J: Clinical report on the treatment of locally advanced lung cancer. Cancer 40:72-77, 1977.

31. Yesner R: Nomenclature of lung cancer as a basis for chemotherapy. J Acad Med Sci, SSSR, 3, 3-6, 1976.

32. Rohwedder J, Sagastume E: Heparin and polychemotherapy for treatment of lung cancer. Cancer Treat Rep 61:1399-1401, 1977.

33. Wolf J: Chemotherapy for carcinoma of the lung. In Advances Chemotherapy, E Greenspan, ed. New York: Raven Press, 1977.

34. Brindley C, Griffin J, Williams JS, Wolf J: An analysis of comparative trials of L-asparaginase, cyclophosphamide and placebo in patients with inoperable bronchogenic carcinoma using corrected survival estimates. Oncology 35, February 1978.

35. Hyde L, Wolf J, Phillips RW, et al: Combined chemotherapy for squamous cell carcinoma of the lung. Accepted by Chest.

VETERAN'S ADMINISTRATION

SURGICAL ADJUVANT CANCER CHEMOTHERAPY GROUP

1960 - 1978

1. Lee L: Cancer chemotherapy in the clinical services of the Veterans Administration. Cancer Chemother Rep 7:46, 1960.

2. VA Surgical Adjuvant Cancer Chemotherapy Study Group: Status of adjuvant cancer chemotherapy - a preliminary report of cooperative studies in the Veterans Administration. Arch Surg 82:466, 1961.

3. Higgins G, Serlin O, Hughes F, Dwight RW: The Veterans Administration Surgical Adjuvant Group - Interim report. Cancer Chemother Rep 16:141, 1962.

4. Higgins G: Evaluation of chemotherapeutic agents as adjuvants to surgery in twenty-two Veterans Administration hospitals: Experimental design. Cancer Chemother Rep 20:81, 1962.

5. Hughes F, Higgins G: Veterans Administration adjuvant lung cancer chemotherapy study progress report. J Thor and Cardio Surg 44:295-308, 1962.

6. VA Surgical Adjuvant Cancer Chemotherapy Study Group: The use of 5-fluoro-2'-deoxyuridine as a surgical adjuvant in carcinoma of the stomach and colon-rectum. Cancer Chemother Rep 24:35, 1962.

7. Humphrey EW, Dietrich FS: Clinical experience with the methyl ester of streptonigrin. Cancer Chemother Rep 33:21, 1963.

8. Higgins G: The use of 5-fluorodeosyuridine (FUDR) as a surgical adjuvant in carcinoma of the stomach and colorectum. Arch Surg 86:926, 1963.

9. Preston F, Nora, PF: Chemotherapy as an adjunct to surgery in the treatment of cancer. Surg Clin N Am, February, 1963.

10. Lawton RL: Jet injection of drugs into malignant neoplasma. Cancer Chemother Rep 37:57, 1964.

11. Lawton RL, Taylor JC, Latourette HB: Metastatic retinoblastoma treated with radiation and continuous intraarterial infusion of triethylenemelamine. Cancer Chemother Rep 38:61, 1964.

12. Lawton RL, Bolton BH, Kaung DT, Woods LA: Hydroxyurea -A Phase I study. Cancer Chemother Rep 39:37, 1964.

13. Dwight RW: Adjuvant chemotherapy in cancer of the large bowel - An interim report of the VA Surgical Adjuvant Cancer Chemotherapy Study. Am J Surg 107:609, 1964.

14. Higgins GA, Flynn T, Gillespie J: The effect of splenectomy on the tolerance to thio-TEPA. Arch Surg 88:627, 1964.

15. Rogers L: Cancer chemotherapy by continuous intraarterial infusion. Cancer 17:1365, 1964.

16. Higgins GA, Souryal T, Gillespie JF: Effect of splenectomy on tolerance to flourinated pyrimidines. Cancer 18:843, 1965.

17. Lawton RL: Cancer chemotherapy of the gastrointestinal tract with reference to intraarterial infusion and irradiation. Am J Surg 109:47, 1965.

18. Serlin O: The use of thio-TEPA as an adjuvant to the surgical management of carcinoma of the stomach. Cancer 18:291, 1965.

19. VA Adjuvant Cancer Chemotherapy Study Group: Adjuvant use of HN and thio-TEPA. Cancer Chemother Rep 44:27, 1965.

20. Lawton RL, Latourette HB, Collier RG: Simultaneous high energy irradiation and chemotherapy: Rationale, technique and results. Arch Surg 91:155, 1965.

21. Preston FW, Nora PF, Kukral JC, Soper T: Intraarterial infusion of streptonigrin in advanced cancer. Cancer Chemo Rep 48:41, 1965.

22. Higgins GA: Chemotherapy and lung cancer. Ann of Thoracic Surg 1:809, 1965.

23. Lawton RL, Rossi NP, Latourette HB, Flynn JR: Preoperative irradiation in the treatment of clinically operable lung cancers. J of Thor and Cardiovas Surg 51:745, 1966.

24. Preston FW, Apostol JV, Nora P: The treatment of solid tumors with vinblastine sulfate administered by arterial infusion. Cancer Chemother Rep 50:573, 1966.

25. Higgins GA, Wolf J: Chemotherapy and lung cancer - present status. J Thor and Cardiovas Surg 51:449, 1966.

26. Hughes FA, Higgins GA, Beebe GW: A report on chemotherapy as an adjuvant to pulmonary resection for lung cancer. JAMA 196:343, 1966.

27. Higgins GA, Beebe GW: Bronchogenic carcinoma - Factors in survival. Arch Surg 94:539, 1967.

28. Higgins GA: Preoperative irradiation for lung carcinoma: The VA national study. In Cancer Therapy by Integrated Radiation and Operation. Springfield, Ill: Charles C Thomas, p.83, 1968.

29. Higgins GA: Preoperative irradiation for colorectal carcinoma: VA national study. In Cancer Therapy by Integrated Radiation and Operation. Springfield, Ill: Charles C Thomas, p.107, 1968.

30. Higgins GA, Lawton RL, Heilbrunn A, Keehn RJ: Prognostic factors in lung cancer. Ann of Thoracic Surg 7:472, 1969.

31. Higgins GA, Dwight RW, Humphrey E, Walsh WS: Preoperative irradiation therapy as an adjuvant to surgery for carcinoma of the colon and rectum. Am J Surg 115:241, 1968.

32. Dwight RW, Higgins GA, Keehn RJ: Factors influencing survival following resection in cancer of the colon and rectum. Am J Surg 117:512-522, 1969.

33. Green R, Humphrey EW, Close H, Patno ME: Alkylating agents in bronchogenic carcinoma. Am J Med Vol. 46, Apr. 1969.

34. Serlin O: Use of FUDR as an adjuvant to the surgical management of carcinoma of the stomach. Cancer 24, No. 2, August 1969.

35. Higgins GA, Humphrey EW, Hughes F, Keehn R: Cytoxan as an adjuvant to surgery for lung cancer. J Surg Oncol 1:221-228, 1969.

36. Higgins GA, White GE: Adjuvant chemotherapy and cancer surgery. In Surgery Annual. New York: Appleton-Century-Crofts, 1969.

37. Higgins GA: The use of fluorinated pyrimidines in conjunction with surgical resection of colon cancer. In Proceedings of the Chemotherapy conference on the Chemotherapy of Solid tumors - An Appraisal of 5-Fluorouracil and BCNU, SK Carter, ed. Washington DC: US Public Health, Education and Welfare, pp.85-94, 1970.

38. Roswit B, Higgins GA, Keehn RJ: A controlled study of preoperative irradiation in cancer of the sigmoid colon and rectum. Radiology 97: 133-140, Oct. 1970.

39. Roswit B, Higgins GA, Shields TW, et al: Preoperative radiation therapy for carcinoma of the lung; report of a national VA controlled study. In Frontiers of Radiation Therapy and Oncology, J Vaeth, ed. New York: S. Karger, p.163-176, 1970.

40. Shields TW, Higgins GA, Heilbrunn A, Keehn RJ: Preoperative x-ray therapy as an adjuvant in the treatment of bronchogenic carcinoma. J Thorac and Cardiovas Surg 59:49-61, 1970.

41. Serlin O, Wolkoff JS, Amadeo JM, Keehn RJ: Use of 5-fluoro-deoxyuridine (FUDR) as an adjuvant to the surgical management of carcinoma of the stomach. Cancer 24:223-228, 1969.

42. Higgins GA: Controlled therapeutic trials. Arch Surg 102:160-161, 1971.

43. Higgins GA, Dwight RW, Smith JW, et al: Fluorouracil as an adjuvant to surgery in carcinoma of the colon. Arch Surg 102:339-344, 1971.

44. Dwight RW, Higgins GA, Roswit B, LeVeen HH, Keehn RJ: Preoperative radiation and surgery for cancer of the sigmoid colon and rectum. Am J of Surg 123:93-103, 1972.

45. Shields TW, Higgins GA, Keehn RJ: Factors influencing survival after resection for bronchial carcinoma. J Thorac and Cardiovas Surg 64:391-399, 1972.

46. Higgins GA: Use of chemotherapy as an adjuvant to surgery for bronchogenic carcinoma. Cancer 30:1383-1387, 1972.

47. Kinne D, Humphrey EW: Combined therapy with cytosine arabinoside and 1,3-bis (2-chlorethyl) -1 nitrosourea in the treatment of advanced solid tumors. Cancer Chemother Rep 56:53-59, 1972.

48. Dwight RW, Humphrey EW, Higgins GA, Keehn RJ: FUDR as an adjuvant to surgery in cancer of the large bowel. J Surg Oncol 5:243-249, 1973.

49. Shields TW, Robinette CD: Long-term survivors after resection of bronchial carcinoma. Surg, Gynecol and Obstet 136:759-762, 1973.

50. Roswit B, Higgins GA, Humphrey EW, Robinette CD: Preoperative irradiation of operable adenocarcinoma of the rectum and rectosigmoid colon. Radiology 108:389-395, 1973.

51. Shields TW, Higgins GA: Minimal pulmonary resection in treatment of carcinoma of the lung. Arch Surg 108:420, 1974.

52. Humphrey EW, Dwight RW, Higgins GA: Preoperative irradiation in the treatment of carcinoma of the colon and rectum. In Surgery of the Gastrointestinal Tract. Miami: Symposia Specialists, pp.503-510, 1974.

53. Higgins GA: Carcinoma of the rectum: Preoperative radiation therapy as an adjunct to surgery. Dis Colon & Rectum 17:598-601, 1974.

54. Higgins GA, Conn JH, Jordan PH, Humphrey EW, Roswit B, Keehn RJ: Preoperative radiotherapy for colorectal cancer. Ann Surg 18:624-631, 1975.

55. Roswit B, Higgins GA, Keehn RJ: Preoperative irradiation for carcinoma of the rectum and rectosigmoid colon: Report of a national VA randomized study. Cancer 35:1597-1602, 1975.

56. Shields TW, Yee J, Conn JH, Robinette CD: Relationship of cell type and lymph node metastases to survival after resection of bronchial carcinoma. Ann Thorac Surg 20:501-510, 1975.

57. Higgins GA, Shields TW, Keehn RJ: The solitary pulmonary nodule (Ten-year followup of Veterans Administration-Armed Forces cooperative study). Arch Surg 11:570-575, 1975.

58. Higgins GA, Humphrey E, Juler GL, LeVeen HH, McCaughan J, Keehn RJ: Adjuvant chemotherapy in the surgical treatment of large bowel cancer. Cancer 38:1461, 1976.

59. Higgins GA, Serlin O, Amadeo JH, McElhinney J, Keehn RJ: Gastric cancer: Factors in survival. Chirugia Gastroenterologica 10:393-398, 1976.

60. Higgins GA: Surgical considerations in colorectal cancer. Cancer 38:891, 1977.

61. Serlin O, Keehn RJ, Higgins GA, Harrower HW, Mendeloff GL: Factors related to survival following resection for gastric carcinoma: Analysis of 903 cases. Cancer 40:1318-1329, 1977.

62. Shields TW, Humphrey EW, Eastridge CE, Keehn RJ: Adjuvant cancer chemotherapy after resection of carcinoma of lung. Cancer 5:2057-2062, 1977.

63. Shields TW, Keehn RJ: Postresection stage grouping in carcinoma of the lung. Surg Gynecol & Obstet 145:725-728, 1977.

64. Matthews MJ, Kanhouwa S, Pickren J, Robinette CD: Frequency of residual and metastatic tumor in patients undergoing curative surgical resection for lung cancer. Cancer Chemother Rep 4:63-67, 1973.

WESTERN CANCER STUDY GROUP

1960-1977

1. Papac RJ, Jacobs E, et al: Clinical experience with 5-FUDR and 5-IUDR in neoplastic diseases. <u>Clin</u> <u>Res</u> 9:79, 1961.

2. Bigley RH, Koler RD, Profsky B, Osgood EE: A comparison of chronic leukemia and lymphocytic sarcoma. <u>Cancer Chemother Rep</u> 16:231, 1962.

3. Papac RJ, Jacobs E, Wong C, Skoog W: Clinical evaluation of the pyrimidine nucleosides 5-fluoro-2'deoxyuridine and 5-iodo-2'deoxyuridine. <u>Cancer Chemother Rep</u> 20:143, 1962.

4. Scott JL, Foye L: Clinical evaluation of 4-propylamino-1-H-pyrazolo (3,4-d) pyrimidine. <u>Cancer</u> <u>Chemother Rep</u> 20:73, 1962.

5. Mass RE: Clinical evaluation of 1-aminocyclopentanecarboxylic acid plasmacytic myeloma. <u>Cancer</u> <u>Chemother Rep</u> 28:17 1963.

6. Scott JL: The effect of nitrogen mustard and maintenance chlorambucil in the treatment of advanced Hodgkin's disease. <u>Cancer Chemother Rep</u> 27:27, 1963.

7. Bigley RH: Treatment of chronic leukemic lymphocytic leukemia with triethylene melamine (TEM) and chlorambucil (CB-1348). <u>Cancer Chemother Rep</u> 32:27, 1963.

8. Papac RJ, Foye L, Jacobs E: Systematic therapy with amethopterin in squamous carcinoma of the head and neck. <u>Cancer Chemother Rep</u> 32:47, 1963.

9. Brook J, Bateman JR, Steinfeld JL: Evaluation of melphalan in treatment of multiple myeloma. <u>Cancer Chemother Rep</u> 36:25, 1964.

10. Bateman JR, Jacobs E, Marsh A, Steinfeld JL: 5-diazuoracil: A Phase I study. <u>Cancer Chemother</u> <u>Rep</u> 41:27, 1964.

11. Bateman JR, Marsh A, Steinfeld JL: Kanchanomycin: A Phase I study. <u>Cancer Chemother Rep</u> 44:25, 1965.

12. Jacobs E, Johnson FD, Wood DA: Stage III metastatic malignant testicular tumors: Treatment with intermittent and combined chemotherapy. <u>Cancer</u> 19:1697-1704, 1966.

13. Bateman JR, Peters R, Hazen JG, Steinfeld JL: Methyl methanesulfonate: Phase I clinical study. <u>Cancer Chemother Rep</u> 50:675, 1966.

14. Steinfeld JL, Soloman J, Marsh A, Hazen JG, Bateman JR: Chemical therapy of patients with advanced metastatic germinal tumors. <u>J Urol</u> 96:933, 1966.

15. Stolinsky DC, Jacobs E, Wood DA, Bateman JR, Hazen JG, Steinfeld JL: Clinical trial of trimethycolchicinic acid methyl ether d-tartrate (TMCA) in patients with advanced cancer. <u>Cancer</u> <u>Chemother Rep</u> 51:25, 1967.

16. Jacobs E, Peters FC, Luce JK, Zippin C, Wood DA: Mechlorethamine HCl and cyclophosphamide in Hodgkin's disease and the lymphomas. <u>JAMA</u> 203:392, 1968.

17. Sadoff L: The nephrotoxicity of streptozotocin. <u>Cancer Chemother Rep</u> 54:457, 1970.

18. Stolinsky DC, Solomon J, Pugh R, Stevens AR, Jacobs EM, Irwin LE, Wood DA, Steinfeld JL, Bateman JR: Clinical experience with procarbazine in Hodgkin's disease, reticulum cell sarcoma, and lymphosarcoma. <u>Cancer</u> 26:5, 1970.

19. Jacobs EM, Reeves WJ, Wood DA, Pugh RP, Braunwald J, Bateman JR: Treatment of cancer with weekly intravenous 5-fluorouracil: Study by the WCCCG. <u>Cancer</u> 27:130, 1971.

20. Bateman JR, Pugh, RP, Cassidy RF, Marshall GJ, Irwin LE: 5-fluorouracil given once weekly: Comparison of intravenous and oral administration. <u>Cancer</u> 28:907-913, 1971.

21. Stolinsky DC, Sadoff L, Braunwald J, Bateman JR: Streptozotocin in the treatment of cancer Phase II study. <u>Cancer</u> 30:61-67, 1972.

22. Stolinsky DC, Bogdon D, Solomon J, Bateman J: Hexamethylmelamine alone and in combination with 5-(3, 3-dimethyl-1-triazeno) imidazole carboxamide in the treatment of advanced cancer. Cancer 30:654, 1972.

23. Stolinsky DC, Jacobs EM, Braunwald J, Bateman JR: Further study of trimethylcolchicinic acid methyl ether d-tartrate (TMCA) in patients with malignant melanoma. Cancer Chemother Rep 56:263, 1972.

24. Solomon J, Bateman JR, Lukes R, Weiner J, Donahue D, Jacobs EM: Vinblastine and mustargen in treatment of lymphomas. Arch Intern Med 131:407-417, 1973.

25. Brook J, Bateman JR, Steinfeld J: Evaluation of chronic low dosage regimen of melphalan in the treatment of multiple meyloma. II. Survival and response rates. Arch Intern Med 131:545-548, 1973.

26. Stolinsky D, Hum G, Jacobs E, Solomon J, Bateman JR: Clinical trial of weekly vinblastine combined with vincristine. Cancer Chemother Rep 57:477-480, 1973.

27. Stolinsky D, Bogdon D, Pugh R, Braunwald J, Hestorff R, Bateman JR: Vinblastine plus vincristine given in intensive three-day courses as therapy for lymphomas, sarcomas and other neoplasms. Cancer Chemother Rep 57:481-484, 1973.

28. Stolinsky D, Bateman JR: Further experience with hexamethylmelamine in carcinoma of the cervix. Cancer Chemother Rep 57:497-499, 1973.

29. Jacobs EM, Goldman R, Solomon J, Hum G, and the Western Cancer Study Group, Los Angeles, California: Cyclophosphamide, vincristine, prednisone and procarbazine: An induction regimen for Stage III and IV lymphomas. Cancer Chemother Rep 53, February 1973.

30. Stolinsky D, Pugh R, Bohannon R, Bogdon D, Bateman JR: Trial of 1,3 bis (2-chloroethyl)-1-nitrosourea (BCNU) combined with vincristine in disseminated gastrointestinal cancer and other neoplasms. Cancer Chemother Rep 58:947-950, 1974.

31. Lewis JP, Linman JW, Marshall GJ, Pajak TF, Bateman JR: Randomized clinical trial of cytosine arabinoside and 6-thioguanine in remission induction and consolidation of adult nonlymphocytic acute leukemia. Cancer 30:84-119, 1977.

32. Reynolds R, Bateman JR: Chromomycin A: Phase I study. Cancer Treat Rep 60:1251-1255, 1976.

33. Kardinal C, Jacobs E, Bull F, Bateman J, Pajak T: Evaluation of a bleomycin adriamycin and vinblastine combination for the therapy of advanced testicular tumors. Cancer Treat Rep 60:953-960, 1976.

34. Durkin W, Pugh R, Solomon J, Rosen P, Bateman J: Intravenous vs. intramuscular bleomycin in far-advanced lymphomatous malignancy. Prospective randomized study. Oncology 33:140-145, 1976.

35. Chlebowski RT, Paroly WS, Pugh RP, Weiner JM, Bateman JR: Treatment of advanced gastric carcinoma with 5-fluorouracil: A randomized comparison of two routes of delivery. Cancer Treat Rep 63:1979-1981, 1979.

36. Chlebowski R, Gota C, Glass A, Weiner J, Bateman JR: Combination chemotherapy with cyclophosphamide plus 5-fluorouracil for treatment of unresectable pancreatic carcinoma. Cancer Treat Rep 63:2119-2121, 1979.

INDEX